Accession no.
36199197

KT-220-248

NURSING SKILLS
FOURTH EDITION

LIS LIBRARY	
Date 6/3/14	Fund nm - Riv
Order No 2485308	
University of Chester	

WITHDRAWN

Commissioning Editor: Mairi McCubbin
Development Editor: Fiona Conn
Project Manager: Sruthi Viswam
Designer/Design Direction: Miles Hitchen
Illustration Manager: Jennifer Rose

Essential
NURSING SKILLS
Clinical skills for caring
Fourth Edition

Maggie Nicol BSc(Hons), MSc(Nursing), PGDipEd, RN
Professor of Clinical Skills, School of Health Sciences, City University London, UK

Carol Bavin DipN(Lond), RN, RM, RCNT
Lecturer, School of Health Sciences, City University London, UK

Patricia Cronin BSc(Hons), MSc(Nursing), PhD, RN
Lecturer in Nursing, School of Nursing & Midwifery, Trinity College Dublin, Ireland

Karen Rawlings-Anderson BA(Hons), MSc(Nursing), DipNEd, RN
Senior Lecturer, School of Health Sciences, City University London, UK

Elaine Cole BSc, MSc, PGDipEd, RN
Senior Lecturer-Practitioner, School of Health Sciences, City University London, UK

Janet Hunter BSc(Hons), MA, PGCert, RN
Senior Lecturer, School of Community & Health Sciences, City University London, UK

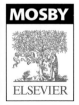

MOSBY

ELSEVIER

Edinburgh London New York Oxford Philadelphia St Louis Sydney Toronto 2012

MOSBY
ELSEVIER

© 2012 Elsevier Ltd. All rights reserved.

No part of this publication may be reproduced or transmitted in any form or by any means, electronic or mechanical, including photocopying, recording, or any information storage and retrieval system, without permission in writing from the publisher. Details on how to seek permission, further information about the Publisher's permissions policies and our arrangements with organizations such as the Copyright Clearance Center and the Copyright Licensing Agency, can be found at our website: www.elsevier.com/permissions.

This book and the individual contributions contained in it are protected under copyright by the Publisher (other than as may be noted herein).

First edition 2000
Second edition 2004
Third edition 2008
Fourth edition 2012

ISBN 978-0-7234-3694-2

British Library Cataloguing in Publication Data
A catalogue record for this book is available from the British Library

Library of Congress Cataloging in Publication Data
A catalog record for this book is available from the Library of Congress

Notices
Knowledge and best practice in this field are constantly changing. As new research and experience broaden our understanding, changes in research methods, professional practices, or medical treatment may become necessary.

Practitioners and researchers must always rely on their own experience and knowledge in evaluating and using any information, methods, compounds, or experiments described herein. In using such information or methods they should be mindful of their own safety and the safety of others, including parties for whom they have a professional responsibility.

With respect to any drug or pharmaceutical products identified, readers are advised to check the most current information provided (i) on procedures featured or (ii) by the manufacturer of each product to be administered, to verify the recommended dose or formula, the method and duration of administration, and contraindications. It is the responsibility of practitioners, relying on their own experience and knowledge of their patients, to make diagnoses, to determine dosages and the best treatment for each individual patient, and to take all appropriate safety precautions.

To the fullest extent of the law, neither the Publisher nor the authors, contributors, or editors, assume any liability for any injury and/or damage to persons or property as a matter of products liability, negligence or otherwise, or from any use or operation of any methods, products, instructions, or ideas contained in the material herein.

ELSEVIER your source for books, journals and multimedia in the health sciences

www.elsevierhealth.com

Working together to grow
libraries in developing countries

www.elsevier.com | www.bookaid.org | www.sabre.org

ELSEVIER   BOOK AID International   Sabre Foundation

The publisher's policy is to use **paper manufactured from sustainable forests**

China

Contents

Contents

Contents

Preface

Throughout your professional life you will constantly be learning new things, and this book is designed to help you. During your pre-registration programme you will be required to achieve the competencies specified in the Standards for Pre-Registration Nursing Education (Nursing and Midwifery Council 2010). These competencies are grouped into four domains: professional values; communication and interpersonal skills; nursing practice and decision-making; and leadership, management and team working. In addition, at various progression points, you will need to demonstrate achievement of specific skills known as the Essential Skills Clusters (NMC 2010). These reflect patients' expectations of newly qualified nurses and relate to:

- Care and compassion
- Communication
- Organisational aspects of care
- Infection prevention and control
- Nutrition and fluid balance
- Medicines management

This book will help you to achieve these skills and all the others that you need in order to become a competent, compassionate and caring nurse. *Essential Nursing Skills* focuses on the skills required by nurses caring for adult patients in a hospital setting, but the skills themselves can be adapted to any clinical setting.

New to this edition

Nursing is a dynamic and rapidly changing profession and the fourth edition of *Essential Nursing Skills* has been completely updated to reflect the changes in nursing and professional and national guidelines. Two new lecturers have joined the author team and this edition is now in full colour with photographs to further enhance your understanding of many of the procedures. It also has a new section listing commonly used biological and haematological values to help you understand your patients' test results. A number of skills have been expanded and several new skills are now included (e.g. assessing the deteriorating patient in Chapter 2, pre- and postoperative care in Chapter 9 and non-invasive ventilation [CPAP and BiPAP] in Chapter 11).

Focus on practical procedures

In order to keep the size of the book small enough to carry around, the rationale for each skill is not included but references and suggestions for further reading are provided at the end of each chapter. The focus is on the practical procedure rather than why the skill is necessary. To provide a clear structure, each skill first describes preparation of the patient, the environment and the nurse, and lists the equipment needed. This is followed by a step-by-step description of the procedure, supported by illustrations and additional information and rationale in the 'Points for Practice'.

Essential Nursing Skills is designed to act as a reminder for skills that you have been taught, and to enable you to prepare yourself for new skills. For example, after observing a registered nurse performing a skill you can refer to *Essential Nursing Skills* to help you understand the preparation required and read a step-by-step description of the procedure.

Points for practice ➡ PFP

Each skill is accompanied by ***Points for Practice (PFP)***, which provide additional guidance and explanation for some aspects of the procedure. *Essential Nursing Skills* is not a textbook and so does not include all the theory and rationale that underpins the various skills. For example, insertion of a nasogastric tube explains how to select, measure and insert the tube; it does not discuss the reasons why such a tube may be necessary. This book is designed to complement your nursing textbooks, not replace them.

Supervised practice

It is vital that you are supervised by a Registered Nurse until you have really mastered each skill and are competent to undertake them alone. As with all aspects of nursing, safety is paramount and you must know your patient's diagnosis and the reason for carrying out the procedure before you perform any skill.

Local policies and procedures

Nursing practice is subject to many local policies and protocols and you will prompted to refer to them throughout the text. Local policies and protocols refer to specific aspects of nursing practice that often vary between clinical areas. These include for example:

- drug-checking procedures (e.g. intravenous drug therapy)
- which nurses are permitted to perform the skill (e.g. male catheterisation)
- cleansing solutions and skin preparation (e.g. intramuscular injection)

Space has been included to enable you to make a note of the local policies and procedures. These must always be adhered to and nurses have a responsibility to update themselves on these regularly. National guidelines (e.g. resuscitation council guidelines) are also reviewed frequently and again it is your responsibility to keep up to date with recent changes. References, suggested reading and useful websites are provided at the end of each chapter.

We hope that you will find this book interesting and that it will become a much used resource to support and enhance your clinical practice. Quality nursing care requires competence but also compassion, respect for patients as individuals and should safeguard their dignity. This provides the foundation for every clinical skill. We are passionate about nursing and hope that this is evident throughout this book.

London, 2012

Maggie Nicol
Carol Bavin
Patricia Cronin
Karen Rawlings-Anderson
Elaine Cole
Janet Hunter

Acknowledgements

The authors would like to acknowledge the valuable contribution by Shelagh Bedford-Turner to the first two editions of this book.

Infection prevention and control

©2012 Elsevier Ltd.

1.1 Standard precautions

The two important principles in infection prevention and control are standard precautions and aseptic non-touch technique.

Standard precautions are the standard infection control procedures that are essential in preventing cross-infection (www.rcn.org.uk). They include the precautions required when contact with body fluids is likely, previously known as universal precautions.

The standard precautions are:

- Hand hygiene (hand washing or hand decontamination with alcohol based hand rubs)
- Safe practice, for example, aseptic technique, care of people with infection or at risk of acquiring infection, risk assessing appropriate placement of patients, including isolation
- Management of invasive devices to reduce the risk of infection to a minimum
- Appropriate use of protective clothing – aprons, gloves, masks, gowns and goggles; sometimes referred to as PPE (personal protective equipment)
- Safe disposal of waste using the national colour-coding system
- Appropriate decontamination of equipment
- Safe provision of food
- Clean, safe environment
- Safe handling of contaminated linen.

1.2 Aseptic non-touch technique (ANTT)

Many healthcare procedures pose an infection risk. For example, in wound care, any break to the continuity of the skin forms a wound, which provides an entry point for any microorganisms to enter, and increases the risk of infection (Dealey 2005). To reduce the risk of microorganisms entering the body, a number of measures can be taken:

- An aseptic technique is the method used to reduce the risk of introducing contamination to the wound or any insertion sites, to protect the patient from the risk of infection.

- Aseptic non-touch technique (ANTT) refers to standardised guidelines for aseptic technique procedures and applies to all healthcare procedures where there is a risk of infection and a healthcare associated infection, e.g. wound care, administration of intravenous medication and catheterisation (Pratt et al 2007). ANTT means that you must avoid touching any part of the equipment that will come into contact with the patient e.g. the centre of a sterile wound dressing, the tip of a needle or intravenous cannula. It is also important to avoid touching the ends of equipment when connecting them e.g. the spike of the intravenous giving set when inserting it into the intravenous fluids (see p. 113). ANTT is designed to maintain asepsis and avoid contamination of wounds or vulnerable sites from microorganisms.

- It is important to assess the risk of contamination before carrying out the aseptic technique as the measures taken will depend on the procedure being undertaken. For example, some procedures will require sterile gloves, sterile dressing pack, sterile towel and dressing e.g. wound care; others may only need sterile equipment and non-sterile gloves e.g. IV cannulation; both will require non-touch methods.

There are a number of considerations for the use of ANTT, including:

1. Explain all procedures and give the patient the opportunity to wash their hands and bathe or shower. This is often possible even with a wound.

2. Use sterile equipment when carrying out procedures where there is a risk of contamination (e.g. sterile dressing pack, intravenous cannula, syringe and needle).

3. Only handle the part of the equipment that is not in contact with the patient or other medical equipment (Pratt et al 2007).

4. Never place sterile equipment on to a non-sterile surface or touch sterile equipment without sterile gloves. Contamination will occur if you touch the outside of a sterile glove with a non- gloved hand or place a sterile staple remover onto a non-sterile surface.

5. All items used for the procedure must be sterile; the packaging must be intact and within the expiry date.

6. Appropriate choice of personal protective equipment, including gloves, aprons, and face masks (p. 9-12)

7. Appropriate choice of hand hygiene to include hand washing, and the use of alcohol hand rub (p. 5)

8. The environment should be clean. Some procedures will be carried out in a clean treatment room (e.g. wound dressing), some in a ward environment (e.g. catheterisation). Surfaces (e.g. dressing trolley) should be cleaned according to local policy, before and after the procedure. It is important to avoid sterile procedures (e.g. wound dressings) during bed making and at mealtimes.

9. All non-disposable equipment (e.g. blood pressure cuff or transfer hoist) should be decontaminated after each patient according to local policy (p. 16).

1.3 Hand washing

Preparation

- The hands should be decontaminated before and after all patient contact ➡ **PFP1**

Equipment

- A sink with elbow-or foot-operated mixer taps is best
- Liquid soap or antiseptic detergent hand washing solution ➡ **PFP2**
- Disposable paper hand towels
- Foot-operated waste bins.

Nurse

- The arms must be bare below the elbows ➡ **PFP3**
- Remove rings, jewellery and wrist watches ➡ **PFP3**
- Cuts or abrasions on the hands should be covered by a waterproof, occlusive dressing
- The fingernails should be short with no nail polish or artificial fingernails ➡ **PFP4**.

Procedure

1. Adjust the taps so that the temperature is comfortable and the water flow is steady and does not splash the surrounding area. Wet the hands.

2. Apply sufficient soap or antiseptic detergent solution to create a good lather.

3. Rub the hands briskly together, making sure that the thumbs, fingernails, fingertips, palms, backs of the hands and the wrists are thoroughly washed ➡ **PFP5** (Figure 1.1).

4. Scrubbing the skin with a brush is not recommended as it causes microabrasions. Only if the fingernails are visibly dirty should a nailbrush be used.

5. Continue to wash the hands for at least 20 seconds, then rinse thoroughly until all traces of soap/antiseptic detergent are removed ➡ **PFP6**.

6. Turn off the taps with your foot or elbow and allow the water to run off your hands by holding them with the fingers pointing upwards. If the taps are not elbow- or foot-operated, leave the water running until after drying your hands and then use a paper towel to turn off the taps.

7. Dry your hands thoroughly using disposable paper towels, working in one direction from your fingertips towards the wrists. Use a separate towel for each hand. Thorough drying is essential to minimise the growth of microorganisms and to prevent the hands becoming sore.

8. Discard the used paper towels according to local policy ➡ **PFP7**.

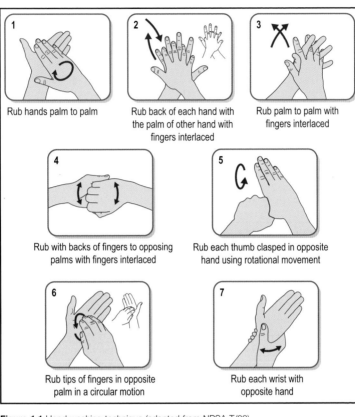

Figure 1.1 Hand washing technique (adapted from NPSA T/09).

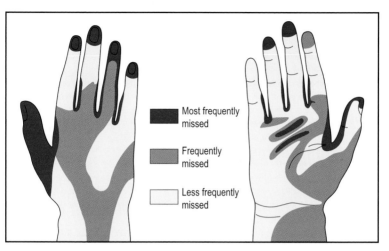

Figure 1.2 Areas often missed when the hands are washed.

Points for practice

PFP1 Methicillin-resistant *Staphylococcus aureus* (MRSA) and *Clostridium difficile* are both important causes of healthcare acquired infection (HCAI). The most important route of transmission is on the hands of healthcare workers. Alcohol hand-rub may be used instead of washing when the hands are socially clean (i.e. not visibly soiled or likely to be contaminated). The alcohol must be applied to all areas of the hands and wrists and the hands then rubbed vigorously until dry. Alcohol effectively reduces microbial counts in clean hands, but it is ineffective if used on hands contaminated with body fluids or excreta. Alcohol-based hand-rub is effective against MRSA but the spores of *C. difficile* can survive in the environment and are not killed by alcohol and so the hands must be washed with soap and water after contact with *C. difficile* patients or their environment (www.dh.gov).

PFP2 Bars of soap should never be used in clinical areas as they provide the ideal environment for growth of micro-organisms when left sitting on the sink in a pool of water. Liquid soap is usually sufficient for hand washing in most situations, but an antiseptic detergent hand washing solution containing chlorhexidine or iodine may be required before invasive procedures such as urinary catheterisation. The local infection control policy will indicate when this is necessary.

PFP3 The forearms must be bare below the elbows because cuffs become heavily contaminated and are likely to come into contact with patients (DoH 2010).

Local policy may permit the wearing of a wedding band. This should be a plain band and loose enough to allow washing and drying underneath it. Wrist watches must not be worn as they prevent effective washing of the wrist area.

PFP4 Winslow and Jaconson (2000) reviewed several studies into the wearing of artificial nails and nail polish. They report that operating theatre personnel with artificial nails harboured gram-negative rods both before and after surgical scrubbing and artificial nails also had higher bacterial loads. Although the evidence about the effect of nail polish is unclear, they found that nurses with chipped nail polish had significantly more organisms than freshly polished or natural nails.

PFP5 Many research studies have shown that hand washing techniques are not always effective. Areas of the hands that are commonly missed are the thumbs, fingernails, fingertips, palms, backs of the hands and the wrists (Figure 1.2), (Wilson 2006).

PFP6 The hand washing technique should take at least 40–60 seconds (NPSA 2009).

PFP7 In some hospitals, hand towels are considered to be clinical waste and so should be discarded in the orange clinical waste bin. In others they are deemed to be household waste and are discarded in the black non-clinical waste bin. Check your local policy.

1.4 Use of masks

Preparation

Patient

- Patients with pulmonary tuberculosis should wear a surgical mask when they leave their single room.
- Ensure the patient understands why staff or the patient is required to wear a mask

Equipment

- **Surgical masks** are recommended for use in the operating theatre and if in contact with patients with pandemic flu ➡ **PFP1**.
- **Respirator masks are** worn to protect healthcare workers from inhaling harmful respiratory particles ➡ **PFP2**.

Nurse

- Staff should wear FFP2 (filtration face piece) or FFP3 masks when caring for patient with pandemic flu. FFP3 masks must not be worn by patients as they are designed to allow expired air to escape via the valve in the mask and therefore will not prevent droplet or aerosol spread.
- The apron or gown should be put on before the mask. Check carefully that you have the right type of mask.

Procedure

1. Secure the ties or stretch the elastic straps over the head. One tie should be above the ears in the middle of the head and the other below the ears at the neck.

2. Adjust the flexible band at the nose to ensure a close fit. Make sure the mask fits snugly over the nose and below the chin

3. Avoid touching the mask when it is being worn ➡ **PFP3**.

4. Remove the gloves, apron or gown and goggles (if worn) and then the mask. If goggles are the reusable type they should be washed in hot, soapy water and dried thoroughly.

5. To remove the mask, untie/break the lower tie first so that the mask stays in place as you unfasten the second tie.

6. Hold the mask by the straps only and away from your body as you discard it into the clinical waste.

7. Wash your hands and dry thoroughly or use alcohol-based hand rub.

➡ Points for practice

PFP1 Surgical masks are worn, by healthcare staff and patients, to prevent droplets being expelled from the mouth and nose into the environment. Eye protection (goggles or a visor) is added when there is a risk of splashing blood or body fluids into the mouth, nose or eyes (Pratt et al 2007).

PFP2 Respirator masks are categorised according to their filtration efficiency and their use will be determined by your institution's Infection Control Policy. FFP2 masks, which offer 95% efficiency, may be required when caring for patients with active pulmonary tuberculosis. FFP3 masks, which offer 98% efficiency, will be required when performing aerosol-producing procedures such as tracheal suctioning (Pellowe 2009).

PFP3 All masks are single use only and cannot be re-used once removed. Surgical masks can be used until they feel moist or humid. FFP2 and FFP3 masks can be worn up to 8 hours if necessary but once removed cannot be re-used.

1.5 Use of aprons

Preparation

Patient

- Aprons should be worn when there is direct patient contact or contact with body fluids. Also when handling bed linen, excreta, equipment etc. from patients with infections such as MRSA, *C. difficile* etc.

Equipment

- Plastic aprons may be available in a variety of colours. In some hospitals, different coloured aprons are used for specific purposes, e.g. for serving meals or performing aseptic dressings.

Nurse

- The apron should be put on after the hands have been washed.

Procedure

1. Wash and dry your hands thoroughly.
2. Pull the apron over your head; avoid touching your hair and clothing with your clean hands.
3. Tie the apron loosely at the back to avoid it becoming gathered at the waist, so that water splashes will run off easily.
4. If gloves are required, put them on after the apron and remove them before the apron is removed at the end of the procedure ➡ **PFP1**.
5. To remove the apron, pull at the top to break the neckband and let the top fold down. Break the waist-ties and carefully fold the apron, touching only the 'clean' side, to prevent the spread of microorganisms ➡ **PFP2**. Do not allow your hands to touch your uniform.
6. Discard the used apron into the clinical waste bag.
7. Wash and dry your hands thoroughly or use alcohol hand rub (see p. 5).

➡ Points for practice

PFP1 Your gloves are likely to be more heavily contaminated than your apron. Removing your gloves before the apron reduces the risk of contamination of your clothing when breaking the neckband and waist-ties to remove the apron.

PFP2 Folding the apron carefully as it is removed reduces the risk of shaking organisms into the air and your hands only touch the 'clean' side of the apron.

1.6 Use of gloves (non-sterile)

Preparation

Patient

- Gloves should be worn whenever patient care involves dealing with blood or body fluids.
- Gloves will also be required when there is contact with patients with infections such as hepatitis, methicillin-resistant *Staphylococcus aureus* (MRSA) or *C. difficile*.
- Check whether the patient has a latex allergy ➡ **PFP1**.

Equipment/Environment

- Seamless, single-use gloves are recommended. These fit either hand ➡ **PFP1**.

Nurse

- The use of gloves does not reduce the need for hand washing. The hands must be washed before and after gloves have been worn ➡ **PFP2**.

Procedure

1. It is important to choose the correct size of glove; otherwise dexterity will be severely impaired.

2. If the gloves are required for a 'clean' procedure (e.g. blood glucose monitoring), they should be taken from those stored in a clean area where they are protected from dust.

3. When removing gloves, do not touch your wrists or hands with the dirty gloves. Using a gloved hand, pinch up the glove of the other hand at the wrist (Figure 1.3A) and pull it off, turning it inside out. With the non-gloved hand, slip your fingers into the wrist of the other glove (Figure 1.3B) and pull it off, again turning it inside out.

4. Used gloves must be discarded in the orange clinical waste bag.

5. Wash and dry the hands thoroughly ➡ **PFP2**.

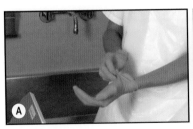
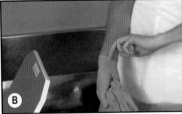

Figure 1.3 Removal of gloves.

Points for practice

PFP1 Latex-free non-sterile gloves are now used more commonly than those containing latex but packs such as dressing or catheterisation packs may still include them. Latex gloves should not be used if the patient has a latex-allergy.

PFP2 If an apron is worn, this should be removed after the gloves, but before the hands are washed (see p. 5). The hands must be washed before and after gloves are worn because the hands sweat within the gloves, creating a warm, moist environment, which encourages microorganisms to multiply (Allen 2005). Also, gloves have been shown to develop tiny punctures that go undetected but allow microorganisms to pass through. For information on the use of sterile gloves see page 287.

1.7 Disposal of waste and care of equipment

Clinical waste

Any waste generated in healthcare settings that has been in contact with blood or other body fluids is classed as clinical waste and must be incinerated. This includes soiled dressings, catheters, urine drainage bags, sputum pots, incontinence pads, etc. Used aprons and gloves are also likely to be contaminated by blood or other body fluids and so these should also be classed as clinical waste. All clinical waste must be placed in **orange clinical waste bags** for incineration (DH 2006).

Non-clinical waste

Waste generated in hospital that poses no risk to others is classed as non-clinical waste and may be disposed of in the same way as normal household waste. This includes waste such as paper hand towels, newspapers, dead flowers, food packaging, etc. Non-clinical waste should be placed in **black plastic bags** for disposal (DH 2006).

Needles and other sharps

Many healthcare procedures involve the use of needles or other devices capable of puncturing the skin, such as scalpels, lancets, etc., which are collectively referred to as 'sharps'. An injury from a needle or other device contaminated with blood or other body fluids poses a high risk to healthcare workers and so special care must be taken when using and disposing of sharps (Blenkharn & Odd (2008)). All sharps must be discarded into special yellow sharps bins, which are rigid, puncture resistant and leak proof (Figure 1.4). They have a special opening that is designed to allow sharps to be dropped easily into the container, but will not allow items to spill out should the container topple over. Sharps bins must not be filled more than three-quarters full, and once closed, they cannot be reopened.

Used needles must never be resheathed and should not be separated from the syringe except if used for venepuncture (see p. 106). If removal of the needle from the syringe is necessary, a sharps bin with a needle-removing facility on the top should be used so that the needle is not handled (Figure 1.4). The safe disposal of needles and other sharps is always the responsibility of the person who used them; they should never be left for anyone else to clear away. Where possible, the sharps bin should be taken to the place where the sharps will be used, as this allows immediate disposal after use. If this is not possible, a rigid tray or receiver should be used to contain the sharps until they can be safely tipped, without further handling, into the sharps bin. Items **must never be forced** into an already full container, as this may result in injury.

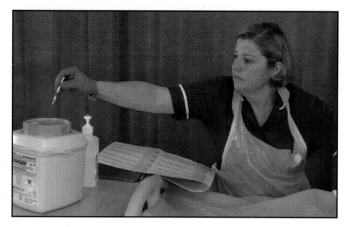

Figure 1.4 Safe disposal of sharps.

Linen

Used linen

This refers to all bed linen, clothing, towels, etc., that has been used by patients, but is not soiled. A plastic apron should be worn when making beds and handling used linen to prevent contact with your uniform, and gloves will be necessary if the patient has an infection, such as MRSA or *C. difficile*, even when the linen is not soiled. Used linen should be placed in a polythene or fabric linen-bag. These bags must not be overfilled and should be securely fastened to prevent spillage of the contents. Check clothing, such as pyjamas, to ensure that objects, such as spectacles or hearing aids, are not in the pocket.

Soiled or fouled linen

This refers to linen contaminated with blood or other body fluids or excreta. To prevent leakage, this linen should be placed in a plastic bag (often red but the colour may vary according to local policy), which should be sealed and then placed in a linen-bag as described above. Personnel wearing protective clothing and gloves will deal with soiled or fouled linen in the laundry.

Infected linen

This refers to linen from patients with infectious conditions, such as salmonella, hepatitis, pulmonary tuberculosis or MRSA. This linen must be placed in a plastic bag with a water-soluble seam and then placed in a special fabric linen-bag, which is often red or has red markings on it. In the laundry, the infected linen is not handled by anyone, but put straight into a high-temperature (95°C) washing machine in its plastic bag. The water-soluble seam will dissolve during the wash, allowing the linen to be laundered (Wilson 2006).

Non-disposable equipment

Although the majority of clinical equipment is now disposable, some items are designed to be reused, and this requires sterilisation in the sterile supplies department of the hospital. Such equipment (e.g. surgical instruments, vaginal speculae, etc.) should not be washed after use, but placed immediately in a clear plastic bag and returned to the appropriate department for decontamination. There is usually a system whereby all such equipment is placed in a particular bin or bag (the colour of this will vary according to local policy), to await collection for cleaning and sterilisation. Items of equipment that are identified as single-use equipment must never be decontaminated and then reused for another patient (Wilson 2006). Item such as nebulisers (see p. 344) can be reused several times by the same patient before being discarded.

General equipment

Equipment such as washbowls, commodes, beds and mattresses must be cleaned thoroughly between patients to avoid cross-infection. These should be cleaned with alcohol wipes or detergent and hot water, and dried thoroughly (refer to local policy). The use of detergent is essential for effective cleaning as it breaks up grease and dirt and improves the ability of water to remove it (Wilson 2006). All equipment should be stored clean and dry between uses. Many hospital wards provide patients with individual washbowls, which are kept in the bedside locker. However, others keep a number of bowls for communal use in the sluice. Abrasive materials should not be used to clean plastic washbowls as this roughens the surface, making it easy for micro-organisms to become trapped. Once washed, bowls should be placed upside down in a pyramid to allow the air to circulate freely and they dry thoroughly (Wilson 2006). The Royal College of Nursing (RCN) has useful guidelines for the decontamination of equipment and a table to help you determine the appropriate decontamination method according to whether equipment is a high, medium or low risk (*www.rcn.org.uk/infectioncontrol*).

1.8 Taking a swab

Preparation

Patient
- Explain the procedure, to gain consent and cooperation
- Ensure comfort and privacy are maintained.

Equipment
- Sterile swab(s) ➡ **PFP1**
- Plastic specimen bag
- Laboratory request form.

Nurse
- Wash and dry hands thoroughly
- Put on apron and gloves.

Procedure

1. Ask/assist the patient to adopt a position that allows access to the appropriate site ➡ **PFP1**.

2. Open the packaging at the handle end and remove the swab, taking care not to contaminate the absorbent tip ➡ **PFP2**.

3. Twist the end of the swab between your finger and thumb to 'roll' the swab so that all areas of the absorbent tip come into contact with the designated area. Avoid touching the surrounding skin ➡ **PFP3**.

4. Open the transport tube and carefully insert the swab. The 'handle' of the swab becomes the stopper or cap of the tube. Repeat for all the swabs required.

5. Label the specimens ➡ **PFP4** and place it in a plastic specimen bag with the laboratory request form and dispatch to the laboratory or refrigerate as soon as possible.

6. Ensure the patient is comfortable

7. Dispose of clinical waste appropriately and remove gloves and apron and wash hands.

8. Document that the swabs have been taken.

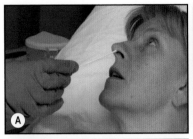

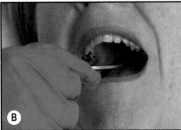

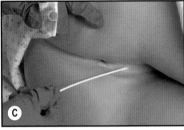

Figure 1.5 Obtaining MRSA swabs.
(A) Nose swab; (B) throat swab; (C)
swabbing the perineum.

Points for practice

PFP1 For MRSA screening, swabs are usually taken from the nose, throat, perineum
(Figure 1.5) and any wounds. A specimen of urine will also be required if the
patient is catheterised (see p. 246). Refer to local policy for the sites to be
swabbed.

PFP2 The swab may come packed inside its transport tube or it may be packed
separately.

PFP3 If the swab is being taken when performing an aseptic dressing technique, this
should be done before cleaning/irrigating the wound with antiseptic solution.
However, some authors suggest that removal of exudate prior to swabbing
allows access to the organisms actually causing the wound infection, which
are different from those in the exudate at the surface of the wound (Santy
2008). If there is no exudate, the tip of the swab may be moistened with
transport medium supplied in the tube (unless it is a charcoal swab) or 0.9%
sodium chloride according to local policy (Santy 2006).

PFP4 The patient's details should include: surname; first name; date of birth;
hospital number; and ward (this is usually available on a self-adhesive label),
date and where the swab was taken from (e.g. axilla).

1.9 Isolation (barrier nursing)

Principles

The 'correct and timely' isolation of infected patients (either suspected or proven) can be very effective in reducing transmission to other patients (DoH 2011). The aim of isolation is to minimise the transmission of micro-organisms from a patient with an infection to others. Isolation, also known as 'transmission-based precautions' and 'barrier nursing', should be used when patients have a known or suspected infection disease or symptoms such as vomiting, diarrhoea or pyrexia of unknown origin (Wilson 2006). Local infection prevention and control policies will indicate which patients need to be isolated. This usually includes patients with infections transmitted by the airborne route (e.g. tuberculosis), those transmitted by respiratory droplets produced during coughing and sneezing (e.g. meningococcal meningitis), and those transmitted by direct contact with patients or their environment (e.g. MRSA, *clostridium difficile*, influenza) (Wilson 2006). Protective isolation (reverse barrier nursing) is used to protect patients from infection. This is appropriate for patients whose immune system is severely compromised e.g. following bone marrow or organ transplant

Healthcare associated infection (HCAI)

The Department of Health (DoH 2011) recommends that all institutions should have a locally agreed 'isolation need risk assessment' to reduce the incidence of HCAI. Where possible, infected patients should be nursed in a single room with en-suite toilet, bath/shower and washbasin. Where single rooms are not available, patients with the same infection should be nursed in isolation wards or dedicated bays and cared for by nurses who are not caring for other patients. Movement of infected patients should only occur when there is a clear clinical need to do so (DoH 2011).

Isolation precautions

Standard precautions (see p. 2) must be used with all patients, including those in isolation (Wilson 2006). The following precautions are recommended by DoH (2011) and Wilson (2006).

Equipment

The isolation room must have a washbasin and ideally an en-suite toilet and shower. Disposable hand towels, liquid soap, plastic aprons, gloves and clinical waste bins should be provided inside or immediately outside the room. Masks and goggles/visor may be necessary (see p. 9). Door signs will be required to alert visitors and staff; however, it is important to maintain patient confidentiality (Prieto and Kilpatrick 2011). Equipment should be single-use only and should not be shared with other patients.

Aprons and gloves

An apron and gloves should be worn for all patient contact. These should be discarded between procedures and before leaving the room. Gloves must be worn when there is contact with body fluids or contaminated items such as dressings. Visitors should also wear aprons and gloves when entering the room/designated isolation area.

Hand hygiene

Hands must be washed (see p. 5) when gloves are removed and before leaving the room. Visitors must also be asked to wash their hands before leaving the room/ designated isolation area.

Excreta

If en-suite facilities are not available, a commode should be left in the room. Excreta (urine, faeces, vomit) should be discarded directly into the toilet, macerator or flushing sluice. Disposable bed pans, vomit bowls and urinals should be used, which are then macerated or incinerated. If reusable bed pans are used these must be decontaminated in the bed pan washer with a temperature of 80°C for at least one minute during the wash cycle.

Linen

All linen must be treated as contaminated and placed in a plastic bag with a soluble seam (alginate bag) and then into another bag, according to local policy (see p. 15). With highly infectious diseases, disposable linen may be used, which is then incinerated with the clinical waste.

Psychological effects of isolation

Patients being nursed in isolation may feel embarrassed or in some way 'dirty' and report feeling shunned, neglected, lonely, abandoned, frustrated and stigmatised. Isolation also limits visual, auditory and sensory cues, creating potential communication barriers between patient and nurse (Cassidy 2006). Thus psychological support and 'social' interaction as well as nursing care is vital.

Bibliography/Suggested reading

Allen, G., 2005. Hand hygiene, an essential process in the OR. AORN 82 (4), 561–562.

Demonstrates that wearing gloves creates a moist, warm, nutrient-rich environment in which bacteria can grow and multiply, and stresses the need for hand washing before and after wearing gloves.

Blenkharn, J.L., Odd, C., 2008. Sharps injuries in healthcare waste handlers. Annals of Occupational Hygiene 52 (4): 281–286.

This article reports a study of healthcare waste handlers who had suffered needle stick injuries due to incorrectly discarded sharps. It stresses the need for careful disposal of sharps to ensure you do not put others at risk.

Bonham, P.A., 2009. Swab cultures for diagnosing wound infections. Journal of Wound, Ostomy and Continence Nursing 36 (4), 389–395.

This article reviews the literature on wound swabbing. It proposes a research-based guideline for wound swabbing technique to standardise practice and ensure that swabs provide useful information that assists diagnostic and therapeutic decision making.

Cassidy, I., 2006. Student nurses' experiences of caring for infectious patients in source isolation. A hermeneutic phenomenological study. Journal of Clinical Nursing 15, 1247–1256.

An interesting study which found that the imposed 'barriers' altered the caring experience and students found balancing the need of the individual whilst preventing the spread of infection difficult.

Dealey, C., 2005. The care of wounds: a guide for nurses. Blackwell Publishing, Oxford.

A comprehensive book that covers the history of wound care, physiology of wound healing, types of dressings and all types of wounds including pressure ulcers and skin care for patients undergoing radiation.

Department of Health. 2006. Technical Memorandum 07-01: Safe Management of Healthcare Waste. Available from the Department of Health website (see below).

A comprehensive document that covers all aspects of waste management in healthcare, within hospitals and in community settings.

Department of Health, 2010. Uniforms and workwear: guidance on uniform and workwear policies for NHS employers. DoH, London.

This provides guidance and rationale for uniform requirements such the 'bare below the elbow' rule for all healthcare practitioners.

Department of Health, 2011. Isolating patients with healthcare associated infection. A summary of best practice. Available from: http://hcai.dh.gov.uk/files/2011/03/Document_Isolation_Best_Practice_FINAL_100917.pdf. [Accessed 6.6.11].

A useful summary of best practice in relation to isolation of patients with HCAI.

Cole, M., 2007. Should nurses take a pragmatic approach to hand hygiene? Nursing Times 103 (3), 32–33.

An interesting article, which argues that recommended practice standards in relation to hand hygiene can be unrealistic and lead to non-compliance. By developing a more pragmatic approach this may lead to better compliance and an overall improvement in standards.

Gould, D., 2002. Hand decontamination. Nursing Times 98 (46), 48–49.

Gould, D., 2002. Preventing cross infection. Nursing Times 98 (46), 50–51.

These two articles outline the hand washing technique and discuss when soap is sufficient and when antiseptic solutions should be used. They also discuss use of gloves, care of the nails and the wearing of rings and wrist watches.

Girou, E., Loyeau, S., Legrand, P., et al., 2002. Efficacy of hand rubbing with alcohol based solution versus standard hand washing with antiseptic soap: a randomised clinical trial. BMJ 325, 362–364.

An interesting study conducted in three intensive care units in France, which found that the reduction in bacterial contamination of the hands was significantly higher when alcohol-based solution was used rather than hand washing.

Hampton, S., 2002. The appropriate use of gloves to reduce allergies and infection. British Journal of Nursing 11, 1120–1124.

This article discusses appropriate and inappropriate use of gloves and the issues surrounding the use of latex and this may impact on the nurse, patient and the environment.

Infection Control Nurses' Association, 2002. Protective clothing: principles and guidelines. Available from ICNA/Fitwise, Drumcross Hall, Bathgate EH48 4JT, UK.

Practical evidence-based guidelines regarding the appropriate use of protective clothing as part of infection prevention and control.

May, D., Brewer, S., 2001. Sharps injury: prevention and management. Nursing Standard 15 (32), 45–53.

A continuing professional development article to help you review the risks associated with needlestick injury and blood-borne viruses and develop safe systems of working. Also discusses what to do if a sharps injury occurs.

National Patient Safety Agency, 2009. Clean you hands campaign. www.npsa.nhs.uk/cleanyourhands/ (accessed 9.4.12).

O'Connor, H., 2000. Decontaminating beds and mattresses. Nursing Times 96 (46):NTPlus, 2–5.

This article defines the terms decontamination, cleaning, disinfection and sterilisation and provides a practical guide to the decontamination of beds and mattresses.

Pellowe, C., 2009. When should staff wear face masks? Nursing Times 105 (34), 16

A useful guide to when to wear surgical masks and when respirator masks are required. It also emphasises the importance of wearing masks correctly and disposing of them safely.

Pratt, R.J., Pellowe, C.M., Wilson, J.A., et al., 2007. epic2: National evidence-based guidelines for preventing healthcare-associated infections in NHS hospitals in England. Journal of Hospital Infection 65, S1–S64.

This article provides evidence-based guidelines for the use of personal protective equipment such as masks, aprons and gloves.

Pratt, R., Pellowe, C., Loveday, H., et al and the *epic* guideline development team, 2001. The EPIC project: developing national evidence-based guidelines for preventing healthcare associated infections. Journal of Hospital Infection 47 (Supplement), S3–S4. Also available from: www.doh.gov.uk/HAI[19.12.11].

Evidence-based guidelines for preventing infections in hospitals and HAIs associated with urethral catheters and central venous catheters.

Prieto, J., Kilpatrick, C., 2011. Infection prevention and control. In: Brooker, C, Nicol, M. (Eds.), Alexander's Nursing Practice, fourth ed. Churchill Livingstone Elsevier, Edinburgh, Ch 16.

This chapter addresses all the key issues of infection prevention and control including how infection is spread, standard precautions and prevention of HCAI.

Raybould, L.M., 2001. Disposable non-sterile gloves: a policy for appropriate use. British Journal of Nursing 10 (17), 1135–1141.

Reports an audit of glove use in which it was found that gloves were sometimes being used inappropriately. Provides a good overview of when they should be worn and a nice diagram, based on work by the ICNA, to show which type of gloves should be worn for which activity.

Royal College of Nursing, 2007. Safe Management of healthcare waste. RCN, London.

Guidance on all aspects of clincal waste management including the classification and the national colour coding system, what to do in the event of spillages and sharps disposal. It also summarises the responsibilities of employers and employees.

Santy, J., 2008. Recognising infection in wounds. Nursing Standard 23 (7), 53–60.

This article provides an overiew of wound healing and reviews the evidence to support whether the wound should be cleaned prior to taking a wound swab and the most effective technique.

Wilson, J., 2006. Infection control in clinical practice, third ed. Baillière Tindall, Elsevier, Edinburgh.

A comprehensive text that explains basic microbiology, types of organisms and how they are spread. It then provides guidance on infection control practices, disposal of waste, decontamination of equipment and advice about all aspects of infection control. It includes a helpful table of major infectious diseases with route of transmission and whether isolation is required.

Winslow, E., Jacobson, A., 2000. Can a fashion statement harm the patient? American Journal of Nursing 100 (9), 63–65.

This article reviews several studies into the effects of artificial and polished nails on hand-hygiene practices. They conclude that artificial nails could contain more bacteria than natural nails and so place patients at increased risk of infection. The evidence regarding the use of nail polish is less clear, but they recommend that if polish is worn it should be freshly applied and clear so that the nails can be inspected for cleanliness.

www.doh.gov

The website of the UK Department of Health has a good overview of MRSA and Clostridium difficile and how they are spread. Also, latest figures on infection rates in hospitals, etc., and good practice guidelines.

www.ips.uk.net/

The website of the Infection Prevention Society, which and has free downloads about hand washing (5 moments) and leaflets explaining MRSA screening in a number of different languages.

www.rcn.org.uk

The Royal College of Nursing website provides a lot of guidance about all aspects of infection control, hand washing technique, standard precautions, management of clinical waste and guidance on uniform. Many of the resources are freely available to non–members.

Chapter 2

Observation and monitoring

©2012 Elsevier Ltd.

2.1 Temperature recording: oral & axillary

Preparation

Patient
- Explain Procedure, To Gain consent and cooperation
- Assess the patient regarding suitable site ➡ **PFP1**
- The patient should be rested

Equipment
- Disposable chemical thermometer, e.g. TempaDot™ ➡ **PFP2** ➡ **PFP3**
- Watch
- Observation chart

Nurse
- Hands must be clean
- Additional protective clothing may be necessary if indicated by the patient's condition (see Ch. 1)

Procedure

Oral

1. Check the patient has not had a hot or cold drink, or smoked a cigarette within the previous 20 minutes as this will lead to an inaccurate measurement (Childs 2011).

2. Check the expiry date of the thermometer and open the packaging. Remove the thermometer taking care not to touch the end with dots.

3. Ask the patient to open their mouth, and gently insert the thermometer under their tongue, next to the frenulum. This is adjacent to a large artery (sublingual artery), so the temperature will be close to core temperature (Figure 2.1A).

4. Ask the patient to close their lips, but not their teeth, around the thermometer, to prevent cool air circulating in the mouth.

5. It is vital to leave the thermometer in position for the recommended length of time (usually 1 minute). However, it does not affect accuracy if it is left for longer than the minimum time.

6. Remove the thermometer, taking care not to touch the part that has been in the patient's mouth. In accordance with the manufacturer's instructions, read the temperature by noting the way that the dots have changed colour (Figure 2.1C).

Axillary

1. Check the expiry date of the thermometer and open the packaging. Remove the thermometer taking care not to touch the end with dots.

2. Ask/assist the patient to expose their axilla. For an accurate recording, the axilla must be dry and free from sweat.

3. With the dots facing the chest wall, position the thermometer vertically between the arm and the chest wall.

4. Ask/assist the patient to keep their arm close against the chest to ensure good contact with the skin (Figure 2.1B).

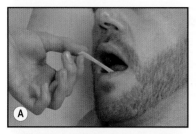
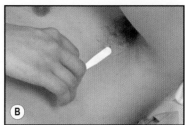
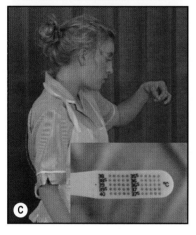

Figure 2.1 A: Positioning the thermometer for oral use; B: positioning the thermometer in the axilla; C: reading the thermometer.

5. It is vital to leave the thermometer in position for the recommended length of time (usually 3 minutes). However, it does not affect accuracy if it is left for longer than the minimum time.

6. Remove the thermometer. In accordance with the manufacturer's instructions, read the temperature by noting the way that the dots have changed colour (see Figure 2.1C).

Oral and axillary

1. Dispose of the thermometer into the clinical waste.

2. Ensure patient comfort; replace clothing etc. as necessary

3. Document the findings according to local policy (see p. 52 for an example of charting) and report any abnormalities. The normal range for adults is 36–37.2° Celsius.

4. Use alcohol rub or wash and dry your hands.

➡ Points for practice

PFP1 The oral site should not be used if the patient is unconscious, extremely breathless (breathing through the mouth), confused, prone to seizures, has mouth sores or has undergone oral surgery. Temperature in the axilla is 0.5° lower than oral temperature. The rectal site is no longer recommended except when an electronic probe is used.

PFP2 Mercury thermometers are no longer widely used as there are risks of breakage. If a mercury thermometer is used, it must be cleaned before and after use or a disposable cover used. The mercury must be shaken down to the bottom of the scale before use.

2.2 Electronic thermometer: oral and axillary

Preparation

Patient
- Explain the procedure to gain consent and co-operation
- Assess patient regarding suitable site for temperature recording ➡ **PFP1**
- Patients should be rested and not had a hot or cold drink or smoked a cigarette within the previous 20 minutes when using the oral site (Childs 2011).

Equipment
- Electronic thermometer with disposable covers
- Check the manufacturer's instructions to ensure safe and accurate use of the electronic thermometer
- Observation chart

Nurse
- Hands must be clean and an apron should be worn
- Additional personal protective clothing may be necessary if indicated by the patient's condition (see Ch. 1).

Oral

1. On the electronic thermometer select 'oral' site.

2. Cover the probe with a disposable cover to prevent contamination.

3. Place the covered probe under the tongue in the same way as a disposable thermometer (Figure 2.2). When the audible signal is heard, remove the probe from the mouth.

4. The temperature is shown in the digital display box.

5. Using a non-touch technique, discard the cover into the locker bag or clinical waste ➡ **PFP2**.

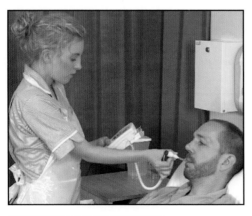

Figure 2.2 Oral electronic thermometer.

Axillary

1. On the electronic thermometer select 'axilla' site.
2. Cover the probe with a disposable cover.
3. Insert the probe horizontally and hold the patient's arm close to the chest to ensure good contact with the skin.
4. When the audible signal is heard, remove the probe from the axilla. The temperature is shown in the digital display box.
5. Using a non-touch technique, discard the probe cover into the clinical waste ➡ **PFP2**.

Oral and axillary

1. Ensure patient comfort and answer any questions regarding the recording.
2. Return the thermometer in the charging point/storage area as appropriate.
3. Document the temperature according to local policy. Report any abnormality. The normal range for adults is 36.0–37.2° Celsius
4. Use alcohol rub or wash and dry your hands.

➡ Points for practice

PFP1 If the patient is unconscious, extremely breathless (mouth breathing) confused, prone to seizures, has mouth sores or has undergone oral surgery, the oral site should not be used for temperature measurement. Temperature in the axilla is 0.5° lower than oral temperature. The rectal site is only used for continuous temperature monitoring in high dependency areas, where a small electronic probe is inserted into the rectum.

PFP2 Most electronic thermometers have a mechanism to eject the probe cover without handling it.

2.3 Temperature recording: tympanic membrane thermometer

Preparation

Patient
- Explain the procedure to gain consent and cooperation
  ➡ **PFP1**
- If the patient has been lying on one side use the other ear as this might lead to an inaccurate reading
- Wax in the ears may lead to an inaccurate reading

Equipment
- Tympanic membrane thermometer with disposable covers
- Check the lens of the thermometer is clean and not cracked
- Observation chart

Nurse
- Hands must be clean
- Additional personal protective clothing may be necessary if indicated by the patient's condition (see Ch. 1).

Procedure

1. Switch on the thermometer
2. Use a non-touch technique to fit a disposable cover.
3. Gently place the covered probe into the ear canal. Ensure a snug fit (Figure 2.3).
4. When the audible signal is heard remove the probe from the ear. The temperature is shown in the digital display box.
5. Use a non-touch technique to discard the cover into the clinical waste bag.
6. Document the findings according to local policy (see p. 52 for an example of charting) and report any abnormalities. Normal range for adults is 36.0–37.2° Celsius.
7. Return the thermometer to the charging point/storage area as appropriate.
8. Use alcohol rub or wash and dry your hands.

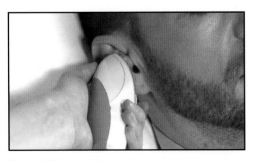

Figure 2.3 Tympanic thermometer.

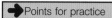

Points for practice

PFP1 Tympanic thermometers measure the temperature by inserting a probe into the outer ear, adjacent to (but not touching) the tympanic membrane. An infrared light detects heat radiated from the tympanic membrane and provides a digital reading. This provides an accurate measure of body core temperature as it is close to the carotid artery.

2.4 Cooling and warming the patient

Cooling the patient

Tepid sponging

Tepid sponging is designed to reduce the patient's temperature. The skin is cooled by applying tepid water with a sponge or flannel to a whole limb or extensive area of the body and then allowing it to evaporate, taking heat with it. With even a slightly raised temperature, this can make the patient feel much refreshed. It is important to maintain dignity and privacy throughout this procedure. Face cloths wrung out in tepid water and placed into the patient's axillae and groins will also assist cooling. Tepid rather than cold water is used, as cold water would cause peripheral vasoconstriction (Childs 2011).

Fan therapy

Cooling the air around the patient, so that the body loses more heat through radiation from the skin, is an effective way of cooling the person. However, it is important that the fan is carefully placed to avoid blowing onto the face of the patient as this can cause drying of the cornea of the eyes, leading to ulceration. The fan should be an oscillating type so that cooling is gentle and covers all areas of the body. As discussed above, cooling the skin too quickly may cause vasoconstriction, resulting in less blood circulating near the surface to be cooled.

Warming the patient

Patients, particularly the elderly, are often cold and may be suffering from hypothermia (a temperature of less than 35°C) on admission to hospital. This may be due to a lack of heating at home, exposure following an accident of some kind, or they may have been lying undiscovered for a period of time. It can also occur following lengthy surgery despite the use of warm air systems, which blow warm air through a disposable blanket onto the patient's body during the operation. A space blanket is made of thin, foil-type material that is designed to reflect back heat to prevent it being lost from the body.

If the patient is receiving intravenous fluids or a blood transfusion, these may be warmed using a blood warmer (see p. 144). If the patient is able to take oral fluids, hot drinks and soup are very effective. Humans lose a great deal of heat through their heads, so covering the head is beneficial. Warming must be managed carefully to prevent warming the patient too quickly, which may lead to shock (Childs 2011).

2.5 Pulse recording

Preparation

Patient
- Explain the procedure, to gain consent and cooperation
- The patient should be resting, either lying down or sitting Allow at least 15 minutes rest after physical activity or emotional upset

Equipment
- A watch with a second hand
- Observation chart

Nurse
- The hands should be clean
- Additional protective clothing may be necessary if indicated by the patient's condition (see Ch. 1)

Procedure

1. Choose a site to record the pulse. For most routine recordings the radial pulse is used (Figure 2.4) ➡ **PFP1**.

2. Using your first and second fingers to feel the pulse, lightly compress the artery. Do not use your thumb ➡ **PFP2**.

3. Count the number of beats for 1 minute. If the pulse is regular, it is sufficient to count for 30 seconds and double the result. If the pulse is irregular, count for a full minute.

4. In addition to the rate per minute, note the rhythm, i.e. whether it is regular or irregular, and the volume/strength of the pulse felt ➡ **PFP3**.

5. Note the colour of the patient's skin and mucous membranes (inside lower eyelid). Pallor may indicate anaemia, while a bluish colour (cyanosis) indicates a lack of oxygen. In dark-skinned patients it is easier to detect this in the nail beds.

6. Document the findings according to local policy (see p. 334 for an example of charting) and report any abnormalities or changes from previous recordings of more than 20 beats per minute. The normal range in adults is 60–80 beats per minute.

7. Use alcohol rub or wash and dry your hands.

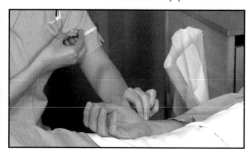

Figure 2.4 Radial pulse recording.

➡ Points for practice

PFP1 The usual site for recording the pulse rate is at the wrist, where the radial pulse is easily felt. Pulses may also be felt at other sites (see p. 61) and these may be used to check tissue perfusion (e.g. following surgery to a limb) or in an emergency.

PFP2 Use light pressure only; pressing too hard can occlude the artery and you will be unable to feel the pulse. Do not use your thumb. You have quite a strong pulse in your thumb and may feel your own pulse rather than the patient's.

PFP3 It is important to feel the patient's pulse even if the pulse rate is shown on the pulse oximeter or automatic blood pressure machine. You need to know the strength and the rhythm of the pulse as well as the rate.

2.6 Assessment of breathing and counting respirations

Preparation

Patient

- The patient should be relaxed and resting, or recent activity should be noted. Get the patient into as upright a posture as is possible and comfortable (see p. 336)
- Do not inform the patient when you will be assessing breathing
  ➡ **PFP1**

Equipment

- Watch with a second hand

Nurse

- The hands should be clean
- Additional protective clothing may be necessary if indicated by the patient's condition (see Ch. 1)

Procedure

1. Observe the movement of the chest wall for symmetry of chest movement – this is best observed in front of the patient rather than at the side ➡ **PFP2**.
2. Observe whether accessory muscles are being used ➡ **PFP3**.
3. Observe the rhythm and depth of respirations ➡ **PFP4**.
4. Count the respirations for 60 seconds.
5. Observe for the following:
   - Difficulty in or struggling with breathing
   - Pain on breathing and its location
   - Noisy respiration – whether there is any wheeze or stridor (high pitched sounds)
   - Cough – whether dry or productive
   - Sputum – amount, colour and consistency (see p. 352).
6. Observe the patient's colour for signs of cyanosis ➡ **PFP5**.
7. Document the respiratory observations according to local policy and report any abnormalities (see p. 52 for an example of charting).
8. Adjust the frequency of observations as necessary.
9. Ensure the patient is comfortable. Breathless patients may be most comfortable sitting in a chair.

PFP1 A more accurate observation is obtained if the patient is unaware that their respirations are being counted. Many nurses achieve this by pretending to be feeling the radial pulse when in fact observing the movement of the chest wall (Figure 11.1 on p. 335).

PFP2 The chest should rise and fall equally or symmetrically. If one side does not move as well as the other this could indicate a pneumothorax (collapsed lung), bronchial obstruction or injury.

PFP3 Accessory muscles are the sternocleidomastoid and trapezius muscles in the neck and shoulders. If these are being used (noticed by movement of these muscles), it indicates that the patient is unable to use the diaphragm and external intercostal muscles adequately (Esmond 2011).

PFP4 If breathing is very shallow and difficult to observe, lightly rest your hand on the patient's chest or abdomen to feel movement. The normal rate for an adult is 12–20 breaths per minute.

PFP5 Cyanosis is a blue discoloration of the skin and mucous membranes and is most noticeable around the lips, earlobes, mouth and fingertips. In dark-skinned patients, signs of poor perfusion or cyanosis may be detected if the area around the lips or nail beds is dusky in colour.

2.7 Blood pressure recording

Preparation

Patient

- Explain the procedure, to gain consent and cooperation
- The patient should be resting on a bed, couch or chair, with their legs uncrossed
- The patient should not have exercised, smoked, had a meal, alcohol or caffeine in the previous 30 minute ➡ **PFP1**

Equipment

- Sphygmomanometer with appropriate size cuff ➡ **PFP2**
- Stethoscope
- Alcohol-impregnated swabs
- Observation chart

Nurse

- The hands should be clean
- Additional protective clothing may be necessary if indicated by the patient's condition (see Ch. 1)

Procedure

1. Ensure the patient is resting in a comfortable position and discourage them from talking during the procedure. If a comparison between lying and standing blood pressure is required, the 'lying' recording should be done first.

2. When applying the cuff, no clothing should be underneath it. If clothing constricts the arm, remove the arm from the sleeve.

3. Apply the cuff such that the centre of the 'bladder' is over the brachial artery (located on the medial aspect of the antecubital fossa) and 2–3 cm above the antecubital fossa ➡ **PFP3**.

4. The arm should be positioned so that the cuff is level with the patient's heart and may be more comfortable resting on a pillow ➡ **PFP4**.

5. The sphygmomanometer should be placed on a firm surface, with the dial clearly visible and the needle at zero.

6. Estimate systolic BP by locating the radial or brachial pulse. Squeeze the bulb slowly to inflate the cuff while still feeling the pulse. Observe the dial and note the level when the pulse can no longer be felt. Open the valve fully to quickly release the pressure in the cuff ➡ **PFP5** (Figure 2.5).

8. If using a communal stethoscope, clean the earpieces with an alcohol-impregnated swab. Curving the ends of the stethoscope slightly forward, place the earpieces in your ears.

9. If the stethoscope has two sides, check that it is turned to the diaphragm side by tapping it with your finger (Figure 2.6).

10. Palpate the brachial artery, which is located on the medial aspect of the antecubital fossa (just to the side of the midline, on the side nearest to the patient).

11. Place the diaphragm of the stethoscope over the artery, and hold it in place with your thumb while your fingers support the patient's elbow and ask the

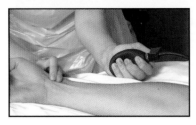

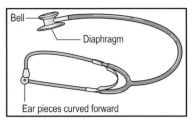

Figure 2.5 Estimating the systolic blood pressure.

Figure 2.6 Stethoscope showing bell, diaphragm and earpieces.

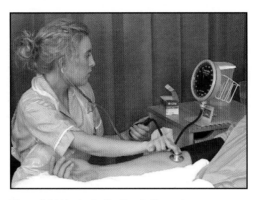

Figure 2.7 Listening for the Korotkoff sounds.

    patient to relax their arm ➡ **PFP6**. You will not hear anything until the cuff is being deflated (step 14).

12. Position yourself so that the dial of the sphygmomanometer is clearly visible.

13. Ensure that the valve on the bulb is closed and inflate the cuff to 30 mmHg above the level noted in step 7. Slowly open the valve to allow the needle of the dial to drop **slowly and steadily** (2–3 mm per second).

14. While observing the needle of the dial as it falls, listen for Korotkoff (thudding) sounds: (Figure 2.7)

    • **Systolic** pressure is the level where these are first heard

    • **Diastolic** pressure is the level where the sounds disappear.

15. Once the sounds have disappeared, open the valve fully, to completely deflate the cuff, and ➡ **PFP7**.

16. Remove the cuff from the patient's arm. Replace clothing and ensure the patient is comfortable ➡ **PFP8**.

17. Document the findings according to local policy (see p. 52 for an example of charting) and report any abnormalities. Report variations from previous recordings. The optimal BP in adults is a systolic pressure of <120 mmHg and a diastolic pressure of <80 mmHg (www.bhsoc.org).

18. Clean the earpieces of the stethoscope and replace equipment. If using an electronic machine, plug it into the mains to charge.

19. Use alcohol rub or wash and dry your hands.

➡ Points for practice

PFP1 The patient should be rested and lying or seated comfortably with the legs uncrossed and should have rested for the previous 5 minutes. If there is a difference between the BP in each arm, use the arm with the higher Bp for measurements (www.bhsoc.org).

PFP2 The sphygmomanometer may be an aneroid or a mercury type. These are used in exactly the same way except that a column of mercury, which must be placed in an upright position, is observed instead of a dial. The bladder part of the cuff must cover at least 80% of the circumference of the upper arm and a sizing guide is usually indicated on the cuff.

    Electronic BP machines are now commonly used. The cuff is positioned in the same way as described in step 4, but no stethoscope is required because the machine provides a digital display of the systolic and diastolic pressures. These machines must be plugged into the mains electricity after use to re-charge the battery.

PFP3 If the patient is receiving intravenous therapy, avoid using the arm that has the intravenous cannula or infusion in progress. Also avoid using the same arm as the pulse oximeter (see p. 350).

PFP4 The arm should be horizontal and supported at the level of the heart. If the arm is too low it could lead to over estimation of the systolic BP by up to 10 mmHg. If the arm is raised above the heart this may lead to under estimation (www.bhsoc.org).

PFP5 By estimating the systolic blood pressure in this way you avoid having to inflate the cuff unnecessarily high during step 13. Some people suggest estimating the systolic BP by pumping the cuff up high and then feeling when the pulse returns; we would argue that this may cause the patient unnecessary discomfort.

PFP6 The arm should not be held rigid as muscle tension may cause a false reading

PFP7 If you do not hear the systolic or diastolic pressure accurately you will need to re-inflate the cuff and repeat the procedure. If still unclear you should allow the patient to rest before repeating the procedure as repeated attempts may affect the accuracy of the reading.

PFP8 If recording lying and standing blood pressure, do not remove the cuff between recordings. The doctor may request that the patient is standing for at least 5 minutes before the standing blood pressure is recorded. Be aware that patients may feel dizzy on getting out of bed (postural hypotension).

2.8 Cardiac monitoring

Preparation

Patient
- Explain the procedure, to gain consent and cooperation
- Explain the need for bed rest while on the monitor ➡ **PFP1**
- Ensure privacy

Equipment
- Cardiac monitor with leads. This should have a maintenance sticker showing that it is safe to use. Check that the cables are in good condition
- Disposable electrodes
- Disposable razor or clippers (if required to remove body hair)

Nurse
- The hands should be clean and an apron worn
- Additional protective clothing may be necessary if indicated by the patient's condition (see Ch. 1)

Procedure

1. Most acute areas will have wall-mounted cardiac monitors. If using a portable monitor, place it on a firm surface, close to an electrical socket. Do not put anything on top of the monitor and keep the patient's drinks etc., away from it.

2. Raise the bed to a safe working height (see Ch. 12, Moving and handling).

3. Expose the patient's chest and examine the sites that will be used for the electrodes.

4. If the chest is very hairy, shave or clip a small patch of hair at each site to allow good contact and adhesion of the electrodes.

5. Check the expiry date of the electrodes and ensure that the gel has not dried out.

6. If the electrode has a small raised patch on the back, use this to roughen the skin slightly where the electrode will be placed. This improves adhesion and contact.

7. Remove the backing paper and taking care not to touch the gel in the middle, stick the electrodes firmly to the chest wall. The electrodes should be placed over bone and not muscle, ➡ **PFP2** avoiding areas that may be used for the placement of defibrillator pads. Electrodes can usually remain in place for 24–72 hours, but may need replacing more frequently if the patient sweats a lot, if the gel dries out or if the patient's skin shows signs of sensitivity.

8. Connect the leads to the electrodes ➡ **PFP3**. This is usually by means of a small clip or press stud. The leads are labelled or colour coded. If using a 3-lead system place the red electrode on the right shoulder, the yellow electrode on the left shoulder and the green electrode on the left lower abdomen (see Figure 2.8) If using a four lead system the additional black lead is placed on the lower, right side of the abdomen. If a 5-lead system is used, place the first 4 leads as detailed above and the white lead is placed in the middle of the chest. ➡ **PFP4**

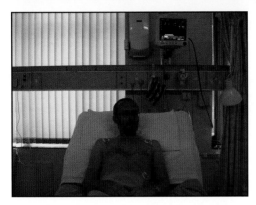

Figure 2.8 Position of electrodes for cardiac monitoring.

9. Turn on the monitor and select lead II, which should produce the most positive (upright-looking) display. If lead II does not produce a good display, try lead I or lead III. If necessary, adjust the 'gain' or size on the monitor to make the display larger and easier to see.

10. Set the alarms to safe parameters, according to the patient's condition and local protocol.

11. Replace the patient's clothing and ensure that the leads are not pulling on the electrodes and that the cables are not under tension or trapped e.g. in bed rails.

12. Explain/demonstrate what will happen if the patient moves or disturbs the electrodes (i.e. abnormal-looking pattern) to prevent unnecessary concern.

13. Lower the bed, adjusting the height for the patient's safety and convenience.

14. Remove apron and wash and dry hands.

15. Document the rhythm shown on the monitor ➡ **PFP5** and report any abnormalities as appropriate.

➡Points for practice

PFP1 In the acute situation, most patients with cardiac monitors are required to rest in bed. However, patients undergoing investigations for cardiac rhythm abnormalities may have a 24-hour tape (Holter monitor) or ambulatory monitoring system (telemetry). The patient may move around with these systems and the rhythm is analysed retrospectively; the ECG trace cannot be viewed in real time. With telemetry a transmitter sends signals to a central monitoring system and the trace can be viewed in real time, though the patient may become 'disconnected' if the patient moves beyond the area where the signal can be picked up. It is vital to know where the patient is at all times, in case of serious arrhythmias.

PFP2 The electrodes should be placed over bone rather than muscle as muscle tremor will cause disruption on the ECG tracing.

PFP3 The leads are referred to as limb leads even though they are attached to the chest. This is because they represent that area of the body, i.e. right arm, left arm and left leg.

PFP4 The 5th (white) lead may be placed in any of the precordial chest lead positions if the monitor is configured to display 2 ECG traces, so that a limb lead and a chest (V) lead can be viewed simultaneously.

PFP5 Most monitors now have the facility to digitally record abnormal rhythms and most record the rhythm whenever the alarm is triggered. If the monitor does not have this facility, it is good practice to printout a rhythm strip at the beginning of each shift and when any abnormal rhythms are noted. The printout should be labelled and signed before being stored in the patient's notes. Some specialist units also have monitors that enable ST segment monitoring.

2.9 Recording a 12-lead ECG

Patient
- Explain the procedure, to gain consent and cooperation
- Explain the need to lie still during the recording in order to gain a good trace
- Close curtains or screens to ensure privacy

Equipment/Environment
- A 12-lead electrocardiography (ECG) machine and leads, and paper for printout
- Disposable electrodes for limb and chest leads (usually disposable, adhesive with clips or press studs)

Nurse
- The hands should be clean and an apron should be worn
- Additional protective clothing may be necessary if indicated by the patient's condition (see Ch. 1)

Procedure

1. Ask/assist the patient to lie in a recumbent or semi-recumbent position.
2. Raise the bed to a safe working height (see Ch. 12, Moving and handling).
3. Expose the patient's ankles, wrists and chest area.
4. Apply the electrodes to the patient's ankles and wrists as shown in Figure 2.9A
   ➡ **PFP1**.

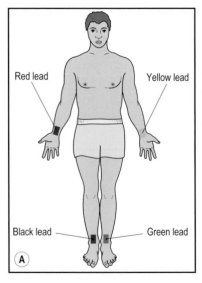

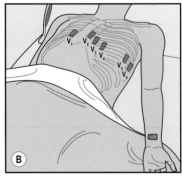

Figure 2.9 12-lead ECG A) position of limb leads; B) position of chest leads.

Table 2.1 Chest lead positions for 12-lead ECG

V1	Right sternal border, 4th intercostal space
V2	Left sternal border, 4th intercostal space
V3	Located directly between V2 and V4 (place V4 prior to V3)
V4	5th intercostal space, mid-clavicular line
V5	5th intercostal space, anterior axillary line
V6	Same plane as V4 and V5, mid axillary line

5. Apply the electrodes to the chest wall as described in Table 2.1 and shown in Figure 2.9B. If necessary, shave the area to ensure good contact/adhesion. In women with large or pendulous breasts it is sometimes difficult to place the chest leads under the breast. The electrodes may be placed over the breast in the appropriate position if this is the case.

6. Connect the ECG leads to the electrodes as labelled or colour coded.

7. Ask the patient to lie still during the recording to avoid artefact being recorded on the trace.

8. Press 'start' on the ECG machine. All 12 leads (views of the heart) will print out on one page. Add the patient's name, ward and hospital number to the printout ➡ **PFP2**

9. Remove the leads and electrodes, wiping away any traces of gel left on the skin.

10. Help the patient to replace their clothing and ensure they are comfortable

11. Lower the bed to a safe level.

12. Remove apron and wash and dry hands.

13. File the ECG in the patient's notes and inform the requesting practitioner that it has been completed.

14. Leave the ECG machine clean, tidy and stocked ready for the next user. Do not tie the leads together as this damages them. Plug the machine into the mains to charge if required.

➡ Points for practice

PFP1 If the patient is an amputee, apply the electrode to the stump.

PFP2 It is usual to note whether the patient has chest pain or is pain free at the time of the ECG recording. In some hospitals it is policy for the person recording the ECG to date and sign the printout.

2.10 Assessment of level of consciousness

Preparation

Patient

- Explain the need for frequent observations, even throughout the night. Neurological observations may need to be monitored every 30 min–2 h depending on the patients condition. Sleeping patients may need to be woken to continue the assessment

Equipment/Environment

- A small, bright torch for assessing pupil size and reactions
- Sphygmomanometer, stethoscope, thermometer and a watch
- Neurological assessment chart (see p. 52)

Nurse

- If the patient is confused and restless, bed rails padded with pillows may be needed. The bed should be at its lowest level
- The hands should be clean
- Additional protective clothing may be necessary if indicated by the patient's condition (see Ch. 1)

Procedure

The Glasgow Coma Scale is an internationally recognised objective tool used to assess and monitor a patient's level of consciousness (Dawes et al 2007). It is used in a wide variety of clinical settings and is a recommended assessment and observation tool for all patients with head injuries (NICE 2007). The patient's level of consciousness is assessed by monitoring their ability to open their eyes (eye opening), talk (verbal response) and move their limbs (motor response). Each of these areas is allocated a score based on the patient's response. The worst total score is 3 and the best 15 (see chart on p. 52). Any reduction in the score is a sign that the patient's consciousness level is deteriorating and should be reported immediately. A patient with a score of 8 or less will usually be in a deep coma.

Assessment of eye opening

Eye opening demonstrates that the arousal mechanisms in the brain are functioning. When assessing this, the scoring system is used as follows:

4 = A score of 4 is given to patients who are conscious, who sense your approach and open their eyes spontaneously or patients who are asleep, but open their eyes in response to a brief verbal stimulus, such as 'hello' or light touch.

3 = A score of 3 is given patients who open their eyes in response to a verbal stimulus such as 'can you open your eyes please?'.

2 = A score of 2 is given to patients who open their eyes only in response to a painful stimulus. This is best applied by a trapezium squeeze (pinching and twisting the muscle where the head meets the shoulder) or supra-orbital pressure (firm pressure in the eye socket just above the eye; Caton-Richards 2010, Dawes et al 2007). Response to centrally applied painful stimulus indicates that the motor pathways are still functioning to some extent (McLeod 2004). Peripheral stimuli, although useful when assessing an individual limb that has not moved in response to central stimulus, could also

be a reflex activity. Other methods (e.g. rubbing the sternum with the knuckles or pressing on nail beds) are not recommended.

1 = A score of 1 is given where there is no eye opening in response to verbal or painful stimuli.

Patients may not be able to open their eyes if there is damage to the oculomotor nerve, which is responsible for movement of the eyelid, or if paralysing medication has been administered. In these situations the nurse should gently open the eyelid (with assistance from another practitioner) when pupil response is to be assessed. If the patient is unable to open their eyes due to swelling, injury or an eye dressing, this is indicated using the letter 'C'.

Verbal response

This assesses whether patients are aware of themselves and their environment. If the patient has a tracheostomy or an endotracheal tube, the letter 'T' can be used to indicate this. The score is used as follows:

5 = A score of 5 is given if the patient is orientated, i.e. able to tell the nurse who they are, where they are, what day, date, month and year it is, and why they are where they are.

4 = A score of 4 is given if the patient is able to hold a conversation, but not able to answer specific questions (i.e. they are confused and not orientated).

3 = A score of 3 is given when the patient can speak, but does so randomly and makes short verbal responses such as swearing or shouting.

2 = A score of 2 is given when the patients speech is incomprehensible, they are grunting or groaning and the nurse may have to use painful stimuli to get a response (as described above).

1 = A score of 1 is given if the patient does not respond to verbal and painful stimuli.

Facial injuries, impairment to speech (e.g. following a stroke), cognitive difficulties (e.g. dementia) or language barriers all need to be considered when scoring the verbal response. Interpreters may be needed and the patient's normal cognitive state should be established as a baseline.

Motor response

This assesses the patient's ability to move purposefully. When assessing motor response, scores are allocated as follows:

6 = A score of 6 is given when the patient can obey commands such as 'lift your arms' or 'squeeze my hands' (where there is no injury or weakness).

5 = A score of 5 is given when the patient can localise to pain. The pain stimulus (see 'Assessment of eye opening' above) is used and patients will usually respond by trying purposefully to remove the source of the pain (brush away the nurse's hand) or 'shrug off' the pain (going 'local' to the pain). Localising to pain means that the patient's brain is receiving sensory information regarding the process of feeling pain and therefore the reduced level of consciousness is not severe.

4 = A score of 4 is given when the patient withdraws from the painful stimulus or moves towards the source of the pain, but does not attempt to remove it. Bending the arms and legs normally and fully in response to pain is known as flexion.

3 = A score of 3 is given when there is an abnormal bending movement such as wrist rotation or bending the ankle joints towards the knees. This is known as abnormal flexion, and usually indicates that the nerve pathways are not functioning normally and in some cases is a sign of deterioration and a poor prognosis.

2 = A score of 2 is given when the patient extends their limbs to pain. This may appear as if the patient is straightening or pointing their arms and legs in a rigid outwards or downwards position. This indicates damage to the brain stem and the prognosis for the patient is very poor.

1 = A score of 1 is given where there is no response to pain.

Pupil response

Raised intracranial pressure causes changes in the size of the pupils and their response to light. Assessment of the pupils (Figure 2.10) evaluates the function of the optic nerve, which causes a reaction to light being shone in the eye, and the oculomotor nerve, which constricts the pupil. A poor reaction in either of these assessments may indicate compression of the nerves and should be reported. When undertaking assessment of the pupils, dim the light in the room and hold the eyelid open (you may need another practitioner to help with this). Before you shine the light in the patient's eye observe the following:

- The resting size of both pupils. The average size is 2–6 mm (Dawes et al 2007), but it varies according to the time of the day and the amount of light available.

- Whether both pupils are equal in size – inequality can be a serious sign of raised intracranial pressure (or the sign of previous eye injury).

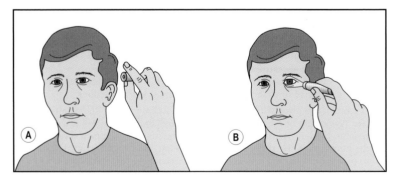

Figure 2.10 Assessment of pupil response.

- The shape of the pupils – they are normally round. Different shapes may indicate damage to the brain.

Bringing the light of the pen torch in from the side of the eye, observe:
- the reaction of each pupil to light.

- the intensity of the reaction, i.e. whether it is brisk, sluggish or absent.

- It is also important to note if the patient has a pre-existing abnormality, or irregularity of the eye/s, for example cataracts, which will affect the response. In addition it is important to note any drugs or medications the patients may have had. Some cause dilation (e.g. atropine) whilst others (opiates, e.g. morphine) cause constriction. Prosthetic eyes will not elicit a pupilliary response.

Vital signs

These are not part of the Glasgow Coma Scale itself but because of their importance, they are usually included on the same chart (Figure 2.11):

- **Temperature** – alterations in patients' temperature may be due to damage of the thermoregulation centre of the brain. A rise in body temperature increases the demand for oxygen by the brain cells, which may already be compromised due to damage. It is usually desirable to keep the body temperature within normal limits, where possible. This may require antipyretic agents such as paracetamol or active measures such as fan therapy (see p. 34). Patients with severe brain injuries may be kept mildly hypothermic in order to reduce metabolic demand in the brain tissue (Cole 2009)

- **Pulse rate and blood pressure** – in patients with severe raised intracranial pressure the blood pressure rises and pulse rate falls. As the brain becomes hypoxic and ischaemic, the body responds by attempting to increase the arterial blood pressure in order to get oxygen to it. As a result there is a need for more blood in each contraction of the heart. This results in a slowing of the heart rate (bradycardia). Respiration rate also decreases and a change in the respiratory pattern occurs (see below). This is known as 'Cushing's reflex' and is a very late response to deteriorating level of consciousness. Careful recording and charting is needed so that a trend in this direction is clearly detectable and reported urgently.

- **Respiration rate** – changes in respiration are a good indicator of the function of the brain stem. This is because there are four respiratory control centres in two parts of the brain stem. Monitoring of respiration rate and pattern is essential as a sudden change, such as Cheyne–Stokes breathing (deep, sighing respirations followed by periods of apnoea for several seconds) or apnoea, is due to a significant rise in intracranial pressure.

Limb movement

In addition to assessing motor response as described above, assessing limb movement can detect weaknesses of one side of the body or limbs. Assessing limb movement and motor power gives an indication of the extent of the damage to the motor cortex that controls motor movement and is graded as follows ➜ **PFP1**:

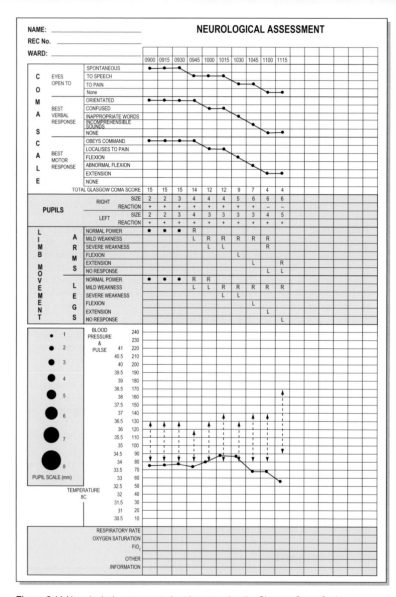

Figure 2.11 Neurological assessment chart incorporating the Glasgow Coma Scale.

- **Normal power** – the nurse applies resistance to any joint movement and this can be matched by the patient, e.g. pulling or pushing whilst holding the hands
- **Mild weakness** – the patient is able to counter the resistance, but is easily overcome
- **Severe weakness** – the patient is able to move the limb but not against resistance
- **Flexion, extension or no response** – there is flexion, extension or no movement in response to central or peripheral painful stimuli.

Other level of consciousness assessment tools

In recent years alternative assessment tools, such as the AVPU (alert, responds to voice, pain or unresponsive) have emerged. The AVPU has a simple structure, which is easy to apply and has been incorporated into the Early Warning Score (also known as Patient At Risk (PAR) score – see p. 76; Palmer & Knight 2006). This is in recognition of the fact that many patients who are critically ill will have altered levels of consciousness. The AVPU can give information quickly about a patient's level of consciousness, which can then be more formally assessed with the Glasgow Coma Scale as necessary ➡ **PFP2**. However, it should not replace the Glasgow Coma Scale as a formal neurological assessment tool (McLeod 2004).

AVPU comprises determining the level of consciousness by assessing (Resuscitation Council UK 2011):

A: Alert – is the patient alert?

V: Verbal – is the patient only responding to verbal stimuli?

P: Pain – is the patient only responding to painful stimuli?

U: Unresponsive – is the patient unresponsive to all stimuli?

➡ Points for practice

PFP1 Assessing motor power requires knowledge of motor nerve anatomy (myotomes) and skill in performing the procedure. If the nurse is to assess more than the presence (or not) of limb weakness then further training in this skill is required.

PFP2 AVPU assessment can be used to assess the conscious level of all patients – and is usually conducted on encountering the patient, noting their response to a greeting such as 'hello', or 'how are you feeling?' Some neurological conditions require a more formal neurological assessment using GCS – namely head- or brain-injured patients; patients with neurological disorders such as a brain tumour, stroke, meningitis; and patients with a reduced level of consciousness following sedation e.g. anaesthetic, opiate analgesia or drug overdose.

2.11 Weighing patients

Preparation

Patient

- Explain procedure, to gain consent and cooperation
  ➡ **PFP1**
- Encourage the patient to empty their bladder
- Weigh the patient on the same scales, at the same time each day/week, and in similar clothing ➡ **PFP2**

Equipment/Environment

- The scales must be on a level surface
- Use the same scales for regular weighing
  ➡ **PFP2**
- Ensure the pointer is at zero or weights are to the left, at zero

Nurse

- The hands should be clean
- An apron should be worn if the patient requires assistance. Additional protective clothing may be necessary if indicated by the patient's condition (see Ch. 1).

Procedure

1. Position the scales for easy access and apply the brakes.

2. Ask/assist the patient to sit on the scales or stand on the platform. If electronic scales are being used, ensure they are charged or plug them in to the mains before the patient sits down.

3. If sitting, ensure that the patient's feet are off the floor (Figure 2.12).

4. Ask the patient to remain still and note the reading.

5. If the scales are electric the weight will be displayed. If manual scales are used check the patient's previous weight to determine the approximate position and move the heavier weight bar (kilograms) to the right until the two pivotal arrows swing (e.g. if the previous weight was 73 kg, move the heavier bar to 70 kg). If the bar is moved too far, the weight will sink and stop swinging. Adjust the lighter weight bar so that the arrows are exactly level and free floating.

6. Note the reading by adding the position of the heavier bar (e.g. 70 kg) to that of the lighter bar (e.g. 3.5 kg; total equals 73.5 kg).

7. If the weight is very different from a recent previous weight, check it again and, if confirmed, report it.

8. Assist the patient back to the bed/chair as necessary.

9. Return the scales to their storage place and clean according to local policy. If electronic, plug them into the mains.

10. Document the weight according to local policy and report any unexpected loss or gain.

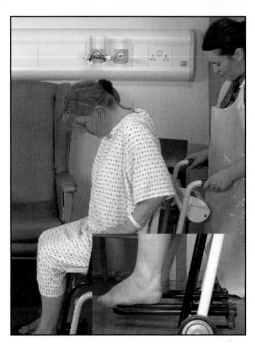

Figure 2.12 Weighing a patient.

➡️ Points for practice

PFP1 Weight measurement may be used to calculate the body mass index (see Ch. 6); to determine weight gain or loss when there is concern over the patient's nutritional status or to determine fluid retention/ fluid loss.

PFP2 It is important to use the same set of scales for regular weighing as there will be variation between sets of scales. The actual weight is usually of less importance than whether the weight is increasing or decreasing; it will not be possible to accurately detect changes unless the same scales are used and the patient is wearing similar clothing at the same time of day.

2.12 Measuring waist circumference

Preparation

Patient

- Explain the procedure to gain consent and cooperation
  ➡ PFP1
- The patient should be standing with their arms hanging freely
- The midriff should be exposed
- Both feet should be together

Equipment/Environment

- A tape measure that does not easily stretch, ideally a disposable paper tape measure, should be used

Nurse

- Hands must be clean and an apron should be worn.
- Additional protective clothing may be necessary if indicated by the patient's condition (see Ch. 1)

Procedure

1. Ask the patient to exhale and measure the waist circumference midway between the lowest rib and the iliac crest.

2. The tape measure should be applied tightly enough that it will not slip, but without putting pressure on the abdomen. Note the measurement in centimetres.

3. Assist the patient back to the bed/chair as necessary.

4. Clean the tape measure according to local policy or discard in clinical waste if disposable.

5. Remove apron and wash hands/use alcohol hand rub.

6. Document the measurement according to local policy and report if above acceptable limits (**➡ PFP2**).

➡ Points for practice

PFP1 Central obesity is linked to an increased risk of cardiovascular disease. Waist circumference measurement is a better predictor of cardiovascular disease than body mass index (see Ch. 6) and is commonly used in predictive scoring systems.

PFP2 A waist circumference above 102 cm in men and above 88 cm in women is considered to confer an increased risk for developing both diabetes and cardiovascular disease. Due to ethnic variations in cardiovascular risk, in the Asian population a waist measurement of above 90 cm in men and above 80 cm in women is considered an increased risk.

2.13 Measuring height

Preparation

Patient	Equipment/Environment	Nurse
• Explain the procedure to gain consent and cooperation ➡ **PFP1**	• Standard height measurement equipment (stadiometer)	• Hands must be clean and an apron should be worn
• The patient should be standing ➡ **PFP2**	• The sliding horizontal rod should move freely on the vertical ruler	• Additional protective clothing may be necessary if indicated by the patient's condition (see Ch.1)
• Shoes should be removed		

Procedure

1. Ask the patient to stand straight with their back and head against the vertical measurement ruler

2. Slide the horizontal rod down until it rests on the top of the patient's head. Note the measurement in centimetres

3. Assist the patient back to the bed/chair as necessary, remembering to replace shoes/slippers to avoid them slipping on the floor

4. Clean the stadiometer according to local policy

5. Remove apron and wash hands/use alcohol hand rub

6. Document the measurement according to local policy.

➡ Points for practice

PFP1 Height measurement is used to calculate body mass index (see p. 152) and for predicting peak expiratory flow rates (see p. 346).

PFP2 If the patient is unable to stand to be measured ask the patient or their family if they know their height.

2.14 Care of the patient having a seizure

Preparation

Patient

- Protecting the patient from injury is of primary concern
- Maintain privacy and dignity ➡ **PFP1**

Equipment/Environment

- Ensure patient safety. This may entail clearing the environment or, on rare occasions, moving the patient from danger

Nurse

- Maintain own safety. Stay with the patient but do not place your fingers in the patient's mouth or try to restrain the patient
- Protective clothing may be necessary if indicated by the patient's condition (see Ch. 1)

Procedure

When the patient has a seizure, ➡ **PFP2** the first phase (the tonic phase) is associated with rigidity of limbs and breath holding. This phase may be brief. In the second phase (clonic phase), there is rhythmical jerking of arms and legs. Characteristically the jerks are unilateral; initially close together and then decreasing in frequency. This phase is followed by a period of deep sleep, when the patient is usually unrousable and their body is limp:

1. Protect the patient from injury, but do not attempt to restrain their limbs
2. Use pillows as necessary to pad hard surfaces, and remove non-essential furniture and equipment
3. Observe the patient continuously, noting the following:
   - duration of each phase of the seizure, including the recovery time (i.e. when able to resume normal activities).
   - limbs involved.
   - whether movement is localised or general.
   - whether the jaw is clenched ➡ **PFP3**
   - whether the patient is frothing at the mouth (saliva) – suction may be needed when the fit has finished.
   - whether the patient has been incontinent of urine or faeces.
   - breathing pattern – this will change. Patients are likely to hold their breath and may become cyanosed or just pale. Loud breathing sounds may indicate the end of the seizure. (The breathing reverts spontaneously and oxygen is not usually required.)
4. During the period of deep sleep following the clonic phase, the patient should be left in the recovery position to maintain an airway and should not be disturbed, allowing the patient to recover in their own time. It can last up to 30 minutes.
5. It is now safe to put your fingers in the patient's mouth to remove food or dentures if necessary.

6. The patient may be disorientated and should be calmly reassured explaining what has happened. Ensure patient comfort by offering a wash, change of clothing etc., as necessary.

7. All seizures must be documented and reported.

If a seizure or seizures occur in rapid succession and last 30 minutes or longer this is called *status epilepticus* (Walker 2005). This requires urgent medical intervention. When fully awake ask the patient whether there was any warning of the seizure (aura) and whether it can be described, e.g. a smell or taste. If there is no previous history of seizures or a change in the pattern/length of seizures, the patient's doctor should be informed.

➡ Points for practice

PFP1 If the seizure occurs in a public place, encourage bystanders to disperse to prevent the patient feeling crowded and possibly embarrassed.

PFP2 The term seizure was previously referred to as 'fitting'. A seizure with tonic and clonic phases was formerly called a grand mal fit.

PFP3 During the tonic phase of the seizure, the patient will clench their jaw and may bite their tongue. Nothing should be inserted into the mouth to try and prevent this.

2.15 Neurovascular assessment

Preparation

Patient
- Explain procedure, to gain consent and cooperation.
- Explain the need for frequent observations ➜ **PFP1**

Equipment
- Screening the bed is not usually necessary, but ensure that dignity and privacy are maintained.
- Raise the bed to a safe working height (see Ch. 12)

Nurse
- Hands must be clean and an apron should be worn.
- Additional protective clothing may be necessary if indicated by the patient's condition (see Ch. 1)

Procedure

Neurovascular assessment involves assessment of the following: ➜ **PFP2**

1. **Movement** – ask the patient to move the toes/fingers and ankle/wrist of the affected limb if possible. If the patient is unable to do so, undertake the movement passively and note any pain that occurs with movement or rest ➜ **PFP3**.

2. **Sensation** – without letting the patient see which toes/fingers you are touching, touch the toes/fingers randomly and ask the patient to tell you which one you are touching. Ask the patient if they feel any altered sensation in the limb such as numbness, tingling or 'pins and needles'.

3. **Perfusion** – in order to assess perfusion observe the following:
   - Temperature – feel the warmth of the limb, both above and below the site of injury. It is best to do this using the back of the hand.
   - Colour – observe the colour of the skin and nail beds. Note any cyanosis, mottling or pallor.
   - Pulse – the pulse should be palpated distal to the injury. It may not always be possible to easily locate a pulse, particularly in the feet. Therefore, once located (Figure 2.13), it is helpful to mark the site to make it easier for subsequent checking ➜ **PFP4**. Note the strength of the pulse. If bandages or a splint prevent you locating a pulse this should be documented ➜ **PFP5**.

4. **Pain/swelling** – if the patient complains of pain or the toes/fingers are swollen, check the bandage, splint or plaster cast for tightness. Note the location, level and characteristics of any reported pain. If swelling is present, note any increase since the last set of observations and consider the removal of tight fitting jewellery and loosening of bandages. Elevation of the limb may help prevent swelling.

5. **Bandage/dressing/splint/plaster cast** – check for bleeding under or around these.

6. Ensure the patient is appropriately covered and comfortable.

7. Remove apron and clean hands prior to completing relevant documentation according to local policy. If more than one limb is affected, separate charts should be used for documentation.

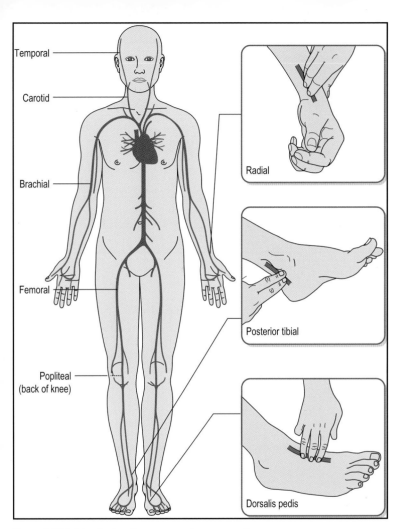

Figure 2.13 Peripheral pulses for neurovascular assessment.

Temporal

Carotid

Brachial

Femoral

Popliteal
(back of knee)

Radial

Posterior tibial

Dorsalis pedis

PFP1 These observations are made following injury or surgery to a limb. The limb may be bandaged, splinted or encased in plaster of Paris.

PFP2 When observing limb perfusion, movement and sensation compare it to the other limb, if that is unaffected. Where possible the pulse on the affected limb should be assessed on admission as a baseline for later comparison.

PFP3 It is important to see all fingers/toes move, particularly as little toes can be covered. Each digit has a separate nerve supply, which may be damaged or compressed.

PFP4 If the dorsalis pedis pulse cannot be located, try to palpate the posterior tibial pulse.

PFP5 If recording 'pulse not felt', take care that it is not confused with 'pulse not able to be located' due to the bandage/splint, etc. If a pulse cannot be located due to a bandage or cast, capillary refill time may be measured to assess perfusion (see p. 82).

2.16 Blood glucose monitoring

Preparation

Patient

- Explain the procedure, to gain consent and cooperation
- Ensure the patient's hands are clean. Do not use alcohol wipes ➡ **PFP1**
- Ask the patient to choose the finger to be used for the procedure ➡ **PFP2**

Equipment

- Blood glucose meter
- Finger-pricking device or lancet
- Gauze swab/cotton-wool ball, according to local policy
- Blood glucose testing strips

Nurse

- Most Trusts require nurses to have undergone formal training in the use of the glucometer –check local policy
- The hands should be clean and apron and gloves should be worn
- Additional protective clothing may be necessary if indicated by the patient's condition (see Ch. 1)

Procedure

1. Ensure all equipment is within easy reach and the patient is comfortable.

2. If necessary, assist the patient with washing and drying of the finger/hand.

3. Use new lancets and platforms for each test ➡ **PFP3**.

4. Check the expiry date of the testing strips and prepare the blood glucose meter and insert the testing strip according to the manufacturer's instructions ➡ **PFP4**.

5. Using the appropriate device, prick the side of the patient's fingertip. Avoid frequent use of the thumbs, index and little fingers where possible ➡ **PFP2**.

6. Allow a drop of blood to fall onto the testing strip – do not smear it (Figure 2.14) ➡ **PFP5**.

7. Ask the patient to press on the site, using the gauze swab/cotton-wool ball, to stem bleeding and reduce the risk of bruising.

8. Wait for the meter to provide a digital display of the result ➡ **PFP6**.

9. Read and document the results according to local policy or use the monitor memory system (if available). Report any abnormalities.

10. Inform the patient of their blood glucose level.

11. Ensure the patient is comfortable and that bleeding has stopped

12. Dispose of all sharps and contaminated waste appropriately (see p. 63) and return equipment as appropriate.

13. Remove gloves and apron and wash hands.

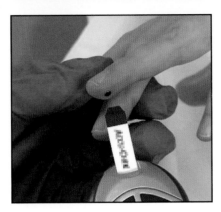

Figure 2.14 Blood glucose monitoring.

➡Points for practice

PFP1 The patient's hands should be clean and washing the hands in warm water will encourage blood flow. If the patient is unable to wash their hands, and there is any possibility that there may have been contact with substances such as fruit juice, the finger should be washed or wiped with a wet tissue and then a dry tissue before pricking (Walker 2004). An alcohol swab must not be used as this may give a false reading and may harden the skin with frequent use (Lawal 2009).

PFP2 The side of the patient's finger is used as it maximises the potential for a sufficient sample and is less painful (Lawal 2009). However, the site should be rotated because even using the side of the finger can be painful, especially if performed several times a day (Hill 2008). This also helps reduce the risk of infection from multiple finger pricks and prevents the area from becoming hardened. The thumb and the forefinger should be avoided as the skin tends to be thicker on these digits (Hill 2008).

PFP3 Use a finger-pricking device, as it is more likely to ensure a good blood flow and is less painful. Before pricking the patient's finger, hold the hand downwards to encourage blood flow, and make a light tourniquet with your hand around the finger to ensure sufficient blood is present in the tip of the finger. Avoid 'milking' blood into the finger as the local blood composition may be disturbed by intermingling with tissue fluid. Taking time to encourage blood flow before pricking the finger will reduce the need for pricking again, which can be distressing for the patient.

PFP4 Preparation of the glucose meter usually involves checking that it has been calibrated for the particular batch of testing strips that are being used. With some glucose meters, the strip is inserted into the monitor after the blood is dropped onto it. Follow the manufacturer's instructions regarding timing and wiping prior to insertion into the machine.

PFP5 The drop of blood should fall onto the strip rather than be 'wiped on', as this may lead to an inaccurate result. Test strips do vary and with some the blood is not dropped directly onto the strip. Always check the manufacturer's instructions.

2.17 Pain assessment

Principles

Pain is often considered to be the fifth vital sign (Lynch 2001) – after temperature, pulse, respirations and BP – which indicates the level of importance that should be placed on assessing and managing pain. This is because pain can have harmful physiological, psychological and emotional effects. Pain is a complex and subjective phenomenon and its successful management has always presented a challenge. There have been significant advances in the management of pain with the development of acute and chronic pain services and improved techniques for administering analgesia, including patient-controlled analgesia (PCA) and epidural analgesia. There is also a greater recognition of the role of non-pharmacological strategies such as transcutaneous electrical nerve stimulation (TENS), physiotherapy, heat pads, massage, relaxation, reflexology, acupuncture and, in some cases, cognitive behavioural therapy (CBT), in the management of pain (Godfrey 2005, Cox 2010).

Effective pain management depends on good interprofessional team working, and the nurse's role is central in ensuring that the patient's pain is assessed, treatment regimens are implemented and their effectiveness evaluated. Successful pain management depends on accurate assessment and reassessment of the patient's pain (Godfrey 2005). Given its complexity, not only must the sensory component be assessed, but also the patient's moods, attitudes, coping efforts, resources and its impact on their life and the lives of their family. This is a continuous process and it is suggested below that there are three key areas for consideration in the assessment of pain. The extent of the assessment will vary with specific circumstances.

1. Who should assess the patient's pain?

Pain is largely a subjective experience and so patients themselves are best placed to assess their own pain accurately (Godfrey 2005). Observation by others involves interpretation of what the patient is feeling and, therefore, can be unreliable. It is vital that nurses accept the patients' estimation of their pain even if it is not accompanied by the usual behaviours (e.g. grimacing, adopting a foetal position, groaning) or alteration to vital signs, e.g. raised pulse. Vital signs can be unreliable as a measure of a person's pain. The way in which different patients respond to pain can be attributed to a multitude of variables, such as age, culture, type of pain and duration. Observation and vital-sign measurement should only be relied upon when the patient is unable to communicate. Assessment of pain is an important aspect of the nurse's role that requires a number of skills, including observation, interpretation and communication skills.

2. When should the patient's pain be assessed?

The frequency of pain assessment is dependent on the individual circumstances. Factors to be considered when determining frequency include:
- The severity of the pain. Pain assessment is often carried out when the patient is resting, but a better indicator of the efficacy of analgesia will be achieved by asking the patient to cough, move or take a deep breath.

- Frequency of assessment should be increased if pain is poorly controlled or treatment regimens are changing.

- Regular pain assessment is important in the postoperative period. Patients with patient-controlled analgesia (PCA – see p. 71) should be assessed each time other vital signs are recorded. For patients with epidural analgesia (see p. 73), the sensory block should be checked approximately 20 minutes after administration of the analgesic.

3. What should be assessed?

Multidimensional pain tools such as the McGill Pain Questionnaire (MPQ) offer a framework for assessment of many of the issues outlined below and include the intensity, sensory, affective and evaluative elements of pain. However, no one tool is adequate for enabling the patient to describe the quality of their pain experience and what is more important is facilitating the telling of their 'story' through open questions, active listening and reflecting (McLafferty and Farley 2008). Initial assessment of a patient's pain should include:

- **The location, duration, intensity and characteristics of the pain.** Defining the nature of a patient's pain is important, as different types of pain will be treated differently. The nurse should establish whether the pain is localised to a particular part of the body or whether it is more generalised. The patient should be asked to describe whether the pain is 'sharp', 'dull', 'intermittent' or 'continuous', and to indicate when it started and how long they have had the pain. The patient's perception of the pain is important and this should be assessed in terms of whether it is 'tolerable', 'unbearable', etc.

- **The underlying condition.** The underlying diagnosis or cause of a patient's pain is central to determining whether the subsequent treatment is curative or palliative. For example, acute pain is often an indicator of disease or injury, which following treatment can be resolved. Conversely, pain may indicate a worsening of the patient's condition, but the overall goal of treatment may be palliative and focus on relieving the symptoms.

- **Is the pain acute, persistent (chronic) or referred?** It is important to establish whether the patient's pain is acute, persistent (chronic) or referred, as this may influence the choice of treatment. For example, pharmacological intervention is the mainstay of acute pain management, whereas chronic pain management often demands a range of treatment options including pharmacological and non-pharmacological regimens. Chronic pain is increasingly being referred to as persistent pain, with some distinguishing between that which is caused by tissue damage (nociceptive) and that which has persisted beyond the original cause as a result of nerve damage or disruption to the normal transmission of pain (neuropathic; Fear 2010). This important physiological distinction has the advantage of informing decision-making about the best way to manage the pain. Referred pain is common in conditions that originate in the viscera. For example, the pain in a myocardial infarction is often referred to the left arm.

- **Any medical/nursing treatment being given?** Any treatment currently being received by the patient should be reviewed in order to determine its effectiveness. Furthermore, current treatment may be an important indicator as to the efficacy of any proposed treatments.

- **Precipitating or exacerbating factors, e.g. mobility/immobility, time of day, eating/drinking.** Determining factors that precipitate or exacerbate the pain facilitates diagnosis and also aids with identification of the goals of care. For example, if a patient develops pain when undertaking a particular activity, the goal of care may be twofold. The patient may be encouraged to either avoid the activity or may undertake a programme that concentrates on maximising their coping potential in that situation. Time of day may also be significant; some patients report higher levels of pain at night.

- **Related symptoms, e.g. nausea, vomiting, breathlessness or sleeplessness.** Related symptoms, such as nausea and vomiting, are often significant in aiding diagnosis, but are also important in that they can cause the patient such distress as to interfere with their ability to cope with pain. A score to indicate the level of nausea and vomiting is often used with patients receiving PCA. This should be assessed and recorded with other vital signs. Pain that causes sleeplessness significantly reduces the patient's ability to tolerate it.

- **Coping strategies used by the patient – pharmacological and non-pharmacological.** When determining the plan of care for a patient in pain, it is important to include any coping strategies the patient may have developed. Medication used by the patient may indicate what 'works' and may subsequently minimise the risk of prescribing treatments that 'do not work'. Non-pharmacological coping strategies (such as use of heat pads or massage) should, whenever possible, be included in the overall plan of care. This will enhance the patient's perception of being involved in their plan of care.

- **Meaning or significance of the pain for the patient.** The patient's perception of the significance of their pain is extremely important. Pain creates fear, anxiety and a sense of loss of control. Fear of death is common. It is essential, therefore, for the nurse to establish how patients perceive their pain.

Self-report pain assessment tools

It is vital that nurses regard pain assessment as a priority. Unless pain is assessed regularly and effectively, patients will continue to suffer unnecessarily. Effective pain assessment is a fundamental part of nursing care and accountability for the accuracy of pain assessment lies firmly within the domain of nursing. However, because of the subjective nature of the pain experience, feedback from patients about the intensity of their pain experiences is essential. Initial and ongoing assessment may be undertaken using a Self-Reporting Pain Assessment Tool, but it is important to remember that they only rate pain intensity, which is only one aspect of the patient's pain experience. The most commonly used are:

- **Visual Analogue Scale (VAS)** uses a 10-cm line with one end-point indicating 'no pain' and the other indicating 'worst pain imaginable' (Figure 2.15). The patient indicates the point on the line that best represents their pain. Some scales include words at set intervals, e.g. 'slight', 'moderate', 'severe'. However, this scale can be difficult to use for patients who have motor ability or visual

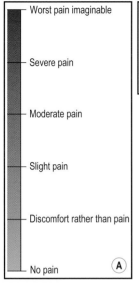

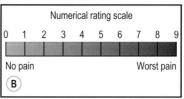

Figure 2.15 A: Visual analogue scale for pain assessment; B: numerical rating scale for pain assessment.

acuity problems as they must be able to indicate the point on the scale that represents their pain.

- **Numerical Rating Scale (NRS).** The Verbal Numerical Rating Scale is similar to the VAS. Using a scale in which 0 is 'no pain' and 10 is 'worst imaginable pain', patients are asked to indicate the number that best represents their pain. As this tool can be administered verbally it is suitable for use with patients with motor ability or visual acuity problems.

- **Verbal Rating Scale (VRS).** These scales ask the patient to consider a series of words that best describes the pain, e.g. 'none', 'mild', 'moderate', 'severe', 'very severe' and 'worst pain imaginable'. Because this scale uses words rather than numbers it is dependent on the patient's understanding and/or interpretation of the words used to describe the pain.

- **Faces Pain Rating Scale** asks the patient to pick a face that best represents their level of pain from a series that range from happy and smiling to grimacing and crying. Each face is numbered and they rise in increments of two with 0 representing the happy face (no hurt) and 10 the saddest face (hurts worst) (McLafferty and Farley 2008). Although this type of rating scale was primarily used with children, it has now been adopted for use with those with communication and language difficulties.

- **The Pain Assessment in Advanced Dementia Scale (PAINAD).** A number of scales have been developed for specific use with cognitively impaired patients and PAINAD is one such tool. Patients who are cognitively impaired may not be able to accurately convey their pain or its intensity with the result that it may be left untreated or undertreated. PAINAD uses five items: Breathing independent of vocalization; negative vocalization; facial expression; body language and consolability (Warden et al 2003). A score of 0, 1 or 2 is given to each item with a possible score of 10 indicating severe pain.

Any of the above scales may be complemented by the use of a body outline that gives a good indication of pain sites. Providing the most appropriate tool is selected for the patient group and the patient is able to understand the tool, there are a number of advantages to using such scales:

- They can be used alone or in conjunction with other pain assessment strategies

- They are relatively simple to use

- They enable the patient to provide a clear picture of pain intensity

- Regular use provides evidence of the efficacy of treatment regimens and indicates an improvement or worsening of the patient's pain experience.

2.18 Patient-controlled analgesia (PCA) and epidural analgesia

Principles

Although patient-controlled analgesia refers to any method or route by which the patient self-administers analgesia, in most clinical settings it is taken to be mean the patient activated intravenous infusion of analgesia via an infusion pump. Patient-controlled analgesia (PCA) became popular as a method of managing postoperative pain in the early 1990s. Today, however, it has a much broader use and have been found to be effective in patients with burns, myocardial infarction, bone marrow transplantation, pancreatitis and sickle cell crisis. It can also be useful with patients who are terminally ill. PCA facilitates active involvement of patients in the management of their pain. Through the use of a syringe driver and a timing device, PCA allows patients to self-administer small doses of an analgesic whenever they feel pain. It has several advantages over intermittent intramuscular or subcutaneous administration of analgesics on an 'as required' basis:

1. PCA gives the patient a sense of control and there is no questioning of the validity of the pain.

2. It enables analgesia requirement to be individualised to a sufficiently high plasma concentration level and stable plasma concentration levels to be maintained thereafter. This prevents the peaks and troughs associated with intermittent injection.

3. Unlike the conventional system of intermittent injection, there is no delay between the request for analgesia and the provision of pain relief.

4. It saves nurses' time.

PCA is usually administered intravenously (although epidural, see below, and subcutaneous infusions are also used) via a syringe driver and timing device. The patient activates the system by pressing a button that releases a small dose of the analgesic into the circulation. There is a 'lock-out' device that prevents further doses being delivered with a specified time interval. The use of the lock-out device allows time for the opioid to start working and although it does limit the amount of analgesia the patient can request it should not be seen as a means of preventing overdose (Chumbley and Montford 2010). Morphine is the most common opiate used and a lock-out period of 5 minutes is normal when it is being administered intravenously. Subcutaneous administration requires a longer lock-out time of 10 minutes (Chumbley and Montford 2010). Morphine administered in 1 mg boluses at 5-minute intervals will provide 12 mg per hour and will normally provide effective pain relief with minimal side effects. However, it is also important to note that patients' requirements for analgesia can vary considerably and 12 mg may be too little or too much. Therefore, it is fundamental that the patient is carefully monitored throughout (see below).

PCA devices

There is a variety of battery or electrically operated PCA devices available. Most will include the following features:

- A lock-out device that prevents the syringe driver delivering more than the maximum preset dose over a set period, e.g. 4 hours.

- Safety features that include alarms for occlusion (blockage), air in the line, low battery or empty syringe.

- A keypad lock and other locking devices that prevent unauthorised access and changes to the programme.

- An electronic microprocessor that allows the flow rate, bolus dose and lockout interval to be set. This will usually record the number of bolus doses requested and administered, which is important when determining the effectiveness of the PCA.

- Anti-syphon valves and anti-reflux valves should be used.

- An alternative is a mechanical system where a 'control module' is worn around the wrist with a connecting pocket-sized infusor. This is less flexible than the electronic pumps as it only delivers a pre-set, non-adjustable volume and has only one lock-out interval and no safety alarms. However, it is much cheaper than the electronic modes and affords the patient greater freedom of movement.

Patient education

The success of PCA is dependent on the patient being willing and able to use it. Therefore, patient education is vital, and with surgical patients this should occur pre-operatively, either in the pre-admission clinic or on the ward. The patient should be encouraged to handle the device and press the buttons etc., in order to become familiar with the device to be used. It is important that the nurse notes the patient's understanding and dexterity in handling the equipment because patients who are unable to manage the device may not receive any analgesia. If a patient is unable to use the system, nurse-administered analgesia will be required.

Monitoring the patient

Regular monitoring is essential for patients with a PCA. This includes the following:

1. Ensuring the machine is placed at or below the level of the patient's heart to prevent any risk of siphoning.

2. Close monitoring of respiration rate, counting for a full minute, particularly immediately after commencement, as respiratory depression is the main side effect of opiate analgesia. Local protocol should be consulted regarding the action to be taken if respirations fall below a certain level; a respiratory rate of less than 8 or 10 respirations a minute usually requires intervention from the pain control nurse, the anaesthetist or doctor. Some protocols stipulate that patients should have oxygen administered whilst the PCA is in progress. Oxygen saturation levels should be recorded with respiratory rate.

3. The patient's blood pressure and pulse should be recorded.

4. Pain should be assessed using a pain assessment tool (see p. 66) to ensure effective pain relief is being achieved.

5. The level of sedation must be monitored; opiates cause sedation and it is important to ensure that the patient is still rousable. Most chart incorporate a sedation score.

6. The incidence/severity of nausea and vomiting should be documented.

7. Where possible, patients' usage (i.e. how often they press the button) should be monitored to determine whether the pain control is effective.

8. The prescribed settings for the PCA system should be checked regularly to ensure proper functioning.

9. All of the above should be monitored at least hourly in the early stages. Some areas have a specially designed pain assessment tool that incorporates all of the above areas.

10. The nurse should monitor the infusion site for signs of inflammation, redness or tissue damage.

11. As with all controlled drugs, the nurse should prepare, administer and document the infusion in accordance with local trust policy. Where possible, and to avoid errors ready-made bags of opioids should be used.

12. The nurse should ensure no other opiates are administered whilst the patient is receiving PCA.

Epidural analgesia

Principles

Epidural analgesia is commonly used for maternal analgesia during childbirth and patients who have undergone vascular surgery, thoracic or abdominal surgery, or orthopaedic surgery to the lower limb. It is also used for patients with intractable cancer pain and those with persistent, neuropathic or visceral pain of a chronic nature. A fine-bore catheter is inserted into the epidural space, which is between the dura mater and the ligaments and bones of the spinal cord. It can be approached at any level of the spine, but is most commonly at the lumbar or sacral level. However, the use of thoracic epidurals is increasing and is seen as the approach that demonstrates improved dynamic pain relief (Wheatley et al 2001). The catheter is usually secured to the patient's back using a sterile fixation device and a clear occlusive dressing, and is then attached to the infusion device.

The drugs most commonly used for epidural analgesia are opioids (e.g. fentanyl, diamorphine) and local anaesthetics (bupivocaine). Dosages vary according to the site of the catheter, the type of surgery and the age and medical condition of the patient. Administration as a continuous infusion is seen as the most effective in the management of postoperative pain. Bolus injections are used less commonly for postoperative pain, but are used for the management of the pain of maternal labour. Patient Controlled Epidural Analgesia (PCEA) is used for postoperative or persistent (chronic) pain as it affords the patient control over their analgesia. It is most effective when used in combination with a low-dose background infusion (Wheatley et al 2001).

Monitoring patients with epidural analgesia

Careful monitoring of the patient is vital and includes the following:

1. The prescribed settings on the epidural device or pump must be checked regularly to ensure it is functioning properly. The device should never be regarded as fail-safe.

2. Single luer-lock connections must be used between the catheter and the administration set. Three-way connectors must not be used to prevent inadvertent administration of other medications.

3. A bacterial filter must be in place at the end of the epidural cannula.

4. The epidural cannula must be clearly labelled so that it cannot be confused with an intravenous cannula.

5. The dressing over the epidural cannula site should be transparent and secure to prevent inadvertently dislodging the catheter and to minimise the risk of contamination. The inspection site should be inspected daily.

6. Close monitoring of sedation levels. Sedation and respiratory depression are known side-effects of opioids. The use of a sedation score is recommended to assist in the early detection of respiratory depression. If the score signifies the patient is becoming unacceptably sedated, the infusion should be stopped and oxygen administered whilst medical or anaesthetic intervention is sought.

7. Close monitoring of respirations should be undertaken alongside sedation scores. Oxygen saturation levels are recorded with respiratory rate, although they should not be used as the primary or only indicator of respiratory depression.

8. The blood pressure and pulse rate should be recorded hourly. Hypotension is associated with the use of local anaesthetics in epidural analgesia and can also occur if the epidural catheter migrates into the subarachnoid space. This would be accompanied by light-headedness, tachycardia (raised pulse) and difficulty with movement. The infusion should be stopped and medical assistance sought immediately if any of these symptoms occur. However, it is important to remember that in postoperative patients hypotension may be due to blood loss.

9. Local anaesthetics can also be toxic to the central nervous systems. The nurse should assess the patient excitation, numbness of the tongue and mouth, slurred speech, twitching, light-headedness and tinnitus (buzzing or ringing in the ears). If central nervous system toxicity occurs the patient may experience respiratory depression, convulsions and is at risk of cardiac arrest. If toxicity is suspected the infusion must be stopped. The priority of medical intervention is the patient's ventilation and oxygen needs.

10. Fluid intake should be monitored to ensure that any reduction in blood pressure is not associated with dehydration. Where possible, oral fluids must be encouraged and intravenous infusion considered.

11. Urinary output must be monitored, particularly in those patients with lumbar epidural analgesia, as it is commonly associated with urinary retention. If the patient has a urinary catheter, hourly measurements should be undertaken. Accurate recording on a fluid balance chart is essential.

12. The height of the epidural block can be assessed by the application of cold to the skin surface. If the patient reports pins and needles in the fingers this should be reported. The hourly rate of the infusion may need to be reduced.

13. Pain should be assessed using a pain assessment tool to ensure effective pain relief is being achieved. Pain should be controlled sufficiently to enable the patient to cough, breathe deeply and mobilise. If the patient reports pain at the site of the infusion, medical staff should be informed as infection or haematoma may be present.

14. Nausea and vomiting (often using a scoring system) should be recorded.

15. Patients receiving opioids can develop pruritus (itching) that is distressing and does not always respond to antihistamines. If the itching does not respond to intervention, the opioid may need to be discontinued.

16. All of the above should be monitored simultaneously and hourly for the duration of the epidural analgesia. Some areas have a specially designed assessment tool.

17. As with all controlled drugs, the nurse must prepare, administer and document the medication according to the local policy (see p. 189). No other opiates should be prescribed or administered while epidural analgesia is in progress.

2.19 Assessment of the deteriorating patient

In addition to routine observations, a number of tools have been developed to assist nursing and medical staff to assess the physiological state of patients in hospital. The National Institute for Clinical Excellence (NICE 2007) have stated that physiological 'track and trigger systems' such as Early Warning Scores (EWS, sometimes known as Patient at Risk Scores) should be used to monitor all adult patients in acute hospital settings. Physiological observations should be monitored at least every 12 hours, unless a decision has been made by a senior nurse or doctor to increase or decrease this frequency for an individual patient.

Early warning scores

EWS add together a number of parameters (see Figure 2.16) based on the patient's observations, level of consciousness and urine output. An overall score is calculated and guidance is provided on the action required, for example, more frequent observations or reporting to a doctor or senior nurse. Abnormalities in physiological parameters of temperature, cardiovascular, respiratory or central nervous system observations and urine output are indicators that the patient may be deteriorating. EWS aim to predict which patients are in need of urgent attention, allow preventive measures to be taken, and identify those patients who might need a step up to higher levels of care (Baines and Kanagasunderam 2008).

Using ABCDE to assess patients

In addition to scoring systems such as EWS, nurses should also use a systematic assessment framework when assessing ill adult patients to detect deterioration or improvement, and after interventions such as administration of oxygen or prescribed medication. One assessment framework is ABCDE: **A**irway, **B**reathing, **C**irculation, **D**isability and **E**xposure (Resuscitation Council 2006). Using this will help to ensure that critical illness is promptly identified and appropriately managed (Jevon 2010). Nurses can use this framework in all clinical settings, whenever there is concern that the patient's condition may be deteriorating.

A: airway

It is important to establish if the patient is responsive and therefore able to maintain his or her own airway. Talk to the patient and note their ability to respond. Ask the patient specific questions such as 'are you in pain?' or 'how are you feeling?' If the patient can talk this indicates a patent airway. An unresponsive patient may not be able to protect their airway; therefore the following are signs of concern and warrant immediate reporting/intervention:

No response – the patient is unconscious and not talking. If no air can be felt from the nose or mouth (see p. 96) this indicates an airway obstruction

Grunting, gurgling, snoring or 'barking' – noises other than talking may indicate a partial airway obstruction caused by swelling, spasm or inhalation of a foreign body

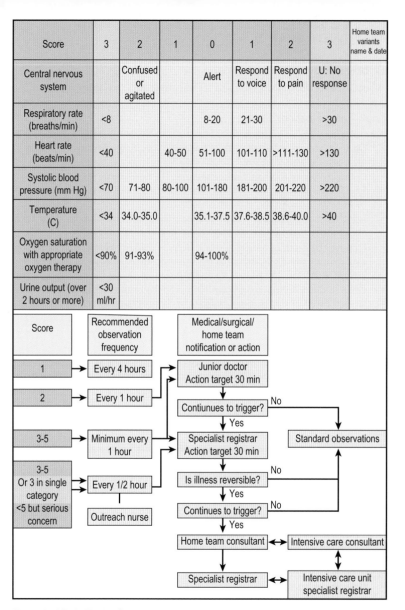

Score	3	2	1	0	1	2	3	Home team variants name & date
Central nervous system		Confused or agitated		Alert	Respond to voice	Respond to pain	U: No response	
Respiratory rate (breaths/min)	<8			8-20	21-30		>30	
Heart rate (beats/min)	<40		40-50	51-100	101-110	>111-130	>130	
Systolic blood pressure (mm Hg)	<70	71-80	80-100	101-180	181-200	201-220	>220	
Temperature (C)	<34	34.0-35.0		35.1-37.5	37.6-38.5	38.6-40.0	>40	
Oxygen saturation with appropriate oxygen therapy	<90%	91-93%		94-100%				
Urine output (over 2 hours or more)	<30 ml/hr							

Score	Recommended observation frequency	Medical/surgical/home team notification or action
1	Every 4 hours	Junior doctor Action target 30 min
2	Every 1 hour	Continues to trigger? → No → Standard observations / Yes
3-5	Minimum every 1 hour	Specialist registrar Action target 30 min
3-5 Or 3 in single category <5 but serious concern	Every 1/2 hour / Outreach nurse	Is illness reversible? → No → Standard observations / Yes → Continues to trigger? → No / Yes → Home team consultant ↔ Intensive care consultant → Specialist registrar ↔ Intensive care unit specialist registrar

Figure 2.16 Early Warning Score.

Urgent help should be summoned and the patients airway should be opened using head tilt/chin lift (see Ch. 3).

B: breathing

When assessing the patients breathing it's important to 'Look, listen and report'.

Look – at the patient's chest

Are they struggling to breathe?
- Do they have an increased work of breathing, i.e using accessory muscles in the neck, the abdomen and between the ribs?
- Count the respiratory rate for one minute. The normal rate for adults is 12–20 breaths per minute. Tachypnoea and bradypnoea should be reported (see p. 334).
- Is the chest rising equally – i.e. is the movement the same on both sides? Lack of symmetry may indicate an underlying lung or rib problem.
- Observe the depth of breathing – is it deep or shallow? Very deep slow breaths may indicate metabolic abnormalities or raised intracranial pressure. Shallow breaths may be due to pain or medication.
- Observe the peripheral oxygen saturation (SpO_2) reading (normal 95–100%; see p. 350). A low SpO_2 could indicate hypoxia or respiratory distress (Jevon 2010).

Listen – for any abnormal noises

Normal breathing is a relatively quiet activity. Noises such as wheezing (a high pitched sound) may indicate narrowed airways and gurgling or rattling may indicate fluid in the lungs. Coughing may be caused by infection or irritation within the lungs or airways.

Report

Any abnormalities found when assessing the patients breathing using 'look' and 'listen' must be reported immediately as they may indicate a serious problem. If the patient's condition allows, help the patient to sit in an upright comfortable position as this will help with lung expansion and breathing.

C: circulation

The cardiovascular system can be affected by many problems such as haemorrhage or acute fluid loss; cardiac events such as myocardial infarction, sepsis, or medication. In circulation, the following should be assessed and any abnormalities should be reported immediately as they may indicate a serious problem.
- Pulse (heart rate) – noting strength, rate and rhythm (p. 35)
- Blood pressure (p. 39).
- Capillary refill time (see p. 82), especially if haemorrhage is suspected.

- Urine output and fluid intake – poor urine output may indicate hypovolaemia.
- Temperature (p. 27).
- Skin temperature – cool skin may indicate peripheral vasoconstriction, hot skin may indicate severe pyrexia.
- Does the patient need an ECG? This is indicated if there is chest pain, collapse or difficulty in breathing.
- Has the patient undergone a surgical procedure? If so, check wound sites, drains etc. for signs of bleeding.
- CVP – if the patient has a central line then a central venous pressure measurement (CVP) may be useful. Low CVP may suggest fluid loss; high CVP may suggest fluid overload or pulmonary oedema.

D: disability (plus diabetes and drugs)

Disability in this context means the patient's neurological state, specifically their level of consciousness. Assess the patient's level of consciousness using the GCS or AVPU (p. 53). A patient with an altered level of consciousness is at risk of airway obstruction and should be observed closely or, if their condition allows, placed in the recovery position. Sudden onset confusion or agitation should be reported.

Diabetes

Low or high blood glucose levels can cause altered levels of consciousness therefore the 'D' assessment should always include a blood glucose measurement if the patient is drowsy or unconscious for an unknown reason.

Drugs

Certain medication (e.g. opiates, sedatives and anaesthetics) can cause an altered level of consciousness. The patient's medication chart should be checked to see if this is the cause of the patient's deterioration.

Any abnormalities found when assessing 'Disability' must be reported immediately as they may indicate a serious problem.

E: exposure (and the environment)

Ensuring patient privacy and dignity, the patient should be undressed to observe for other signs or causes of deterioration such as rashes, wounds, leg swelling or infected tissue. At this point the patients overall skin integrity can be noted:
- Is it dry and flaky or warm and well perfused?
- Is the patient at risk of pressure ulcer formation? Is a further risk assessment needed (see p. 377)
- Has the patient been incontinent when they are usually continent?

At this stage consider 'Have I missed anything in my assessment?' If a temperature has not yet been recorded this should be done for every patient.

Any abnormalities found when assessing 'Exposure' must be reported immediately as they may indicate a serious problem.

Communicating your assessment using SBAR

Following assessment of the patient using ABCDE and/or EWS, it may be necessary to report your assessment to a doctor/senior nurse so that the patient can receive urgent care and treatment. Situation, Background, Assessment and Recommendation (SBAR) is an easily remembered mnemonic that provides a structure for such conversations. It is especially useful when trying to communicate in challenging or critical clinical situations where accuracy and time are critical. When used correctly, SBAR enhances patient safety and has been shown to improve outcomes for patients (Christie and Robinson 2009). The NHS is committed to adopting SBAR communication in all NHS Trusts, especially for accessing medical help, patient handovers and in critical situations. When communicating with other healthcare professionals, a polite and professional approach is essential, no matter how stressed you may be feeling. Using a framework such as SBAR helps to achieve this, and to obtain the optimal care and treatment for patients.

The following example has been adapted from NHS Institute for Innovation and Improvement (2008). All names and wards are fictitious. Each section of SBAR is broken down and used sequentially:

Situation

- Identify yourself by name and the ward/unit you are calling from
- Identify the patient by name and the reason for your call
- Describe your concern or the problem.

For example:

This is Elaine, staff nurse on Ward 16. I am calling about Mr Ahmed in bed 34. Mr Ahmed has suddenly become short of breath and his respiration rate has increased to 24 breaths per minute. His oxygen saturations dropped to 88 per cent on room air so I started him on 24% oxygen but there has been no improvement in the last 5 minutes.

Background

- Give the patient's reason for admission and when he was admitted
- Explain any significant medical history (you may need the patient's notes for this).

He was admitted yesterday under the care of Dr Sharp with an exacerbation of COPD. After a chest X-ray this morning he was started on IV antibiotics. He has been admitted a number of times with COPD and he also has angina and prostate cancer.

Assessment

- Report any other important vital signs
- If you have found other clinical concerns or signs during your assessment state them here.

When I assessed him just now his heart rate is up to 110 and blood pressure is 85/50. He isn't pyrexial but he looks flushed and unwell. He is really struggling to breathe and says that he has bilateral chest pain.

Recommendation

Explain what you need – be specific about your request and time frame, for example:

I am very concerned about Mr Ahmed and would like you to come to see him immediately. Should I keep him on 24% oxygen?

- Make suggestions, for example '*Shall I do an ECG?*'
- Clarify your expectations, for example '*I will tell the family that you will be here within 30 minutes*'.
- If the person you call is unable to help, clarify who you should call next.

2.20 Measuring capilliary refill time

Preparation

Patient
- Explain the procedure to gain consent and cooperation

Equipment
- If the patient is wearing nail polish and the capilliary refill time is to be measured peripherally then the polish should be removed from one fingernail ➡ **PFP1**

Nurse
- The hands should be clean
- Additional protective clothing may be necessary if indicated by the patient's condition (see Ch. 1).

Procedure

Capilliary refill time (CRT) refers to the time it takes for blood refill compressed capilliaries. It is often used in paediatric and neonatal care and, more recently, in adult practice to assess dehydration and the haemodynamic status of the patient. It is a simple test that can be performed quickly; however, many factors can affect the result ➡ **PFP2** therefore CRT should be used in conjunction with other cardiovascular observations (e.g. blood pressure and pulse measurement, urine output etc.) (Lewin and Maconochie 2008).

1. Holding the patient's hand above the level of their heart, press on a finger nail for 5 seconds – this forces the blood out of the capilliaries and causes 'blanching' where the tissue beneath the finger nail looks pale (Figure 2.17).

2. After 5 seconds remove the pressure and count the number of seconds it takes for the normal nail bed colour to return.

3. In patients with normal peripheral perfusion ➡ **PFP3**, capilliary refill should take 2 seconds. It can take longer, i.e. is *delayed*, if the patient is hypovolaemic (blood or fluid loss), dehydrated or has peripheral vascular disease.

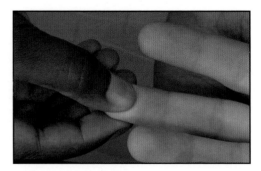

Figure 2.17 Capillary refill time.

4. A delayed capilliary refill time should be reported as it may indicate a problem with the patient's blood volume. Other cardiovascular observations should be performed as necessary.

5. Capilliary refill time is documented using a timeframe, e.g. 'CRT=2 seconds', 'CRT <2 seconds' or 'CRT is delayed at 4 seconds'.

➡ Points for practice

PFP1 Capilliary refill time can be measured peripherally, in the finger or toe nails. This measures the blood perfusion in the areas furthest from the heart. In small children or patients with normally altered peripheral perfusion, e.g. adults with peripheral vascular disease, the test is sometimes performed centrally. Here the skin over the sternum (breastbone) or forehead is pressed for 2 seconds as described above.

PFP2 Factors that may affect the speed of CRT include gender (with males having a slightly faster CRT than females), ambient (external) temperature and patient temperature (hypothermia will slow the CRT).

PFP3 The term 'normal peripheral perfusion' suggests that the patient is free of any disease which may hinder blood flow to the extremities. Patients with poor peripheral blood flow due to disorders such as peripheral vascular disease, Raynaud's disease etc. will have slower CRT even if they are not hypovolaemic or dehydrated. Therefore this test is not suitable or reliable for these groups of patients.

Bibliography/Suggested reading

Cardiac monitoring and ECG

Crawford, J., Doherty, L., 2008. Recording a standard ECG: filling the gaps in knowledge. British Journal of Cardiac Nursing 3 (12), 572–576.

This article focuses the knowledge required to improve understanding and practice in relation to 12-lead ECG recording.

Crawford, J., Doherty, L., 2009. Recording a standard ECG: filling the gaps in quality. British Journal of Cardiac Nursing 4 (4), 162–166.

This article outlines the steps required to improve the quality of ECG recording.

Kucia, A., Quinn, T., 2010. Acute cardiac care: a practical guide for nurses. Blackwell, Chichester.

This book has useful chapters on Cardiac electrophysiology (Ch. 3); Electrocardiogram interpretation (Ch. 10); Cardiac monitoring (Ch. 11) and Arrhythmias (Ch. 23).

Woodrow, P., 2009. An introduction to electrocardiogram interpretation: part 1. Nursing Standard 24 (12), 50–57.

This article describes cardiac electrophyisiology and how to intepret the single lead ECG.

Woodrow, P., 2009. An introduction to electrocardiogram interpretation: part 2. Nursing Standard 24 (13), 48–56.

This article outlines the main indications for recording a 12-lead ECG, what each of the 12 leads represents and likely causes of errors.

Neurovascular observation

Judge, N.L., 2007. Neurovascular assessment. Nursing Standard 21 (45), 39–44.

This article discusses the importance of undertaking neurovascular observations with particular emphasis on identifying acute compartment syndrome.

Height, weight and waist circumference measurement

Ness-Abramof, R., Apovian, C., 2008. Waist circumference measurement in clinical practice. Nutrition in Clinical Practice 23 (4), 398–404.

Whilst this article is based on data from the USA it gives a good summary of the rationale for using waist measurement as an accurate predictor of cardiovascular disease.

Blood glucose monitoring

Hill, J., 2008. Home blood glucose monitoring. British Journal of Cardiac Nursing 3 (3), 105–109.

Although this article focuses on home monitoring of blood glucose, it addresses useful aspects for procedure such as rationale for blood glucose monitoring, the practicalities of undertaking the procedure and the equipment patients may be using. The article concludes with a discussion of how patients can use the results to improve control of their blood glucose.

Lawal, M., 2009. Diabetes: a guide to glucose meters. British Journal of Healthcare Assistants 3 (4), 171–175.

This article is directed at education and training for healthcare assistants. However, the content is useful for students new to monitoring blood glucose as it is presented in a readable and easily understood manner. The article addresses the assessment, planning, implementation and evaluation of glucose estimation with a particular focus on members of the multidisciplinary team who have day-to-day responsibility for monitoring of blood glucose.

National Collaborating Centre for Chronic Conditions, 2008. Type 2 diabetes: national clinical guideline for management in primary and secondary care (update). Royal College of Physicians, London [online]. [Accessed 04.01.12]. Available from: www.nice.org.uk/CG66.

NICE clinical guideline 66 updated NICE clinical guidelines E, F, G and H (2002) and updated and replaced the recommendations on type 2 diabetes in NICE technology appraisal guidance 53 (2002), 60 and 63 (2003).

National Institute for Health and Clinical Excellence, 2009. Type 2 diabetes: newer agents for blood glucose control in type 2 diabetes [online]. [Accessed 04.01.12] Available from: www.nice.org.uk/CG87ShortGuideline.

This short guideline is a partial update of NICE CG66, which together form the full guidelines on type 2 diabetes.

Walker, R., 2004. Capillary blood glucose monitoring and its role in diabetes management. British Journal of Community Nursing 9 (10), 438–440.

This article addresses context and target blood glucose levels, when and by whom testing needs to be undertaken, frequency of testing, application of results, obtaining accurate and reliable results and quality control and assurance.

Pain assessment

Chamley, C., 2011. Pain management. In: Brooker, C., Nicol, M. (Eds.), Alexander's Nursing Practice, fourth ed. Churchill Livingstone Elsevier, Edinburgh.

This chapter provides an overview of a wide range of issues related to pain management. It addresses theories of pain, pain physiology, classification of pain types and the management of pain.

Chumbley, G., Mountford, L., 2010. Patient-controlled analgesia pumps for adults. Nursing Standard 25 (8), 35–40.

This is a further article in the series presented by the group of pain nurse specialists and specifically examines the main features of opioid patient-controlled analgesia. Risks and potential side-effects are explored as is the importance of educating patients in the safe use of PCA.

Cox, F., 2010. Basic principles of pain management: assessment and intervention. Nursing Standard 25 (1), 36–39.

This article is the first in a comprehensive series in which a group of pain nurse specialists examine a wide range of issues related to pain and its management. This first article provides an overview of the nature, causes and structured management of acute, chronic and neuropathic pain. It also explores the physiological basis of pharmacological and non-pharmacological interventions.

Fear, C., 2010. Neuropathic pain: clinical features, assessment and treatment. British Journal of Nursing 25 (6), 35–40.

This article, the sixth in a series on pain, specifically examines neuropathic pain, its causes, presentation and approaches to treatment.

Godfrey, H., 2005. Understanding pain, part 2: Pain management. British Journal of Nursing 14 (17), 904–909.

This article is the second of two that examine understanding pain from a physiological perspective. This article focuses on the importance of pain assessment in ensuring effective management of pain. It also explores the physiological basis of pharmacological and non-pharmacological interventions.

Lynch, M., 2001. Pain as the fifth vital sign. Journal of Intravenous Nursing 24 (2), 85–94.

Although old, this article supports the contention that assessment of pain is important enough for it to be considered the fifth vital sign.

McLafferty, E., Farley, A., 2007. Assessing pain in patients. Nursing Standard 22 (25), 42–46.

This article defines pain and discusses options for its assessment. Unidimensional and multidimensional pain assessment scales are examined.

Warden, V., Hurley, A.C., Volicer, V., 2003. Development and psychometric evaluation of the Pain Assessment in Advanced Dementia (PAINAD) Scale. Journal of the American Medical Director's Association 4, 9–15.

This article presents the development of a pain assessment tool for those with advanced dementia.

Wheatley, R., Schug, S., Watson, D., 2001. Safety and efficacy of postoperative epidural analgesia. British Journal of Anaesthesia 87 (1), 47–61.

This article examines issues of safety and efficacy of post-operative epidural analgesia. Efficacy issues include the choice of drug, site of insertion, pre- or post-incisional epidural analgesia and method of drug delivery. Safety issues addressed include incidence of neurological complications due to epidural analgesia, adverse events due to the insertion and presence of the epidural catheter in the epidural space, adverse events related to epidural drug administration, and organisational issues.

Temperature, pulse, respirations and blood pressure

Childs, C., 2011. Maintaining body temperature. In: Brooker, C., Nicol, M. (Eds.), Alexander's nursing practice. Churchill Livingstone Elsevier, Edinburgh, Ch 22.

This chapter includes regulation of body temperature, measurement of body temperature and nursing care of patients with pyrexia and hypothermia.

Esmond, G., 2011. Nursing patients with respiratory disorders. In: Brooker, C., Nicol, M. (Eds.), Alexander's Nursing Practice, Churchill Livingstone Elsevier, Edinburgh, Ch 3.

This chapter provides an overview of the relevant anatomy and physiology and addresses all aspects of respiratory nursing from counting respirations to caring for patients with respiratory failure, TB and lung cancer.

Kisiel, M., Perkins, C., 2006. Nursing observations: knowledge to help prevent critical illness. British Journal of Nursing 15 (19), 1052–1056.

Discusses the importance of nursing observations and early warning systems. The article uses a clinical scenario to explain the physiological processes and explain the stages of shock and how this will be reflected in the patient's observations. There is a useful diagram summarising the angiotensin pathway and its effect on blood pressure.

McMillen, R., Pitcher, B., 2010. Patient observations: a guide for support workers. British Journal of Healthcare Assistants 4 (9), 434–437.

Although aimed at healthcare assistants, this article will be very useful for students. The article provides an overview of temperature, pulse, BP, respirations and oxygen saturations and includes normal and abnormal values. The rationale for the use of early waning systems is also included.

O'Brien, E., Petrie, J., Littler, W., 1997. Blood pressure measurement: recommendations of the British Hypertension Society, third ed. BMJ Publishing Groupm, London.

*Although now several years old this still provides an excellent guide to the correct technique for BP recording (cuff sizes, equipment, position, etc.) and the factors that can affect it. The British Hypertension Society website is also a good source of information and includes a useful tutorials about BP measurement and hypertension (**www.bhs.org**).*

Parkes, R., 2011. Rate of respiration: the forgotten vital sign. Emergency Nurse 19 (2), 12–18.

This article stresses the importance of recording respiratory rates as a highly sensitive marker of the patient's condition and of early signs of deterioration. Good review of the relevant anatomy and physiology.

Scrase, W., Tranter, S., 2011. Improving evidence-based care for patients with pyrexia. Nursing Standard 25 (29), 37–41.

A literature review that includes definitions of fever and hyperpyrexia and why the body produces a rise in temperature. It discusses the pros and cons of using antipyretics to control pyrexia.

Skinner, S., 2005. Understanding clinical investigations: a quick reference manual, second ed. Baillière Tindall, Edinburgh.

This excellent book provides information about a wide range of clinical investigations, including temperature, pulse respirations and BP. It includes the implications for nurses and provides a quick summary of the relevant physiology.

Assessing deteriorating patients (ABCDE and SBAR)

Baines, E., Kanagasunderam, N.S., 2008. Early warning scores. Student BMJ [online]. [Accessed 06.06.11] Available from: http://archive.student.bmj.com/issues/08/09/education/320.php.

This article is aimed at medical students but is also of interest and relevance to nurses. It describes how and why early warning scores were developed and gives a clinical example of their use.

Christie, P., Robinson, H., 2009. Using a communication framework at handover to boost patient outcomes. Nursing Times 105 (47), 13–15.

This article describes how SBAR has been successfully used in one healthcare Trust to improve patient safety and outcomes.

National Institute for Health and Clinical Excellence, 2007. Acutely ill patients in hospital. NICE, London. (Clinical guideline 50.) [online]. [Accessed 04.01.12] Available from: www.nice.org.uk/Guidance/CG50.

NICE have produced a clinical guideline with a comprehensive evidence base. This long document explains how and why staff need to recognise and respond to acutely ill adults in hospital. A summary is available and a number of interesting references.

NHS Institute for Innovation and Improvement, 2008. SBAR. [online]. [Accessed 04.01.12] Available from: http://www.institute.nhs.uk/quality_and_service_improvement_tools/ quality_and_service_improvement_tools/sbar_-_situation_-_background_-_assessment_-_ recommendation.html.

This website gives a comprehensive example of using SBAR and includes NHS recommendations

Odell, M., 2010. Are early warning scores the only way to rapidly detect and manage deterioration? Nursing Times 106 (8), 24–26.

This article discusses the use of EWS and also other ways that nurses can assess deteriorating patients. Communication with patients, families and the medical teams is emphasised.

Care of seizures

Walker, M., 2005. Status epilepticus: an evidence based guide. BMJ 331:673–677.

This is an interesting article that looks at who is at risk of status epilepticus, how it is diagnosed and the various drug treatments available with their benefits and side effects. Although aimed at doctors it makes interesting reading and explains concepts clearly.

Assessment of level of consciousness

Blows, W.T., 2005. The biological basis of nursing: clinical observations. London: Routledge.

Three chapters in this book explore the biological basis of neurological observations including consciousness, eyes and movement.

Caton-Richards, M., 2010. Assessing the neurological status of patients with head injuries. Emergency Nurse 17 (10), 28–31.

This article is written for Emergency Nurses who assess patients with reduced levels of consciousness of unknown cause. It emphasises the need for standardised, continuous assessment.

Cole, E., 2009. Initial assessment and management of the trauma patient in the emergency department. Oxford: Wiley Blackwell.

This book has a chapter which specifically looks at traumatic head and brain injuries, and the essentials of assessment and management.

Dawes, E., Lloyd, H., Durham, L., 2007. Monitoring and recording patients' neurological observations. Nursing Standard 22 (10), 40–45.

This article clearly discusses the use of the Glasgow Coma Scale and the associated observations necessary for neurological assessment.

McLeod, A., 2004. Intra- and extracranial causes of alteration in level of consciousness. British Journal of Nursing 13 (7), 354–361.

This article examines the concepts of consciousness and intracranial pressure and what is meant by 'altered level of consciousness'. Assessment strategies are identified and AVPU, a simple alternative to the Glasgow Coma Scale, is presented as an alternative initial assessment tool.

National Institute for Health and Clinical Excellence, 2007. Head injury: triage, assessment, investigation and early management of head injury in infants, children and adults. NICE, London (Also available: www.nice.org.uk).

This provides evidence-based recommendations on the management of patients with head injury. It addresses all aspects of care from pre-hospital assessment and immediate management at the scene, through assessment in A&E and admission and observation to discharge and follow-up. The document is nearly 250 pages long but it is available on the website and the recommendations are summarised from pages 6–23.

Palmer, R., Knight, J., 2006. Assessment of altered conscious level in clinic al practice. British Journal of Nursing 15 (22), 1255–1259.

This article critically appraises the literature focusing on the use and application of the Glasgow Coma Scale (GCS). The paper reviews the anatomical basis of consciousness and considers some of the issues of application of GCS in practice, including painful stimuli.

Resuscitation Council UK, 2011. Advanced Life Support. [online].[Accessed 04.01.12] Available from: http://www.resus.org.uk.

This website discusses the use of AVPU and the assessment of consciousness.

Capillary refill

Lewin, J., Maconochie, I., 2008. Capillary refill time in adults. Emergency Medical Journal 25:325–326.

This paper reviews the evidence base and describes some of the potential factors that can affect the accuracy of measuring CRT in adult patients.

Chapter 3

Resuscitation

©2012 Elsevier Ltd.

3.1 Assessment of collapsed person and recovery position

Preparation

Patient	Equipment	Nurse
• The person is collapsed and unresponsive when called or shaken	• No equipment is necessary.	• Annual CPR updates are vital to maintain skills • Check www.resus.org.uk regularly for the most recent guidance

Procedure (DRSABC) ➜ PFP1

Danger

Approach the person/surroundings carefully to exclude any risk of danger to yourself, e.g. electrical cable. There may be something to indicate the possible cause of collapse (e.g. fall or injury). Kneel beside the person.

Response

Assess the person's conscious state. Shake their shoulders (unless there is possibility of neck injury) and shout (in both ears) to see if they respond.

Shout for help

If the person is unconscious (i.e. totally unresponsive) call for help from a bystander. Ask the bystander to wait while you complete your assessment. If you are completely alone **do not** go for help yourself until you have checked the **airway** and **breathing**.

Airway

With one hand tip back the forehead (unless there is neck injury) and with two fingers of your other hand lift the chin to raise the tongue from the back of the throat to open the airway (Fig. 3.4 on p. 96). Look for any obvious obstruction in the mouth ➜ **PFP2**. Keep the chin raised.

Breathing

Place your cheek near the person's nostrils to **feel** for any breathing. **Look** for chest movement and **listen** for breath sounds. Observe for no more than 10 seconds. If breathing is present, place the casualty in the recovery position (see below). If no breathing is detected ➜ **PFP3** start basic life support (see p. 95).

Recovery position

1. Continue to kneel beside the person
2. If the person is wearing spectacles remove these and place on one side ➜ **PFP4**

3. Position the person's nearest arm at 90° to their shoulder with the elbow bent

4. Hold the back of the person's other hand against their cheek that is nearest to you and keep holding it in position

5. Take hold of the leg furthest from you at the knee and raise it until the foot is flat on the floor.

6. Place your hand on the knee and pull towards you so that the person turns onto their side ➡ **PFP5**

7. Draw the person's knee towards their chest to prevent them rolling onto their stomach (Fig. 3.1)

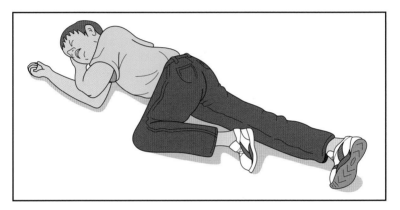

Figure 3.1 Recovery position.

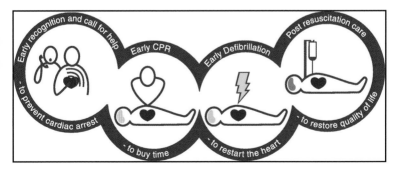

Figure 3.2 Chain of survival. From Langhelle, et al. 2005. Reproduced with permission from Laerdal.

8. Tilt the chin again to maintain an open airway
9. Send for help ➡ **PFP6** and continue to observe the person closely to ensure that breathing and circulation are being maintained
10. If the ambulance has not arrived by 30 minutes, turn the person to their other side to prevent pressure ulcers.

➡**Points for practice**

PFP1 The mnemonic DRSABC (Doctor's ABC – **D**anger, **R**esponse, **S**hout for help, **A**irway, **B**reathing and **C**irculation) will help you remember the correct procedure for assessing a collapsed person. The Resuscitation Council (www.resus.org.uk) describes the interventions that contribute to a successful outcome after cardiac arrest as a Chain of Survival (Fig. 3.2).

PFP2 Only attempt to remove an obstruction if it is visible and easy to remove. Feeling inside the mouth with your finger is **no longer recommended** as you may push the obstruction further into the airway.

PFP3 If the person is gasping this does not indicate breathing and so basic life support should be started.

PFP4 Spectacles may get broken and cause discomfort when the person is turned onto their side in the recovery position.

PFP5 Before turning the person onto their side check to see that there is nothing large in the pocket (e.g. large bunch of keys) that might cause damage if lying on it for a period of time.

PFP6 If the collapse has occurred in the street or someone's home, dial 999 for an ambulance. In a hospital or nursing home, refer to local policy. Ask the bystander to return to let you know that help is on the way. At this point you can go for help yourself if no one else is available.

3.2 Basic life support with cardiopulmonary resuscitation (CPR)

Preparation

Patient

• The patient is unresponsive when called and shaken

Equipment

• Some people carry a pocket resuscitation mask, which may be used to prevent contact with the person's saliva during mouth-to-mouth respiration in an emergency (Fig. 3.3). Some nursing homes/clinics also have these ➡ **PFP1**

Nurse

• Yearly updating in resuscitation techniques is vital to maintain these skills.
• Check the Resuscitation Council website regularly (www.resus.org.uk) for the most recent guidance

Procedure

Danger

Approach the person/surroundings carefully to exclude any risk of danger to yourself, e.g. electrical cable. There may be something to indicate the possible cause of collapse (e.g. fall or injury). Kneel beside the person.

Response

Assess the person's conscious state. Shake their shoulders (unless there is the possibility of neck injury) and shout (in both ears) to see if they respond.

Shout for help

If the person is unconscious (i.e. totally unresponsive) call for help from a bystander. Ask the bystander to wait while you complete your assessment.

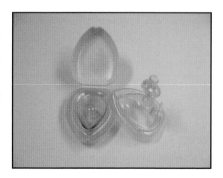

Figure 3.3 Pocket mask.

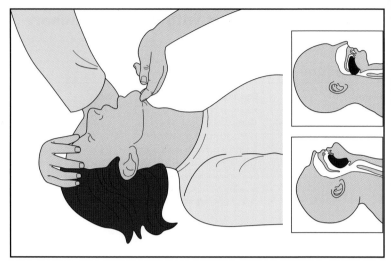

Figure 3.4 Chin lift to bring tongue forward from back of throat.

Airway

With one hand tip back the forehead (unless neck injury) and with two fingers of your other hand lift the chin to raise the tongue from the back of the throat to open the airway (see Fig. 3.4). Look for any obstruction in the mouth. Keep the chin raised.

Breathing

Place your cheek near the person's nostrils to **feel** for any breathing. **Look** for chest movement and **listen** for breath sounds. Observe for no more than 10 seconds.

If the person is **not breathing** normally send for help ➡ **PFP2**. If no-one else is around ring/go for help ➡ **PFP3** and then commence **cardiopulmonary resuscitation** (CPR; see below) ➡ **PFP4**.

Cardiopulmonary resuscitation

1. With the person lying flat on their back commence external cardiac compressions.

2. **Hand position.** Identify the middle of the sternum (breast bone) and place the heel of one hand in the middle of the lower half of the sternum. Place your other hand on top and interlock the fingers (Fig. 3.5) ➡ **PFP5**.

3. Keeping your arms straight and your shoulders in line with your elbows and heels of your hands give 30 compressions at a rate of 100–120 per minute.

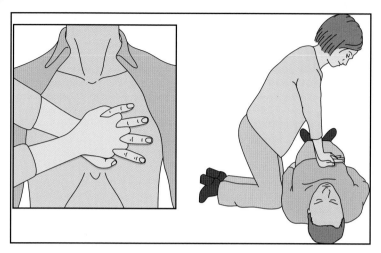

Figure 3.5 Hand position for cardiac compressions.

You should press hard enough to compress the chest wall by 5–6 cm (Resuscitation Council UK 2010 ➡ **PFP6**).

4. **Mouth-to-mouth breathing** ➡ **PFP1.** Keeping the chin lifted, pinch the soft part of the person's nose. Take a normal breath in and place your lips around the person's open mouth and ensure a good seal. Blow steadily into the person's mouth whilst watching from the corner of your eye to see the chest rise. Take your mouth away as the chest falls and air comes out. Repeat once ➡ **PFP7**.

5. Continue giving cycles of 30 compressions and two breaths until help arrives ➡ **PFP8**.

6. Once help arrives, the experienced professionals will take over from you ➡ **PFP9**.

➡ Points for practice

PFP1 Although no longer emphasised when training lay people, mouth-to-mouth breathing should be carried out by those who have been taught to do so (Resus Council, 2010).

PFP2 Ask the bystander to return to let you know that help is on the way. If you are in a location that has an Automated External Defibrillator (AED; p. 102) ask the bystander to get it.

PFP3 If there is no-one to send for help, it is important to go yourself before you start cardiopulmonary resuscitation so that help will be on its way. However, it is important to check the airway and breathing before you do so (see step 4).

PFP4 Feel for the carotid pulse if you have been trained to do so and look for general signs of circulation such as movement, coughing, groaning, etc. The carotid pulse is nearest to the heart. If no pulse can be felt here, there is no cardiac output. If this is a respiratory arrest (i.e. circulation is present, but the person is not breathing) go to step 4 and give 10 breaths per minute.

PFP5 The person's clothing may need to be adjusted to ensure the correct positioning of the hands.

PFP6 Resuscitation procedures are reviewed regularly. It is important to ensure that you have knowledge of the most up-to-date guidelines.

PFP7 The chest should rise with every breath. If it does not, check the mouth again for visible obstruction and make sure the chin is still lifted to bring the tongue forward. Do not over-breathe as this may inflate the stomach and cause vomiting. Wait for the chest to fall after each breath before giving another breath. Each breath should take 1 second and the 2 breaths no more than 5 seconds.

PFP8 If more than one person is present alternate between compressions and mouth-to-mouth breathing every 2 minutes. Do not stop CPR to check for circulation unless the casualty shows signs of regaining consciousness or starts to breathe normally.

PFP9 Despite your best efforts, the person may not survive. Cardiopulmonary resuscitation is physically and emotionally exhausting. Try to talk through what happened with someone afterwards

3.3 Ward-based cardiopulmonary resuscitation

Preparation

Patient

Check:

- Unconscious
- Not breathing
- No pulse
- Is the patient for resuscitation?
  ➡ **PFP1**

Equipment

- Emergency equipment box or trolley including emergency drugs box
  ➡ **PFP2**
- Gloves, goggles and plastic aprons (usually kept with emergency equipment)
- Oxygen cylinder (if piped oxygen is not available)
- Suction machine (if piped suction is not available)
- Intravenous infusion stand
- Cardiac monitor and defibrillator

Nurse

- Screen bed area to maintain privacy
  ➡ **PFP3**
- Summon help ➡ **PFP4**
- The most experienced nurse should coordinate the activities of other staff
- If sufficient staff is available, delegate someone to care for the other patients

Procedure

1. Lay the patient flat. If in bed, remove pillows and the head of the bed ➡ **PFP5**.

2. If there is no carotid pulse, commence cardiopulmonary resuscitation at a ratio of 30 compressions to two breaths (see p. 96).

3. Once available, insert an appropriate sized oropharyngeal (Guedel) airway ➡ **PFP6**. Insert it into the mouth upside down and then turn it into position over the back of the tongue (Fig. 3.6).

4. Attach the oxygen tubing to the mask/valve bag (e.g. Ambu bag) and set oxygen flow to 15 litres per minute ➡ **PFP7**.

5. Holding the chin up and the face mask tight against the face (Fig. 3.7), compress the bag at a steady speed. Check that the chest is rising with each compression of the bag ➡ **PFP8**.

6. Continue giving 30 external cardiac compressions to every 2 'breaths'. Continue cardiac compressions with as few interruptions as possible.

7. When the medical/senior nursing team arrives the following may be instigated according to the condition of the patient:

    - Endotracheal intubation – check the suction machine is working and has an oral (Yankauer) sucker attached. Once the patient is intubated, a tracheal suction catheter will be required.

    - Intravenous cannulation (often internal/external jugular) to enable drugs such as epinephrine (adrenaline) to be given intravenously.

    - Cardiac monitoring/recording.

    - Defibrillation, within 3 minutes of cardiac arrest if possible. Continue cardiac compressions while it is charging.

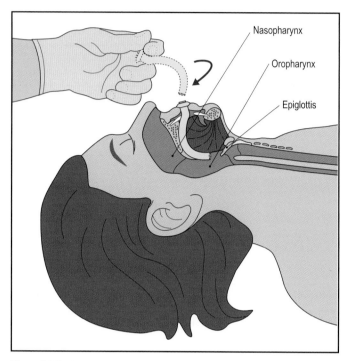

Nasopharynx

Oropharynx

Epiglottis

Figure 3.6 Position of the oropharyngeal (Guedel) airway.

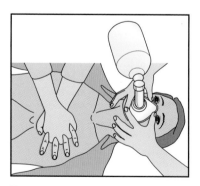

Figure 3.7 Use of bag-valve-mask.

8. The timing of each event and the administration of any drugs must be documented according to local policy.

9. If resuscitation is successful, close monitoring of the patient's condition will be necessary. The patient may be transferred to an intensive care unit. If resuscitation is unsuccessful, ensure privacy and dignity are maintained and prepare the patient to be seen by the family ➡ **PFP9**.

10. Clean equipment and re-stock all disposable items immediately. Dispose of used equipment according to local policy ➡ **PFP10**.

➡ Points for practice

PFP1 Resuscitation is not appropriate for some patients. The situation must be discussed with the patient and/or the family and if a decision has been made not to resuscitate, this must be written in the medical notes by the patient's medical consultant. It should also be written in the nursing documentation and communicated at every shift handover.

PFP2 When starting work or placement in a new clinical area it is important to note the location of emergency equipment and the emergency telephone numbers.

PFP3 If this is not easily achieved then screen other patients to ensure privacy and reduce their distress at seeing what is happening.

PFP4 In a hospital, there will be a Resuscitation Team, who can be summoned urgently by phoning a special number. It is vital to check that you know the emergency number in every area that you work. The ward may also have an emergency buzzer system to summon help.

PFP5 Most hospital beds have a CPR lever to quickly flatten the bed in an emergency. If the patient is on a pressure-relieving mattress, it will have a quick-release mechanism to enable rapid deflation in an emergency.

PFP6 The Guedel airway is designed to hold the tongue forward to prevent it obstructing the airway. The correct size is determined by choosing an airway that is the same length as the distance from the tip of the patient's ear to the corner of his/her mouth.

PFP7 Oxygen may be given without prescription in an emergency situation.

PFP8 Two people will be required for this; one to hold the face mask in position and the other to squeeze the Ambu bag.

PFP9 Make sure that all the equipment has been cleared away and that the bed area is tidy. One pillow should be placed under the head and the bed made as usual with sheets and a counterpane.

PFP10 Despite your best efforts resuscitation may be unsuccessful. This can be distressing for all involved (including other patients) and time should be made available to provide support.

3.4 Automated external defibrillator (AED)

Preparation

Patient	Equipment	Nurse
• Unconscious	• Automatic External Defibrillator	• Trained in use of AED
• Not breathing	➡ **PFP1**	• Attend annual update
• No palpable pulse		

Procedure

1. Send for help and locate/ask the person to bring the AED ➡ **PFP2**.

2. Lay the patient flat. If in bed, remove the pillows and the head of the bed.

3. If there is no palpable pulse, commence CPR at a ratio of 30 chest compressions to 2 breaths (see p. 96).

4. Switch on the AED and follow the voice prompts. **Continue cardiac compressions** if another person is present to attach the AED ➡ **PFP3**.

5. Expose the chest fully. If necessary shave the sites before applying the pads (a razor is supplied with the AED). Ensure that the chest is dry.

6. Remove any metal objects e.g. neck chains and under-wire bras ➡ **PFP4**. Remove any medication patches (e.g. nicotine patch) on the front of the torso. If in doubt, remove it.

7. Firmly apply the pads, as indicated in the diagram on the pad. **Chest compressions should continue during this process**. (Fig. 3.8)

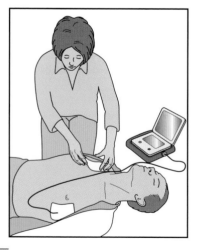

Figure 3.8 Use of automatic external defibrillator (AED).

8. The machine will prompt you when it is about to 'Analyse'. Instruct everyone to stand back while the machine analyses the heart rhythm ➡ **PFP5**. A trace will be stored in the memory for later retrieval.

9. If the machine detects either Ventricular Fibrillation (VF) or Ventricular Tachycardia (VT), it will prompt 'Shock advised' and 'Charging'. **Compressions should continue while the machine is charging**.

10. When the machine is charged, it will prompt 'Stand clear' and 'Press to shock now'. Before the shock is delivered the operator MUST ensure that all personnel are clear, and that any oxygen being administered is removed. The casualty may 'jump' as the shock discharges ➡ **PFP6**.

11. **Re-commence CPR as soon as the shock has been delivered**. It may take several seconds for the heart to begin to function again. Unless the casualty recovers, continue CPR. The machine will run another cycle after 2 minutes, analysing, and if required charging for a shock. Repeat the process until either the casualty recovers or expert help arrives.

12. If the outcome is successful, the patient will be transferred to a High Dependency Unit. If unsuccessful, tidy away any equipment and prepare the person to be seen by their family.

13. Document all activities, the timing of events and, if resuscitation was unsuccessful, whether circulation was restored at any point during the resuscitation.

14. Replenish equipment and return the AED. Any stored tracings may be useful to the healthcare team and so should be downloaded onto a computer.

15. Despite your best efforts, the person may not survive. Cardiopulmonary resuscitation is physically and emotionally exhausting. Try to talk through what happened with someone afterwards.

➡ Points for practice

PFP1 AEDs are usually available at public places such as railway stations and shopping centres, as well as health centres and nursing homes. Regular checks of expiry dates and battery condition are required to maintain an efficient unit. Modern machines run an automatic self-check daily to detect any faults.

PFP2 The sooner the patient is assessed and a shock delivered, the better the chance of restarting the heart.

PFP3 Research indicates that the fewer interruptions, and the shorter the duration of interruptions in chest compressions, the better the chances of survival (Resuscitation Council UK 2010).

PFP4 Metal is a conductor, contact with which can cause a false conduction path, resulting in burns and/or electrocution.

PFP5 If the patient is touched during the machine's 'Analyse' phase it may detect (and act upon) a false rhythm. Some machines produce a paper print out.

PFP6 The shock stops the heart and halts the arrhythmia. When the heart restarts it is hoped that it will return to normal sinus rhythm.

Bibliography/Suggested reading

Bosson, N., 2009. Tracheal intubation, laryngeal mask airways [online]. [Accessed 14.4.11]. Available from: http://emedicine.medscape.com/article/82527-overview#a03.

A good overview of the design and indications with clear diagrams to show insertion technique and positioning

Gallimore, D., 2006. Understanding the drugs used during cardiac arrest response. Nursing Times 102 (23), 24–26.

A useful guide to the drugs used in a cardiac arrest and their actions

Jevon, P., 2006. Resuscitation skills part 1: recovery position. Nursing Times 102 (25), 28–29.

Jevon, P., 2006. Resuscitation skills part 2: clearing the airway. Nursing Times 102 (26), 26–27.

Jevon, P., 2006. Resuscitation skills part 3: basic airway management. Nursing Times 102 (28), 26–27.

Jevon, P., 2006. Resuscitation skills part 4: chest compressions. Nursing Times 102 (28), 26–27.

This clearly written series of articles gives an overview of the whole resuscitation procedure with detailed discussion and clear diagrams to show each stage

Langhelle, A., Nolan, J., Herlitz, J., et al, 2005. Recommended guidelines for reviewing, reporting, and conducting research on post-resuscitation care: the Utstein style. Resuscitation 66:271–283.

Moule, P., Albarran, J., 2005. Practical resuscitation, recognition and response. Oxford: Blackwell.

An excellent resource that covers all aspects of resuscitation including professional and ethical/legal issues, recognising the sick patient and preventing cardiac arrest, basic and advanced resuscitation, and post-resuscitation care

Resuscitation Council UK, 2010. [online]. [Accessed 04.1.12]. Available from: www.resus.org.

This website has the most up-to-date guidelines and you should check it regularly for updates

Chapter 4

Vascular access and intravenous therapy

©2012 Elsevier Ltd.

4.1 Venepuncture

Preparation

Patient	Equipment	Nurse
• Explain the procedure, to gain consent and cooperation • The patient should be sitting or lying comfortably, with the appropriate arm supported • If clothing is tight or restrictive remove the arm from the sleeve.	• Vacuum tube sampling system (includes tube holder and needle adaptor, usually 21- gauge or winged infusión device) ➡ **PFP1** • Blood sample tube(s) as appropriate • Skin-cleansing agent (e.g. chlorhexidine in alcohol) according to local policy • Tourniquet (disposable) • Gauze swabs • Small self-adhesive dressing • Sharps bin	• Hands must be washed and dried thoroughly • Non-sterile gloves (close-fitting to allow dexterity) and apron should be worn • Additional protective clothing may be necessary if indicated by the patient's condition (see Ch. 1) • Adopt a comfortable position to avoid stooping • Some Trusts may require additional training for venepuncture

Procedure

1. Check the patient's identity with the blood test request form and ask/assist patient to adjust clothing as necessary.

2. Assemble all equipment. Do not label the sample tubes until the blood specimen is in them ➡ **PFP2**.

3. Apply the tourniquet using a quick release knot ➡ **PFP3** and inspect the arm to select a suitable vein ➡ **PFP4**. Palpate the vein to locate its position and ensure that it is not an artery (which will pulsate) or a tendon. If necessary, palpate the vein without gloves and then put them on once the vein is identified.

4. Clean the skin with the skin-cleansing agent and allow it to dry completely ➡ **PFP5**. Do not touch the area once the skin is cleaned.

5. With the patient's arm straight and well supported, use your non-dominant hand to pull the skin tight over the vein to 'anchor' the vein. This should be just below the selected insertion site

6. Take the plastic tube holder and needle of the vacuum system in your dominant hand. With the bevel of the needle upward and directly over the vein, insert the needle at an angle of about 15°–30° through the skin and into the vein (Fig 4.1A). When the vein is punctured, reduce the angle of the needle to avoid damaging the vein wall.

7. **Vacuum system** – hold the needle and plastic holder securely in place (no blood is visible until the sample tube is attached) and attach the sample tube by pushing it firmly onto the needle attachment inside the holder

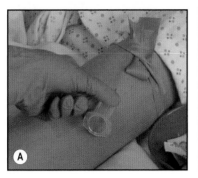 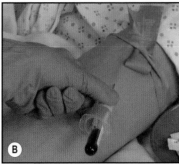

Figure 4.1 A:Venepuncture using vacuum system: insertion into the vein; B: venepuncture: attaching the blood sampling tube.

(Fig. 4.1B). The tube will then automatically fill with blood to the required amount. If additional samples are required, remove the tube when full (no blood will leak out) and attach another ➡ **PFP6**.

Needle and syringe – blood will appear at the tip of the syringe to indicate that the vein has been punctured. Hold the needle in position with one hand and, with the other, steadily pull back the piston of the syringe until the required amount of blood is obtained. Do not pull too vigorously or the vein may collapse.

8. Remove the tourniquet, hold the gauze swab over the puncture site and remove the needle. Do not press until the needle is out of the vein as this is very painful. Continue to apply pressure (or ask the patient to do this) for 2–3 minutes until the bleeding stops, to prevent bruising. Ask the patient not to bend their arm as this may cause a haematoma.

9. **Needle and syringe** – using the non-touch needle-removing device on the sharps bin remove the needle from the syringe before transferring the blood to the sample tube ➡ **PFP7**.

    Vacuum system – using the non-touch needle-removing device on the sharps bin (Fig. 4.1b). Remove the needle and discard immediately. If appropriate, retain the plastic tube holder for future use ➡ **PFP8**.

10. Gently invert each blood bottle a few times, to mix the blood sample with any additives.

11. Inspect the puncture site; once the bleeding has stopped, apply a small self-adhesive dressing, if required.

12. Assist the patient to replace clothing as necessary; readjust the height of the bed

13. Remove gloves and discard with other waste and wash and dry hands thoroughly

14. Label specimens with the patient's surname, first names, hospital number, date of birth, ward/clinic and the date of the sample. A printed adhesive label with these details is usually available.

15. Place samples in the appropriate collection point for transportation to the laboratory.

16. Document the blood samples taken.

➡Points for practice

PFP1 There are a number of blood collection systems available for venepuncture, with integrated safety devices and needless systems (e.g. vacutainer). These safety devices can reduce the risk of needlestick injury, and contamination from the blood sample, and so should be used whenever possible (Gabriel 2009).

PFP2 Do not label the sample tubes in advance in case venepuncture is unsuccessful and the tubes are mistakenly used for another patient.

PFP3 The tourniquet should be applied 5–10 cm above the intended venepuncture site. It should not be applied for longer than 1 minute before collecting the blood specimen. Prolonged use will cause intravascular fluid to leak into the tissues and may affect the accuracy of the blood test (Lavery and Ingram 2005).

PFP4 The best veins are usually found at the elbow, in the antecubital fossa. These veins are less mobile, easier to puncture and less painful than veins in the hand or lower arm. To increase blood flow to the arm, ask the patient to clench and unclench a fist several times. If very cold, ask the patient to warm their hands in warm water for a few minutes. Gently tapping the vein may also increase vasodilation by causing histamine release at the site. This must be gentle, as vigorous tapping may cause venous spasm. It may also help to lower the patient's arm below heart level to increase the blood supply to the veins.

PFP5 The skin-cleansing agent is usually alcohol-based and must be allowed to dry completely before proceeding. Any residual alcohol causes pain for the patient and may damage the cells and affect the blood specimen.

PFP6 Blood bottles are colour-coded, and filled in order as they appear on the manufactuer's colour guide. Refer to local policy regarding the blood bottles used in your practice área.

PFP7 Cells may be damaged if the blood is squirted through the needle into the sample tube. Damage can cause them to leak potassium and may lead to an inaccurate result.

PFP8 Refer to local policy regarding re-use of the plastic holder. It should always be discarded if it becomes contaminated with blood or the patient has an infection such as hepatitis or MRSA.

4.2 Intravenous cannulation

Preparation

Patient

- Explain the procedure, to gain consent and cooperation
- The patient should be sitting or lying comfortably, with the appropriate arm (non-dominant if possible) supported. If the cannula is for an intravenous infusion or the clothing is tight or restrictive, remove the arm from the sleeve
- Local anaesthetic cream, if used, must be applied at least 1 hour prior to the procedure ➡ **PFP1**
- Cannulation will be easier if the patient's arms and hands are warm and well perfused

Equipment

- Disposable tourniquet
- Skin-cleansing agent (e.g. chlorhexidine in alcohol) according to local policy
- Cannula of appropriate size
  ➡ **PFP2** – check the expiry date and that the packaging is intact
- Sterile cannula dressing according to local policy
  ➡ **PFP3**
- Ten millilitres of 0.9% sodium chloride to flush the cannula (check expiry date)
- Injectable cap or prepared infusion ready to connect (see p. 113)
- Disposable pad or towel to place under the arm to protect the bed linen
- Sharps bin

Nurse

- Hands must be washed and dried thoroughly
- Gloves (close-fitting to allow dexterity) and an apron should be worn
- Additional protective clothing may be necessary if indicated by the patient's condition (see Ch. 1)
- Adopt a suitable position to avoid stooping
- Some Trusts may require additional training for intravenous cannulation

Procedure

1. If possible, choose the patient's non-dominant arm for cannulation. Place the towel or pad under the arm and check expiry dates on all equipment.

2. Apply the tourniquet 5–10 cm above the proposed site of cannulation, using a quick reléase knot, ➡ **PFP4** and check for arterial blood flow. If the tourniquet is so tight that it prevents arterial blood flow, the veins will not fill.

3. Ask the patient to clench and unclench their fist several times to encourage venous filling. It may also help to lower the arm below the heart level to increase venous filling. Gently tapping the vein may also encourage vasodilation by causing histamine release at the site. Select a vein by palpation, not just visually, to ensure that it is suitable (i.e. bouncy not hard) and is not an artery (which will pulsate) or a tendon ➡ **PFP5**. You can palpate the vein without gloves and then put them on once the vein is selected.

4. Clean the site with cleansing agent and allow it to dry. Do not touch the site again with your fingers.

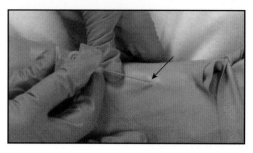

Figure 4.2 IV cannulation: winged cannula with bevel upwards.

5. Take the cannula and check that the needle can be removed easily, but do not remove it. Hold the cannula in your dominant hand with the sharp bevelled end facing upwards (Fig. 4.2).

6. With your other hand, hold the patient's arm and 'anchor' the vein with your thumb, just below the selected insertion site, to prevent it moving when punctured.

7. Holding the cannula at an angle of 20–30° either directly over the vein or just to one side of it, insert the cannula through the skin and into the vein ➡ **PFP6**.

8. Stop advancing the cannula as soon as blood appears at the end of the cannula, which indicates that it has entered the vein and lower the angle of the cannula.

9. Holding the needle part of the cannula with one hand to stop it advancing any further (and going right through the vein), slide the cannula off the needle and into the vein with the other hand.

10. Hold the cannula in place to prevent dislodgement and release the tourniquet. Place a piece of sterile gauze under the end of the cannula to contain any drops of blood during removal of the needle (step 13).

11. If an injectable cap is being used, open the packaging (taking care not to contaminate the sterile end) and hold it between the thumb and forefinger of your dominant hand. If an infusion is to be connected omit this step and follow the procedure in 'Preparing an infusion' (see p. 113).

12. With your other hand, apply pressure to the vein immediately above the end of the cannula to minimise blood flow (Fig. 4.3).

13. Remove the needle and swiftly insert the injectable cap or the administration set of the infusion. Discard the needle into the sharps bin.

14. Clean up any blood and apply the sterile dressing, ➡ **PFP7** ensuring that the cannula is held securely in place.

15. Flush the cannula with 0.9% sodium chloride to ensure patency.

16. Discard sharps any other clinical waste safely.

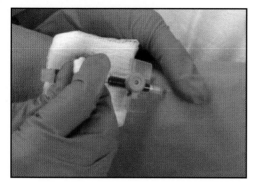

Figure 4.3 IV cannulation: applying pressure to the vein before withdrawing needle.

17. Remove gloves and apron and discard in clinical waste.
18. Wash and dry hands throughly.
19. Return sharps bin and any unused equipment to the appropriate places.
20. Document the date and time of cannulation, the location, type and gauge used in the nursing records. Apply sticker to indicate date of cannulation on the dressing.
21. Ensure the patient is comfortable and explain any restrictions to mobility and the need to protect the cannula site. Ask the patient to report any swelling, redness or pain.
22. The cannula site should be monitored using the Visual Infusion Phlebitis Score (p. 122).

➡Points for practice

PFP1 Although most adult patients will not require it, local anaesthetic may be desirable with patients who are extremely anxious or needle-phobic. Local anaesthetic cream must be applied at least 1 hour in advance to be effective and the possibility of allergy must be considered. The use of injected local anaesthetic is debatable as this requires a needle-prick and may make the selected vein more difficult to see (Lavery and Ingram 2005).

PFP2 The size of cannula required will be determined by the type of fluid to be infused and the size and condition of the patient's veins. The smallest gauge capable of achieving the required flow rate should be used (RCN 2010).

PFP3 The dressing must be sterile. Transparent moisture permeable dressing and those that are gauze and transparent membrane are ideal as they permit visual inspection of the site without removal of the dressing.

PFP4 Site selection should avoid areas of flexion if at all possible and the distal areas of the upper limbs should routinely be used first. This allows subsequent cannulation to proximal to the previously cannulated site (RCN 2010).

PFP5 If it is difficult to palpate the vein with gloves on, do this without gloves and then put them on once the vein is identified.

PFP6 Despite 'anchoring' with the thumb, the vein sometimes moves when directly punctured from above. Consequently, many people prefer to insert the cannula through the skin slightly to one side of the vein and then direct it into the vein.

PFP7 The type of dressing used will be dictated by local policy. Non-sterile tape should not be used to secure the cannula as this has been shown to increase the risk of infection.

4.3 Preparing an infusion

Preparation

Patient
- Explain the reasons for intravenous infusion and any limitations to mobility
- Patient will already have an intravenous cannula

Equipment
- Intravenous infusion fluid according to the prescription
- Intravenous administration set of appropriate type ➡ **PFP1**
- Intravenous infusion stand
- Sterile gauze squares

Nurse
- Wash and dry hands thoroughly, and put on apron
- Non sterile gloves should be worn when connecting the infusion to the cannula
- Additional protective clothing may be necessary if indicated by the patient's condition (see Ch. 1).

Procedure

Intravenous fluid

1. Check the '6 rights' as described on page 183. The intravenous fluid to be administered must be checked by a registered nurse ➡ **PFP2**. Blood transfusions require special checking procedure (see p. 144).
2. Check the outer wrapper is intact and not damaged in any way
3. Open the outer wrapper and remove the bag
4. Check the fluid bag for leakage, particles, cloudiness, expiry date and batch number.

Administration set

1. Check the contents are sterile, i.e. the outer wrapper is not damaged or wet.
2. Check the expiry date/date of sterilization.
3. Open the packaging and remove the administration set. Both ends should be covered with protective caps to maintain sterility.
4. Close the flow control clamp on the administration set.

Assembly

1. Remove the protective cap from the insertion port on the bag of fluid and hold carefully to maintain sterility.
2. Remove the protective cover from the spike of the administration set (just above the drip chamber).
3. Taking care to maintain sterility, insert the spike into the bag, pushing and twisting until fully inserted (Fig. 4.5).
4. Hang the bag on the infusion stand. Squeeze and release the drip chamber until it is half-full of fluid.

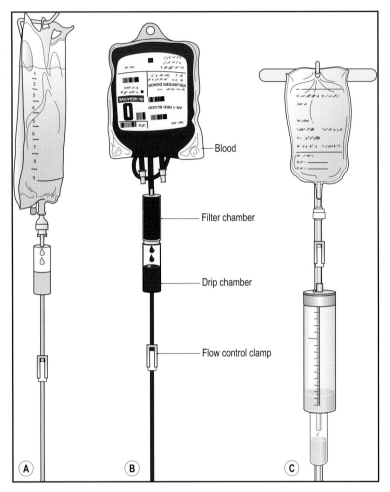

Blood

Filter chamber

Drip chamber

Flow control clamp

(A)   (B)   (C)

Figure 4.4 Types of administration set.

5. To expel the air from the administration set, partially open the roller clamp to allow fluid to run through the set; not too quickly or it will draw in air from the drip chamber.

6. When all the air has been expelled, close the roller clamp. The infusion is now ready for use.

Connecting the infusion

1. Inspect the cannula site using a visual infusion phlebitis score (see p. 122). Do not continue with administration if phlebitis is noted.

2. If the cannula is healthy, put on gloves and place a folded gauze square under the end of the cannula to catch any spillage.

3. Taking care to maintain sterility, remove the protective cap from the administration set and the cap from the cannula. Swiftly connect the set and 'lock' into position ➡ **PFP4**.

4. Secure the tubing with tape to prevent pulling (Fig. 4.7) and adjust the roller clamp to set the infusion to the prescribed rate (Fig. 4.6).

5. Ensure the patient is comfortable and understands about the infusión, and instruct the patient to report any swelling, redness or pain.

6. Discard all packaging and remove gloves and apron; discard in clinical waste and wash hands.

7. Record the time the infusion started and the batch number of the intravenous fluid according to local policy.

8. Document the infusion and monitor fluid balance according to local policy.

➡ Points for practice

PFP1 The type of administration set used will depend upon the type of fluid being administered. Blood requires an administration set with a filter (Fig. 4.4B) that incorporates a 170 mm filter to remove microaggregates that are formed during storage of the blood (Bradbury and Cruickshank 2000). Clear fluids require a simple administration set without a filter chamber (Figure 4.4A).

PFP2 In most cases, all intravenous fluids must be checked by a registered nurse, although in some institutions two nurses are required to check intravenous fluids. Procedures for checking blood transfusions are detailed on page 144.

PFP3 Infusions requiring great accuracy will be controlled through an intravenous pump or syringe driver. A burette (Figure 4.4C) may be used to administer small amounts of fluid or drugs.

PFP4 All administration sets should be fitted with a luer lock device that can be twisted to lock the tubing in place. This is to prevent an accidental disconnection and prevent the entry of micro-organisms. Replacing administration sets every 72 hours has been shown to be safe; however, they should be changed more frequently if used to administer blood (see p. 147) or parenteral nutrition (see p. 136). Apply a sticker to the administration set to indicate the start date, if required.

4.4 Changing an infusion bag

Preparation

Patient	Equipment	Nurse
• Explain the procedure	• Intravenous infusion fluid as prescribed For blood transfusions see Ch. 5	• Wash and dry hands • The infusion fluid must be checked by a registered nurse

Procedure

1. Inspect the cannula site using a visual infusion phlebitis score (see p. 122). If phlebitis is noted, do not continue with the administration.

2. Remove the infusion fluid from its outer wrapper and check the fluid bag for leakage, particles, cloudiness, expiry date, volume and batch number.

3. Check the '6' rights as described on page 183 to ensure that it is the correct infusion fluid (NB This must be checked by a registered nurse, see p. 184).

4. Close the roller clamp on the administration set.

5. Remove the empty infusion bag from the stand and pull out the spike of the administration set, taking care not to contaminate it.

6. Remove the protective cover from the inlet port of the new infusion bag and insert the spike of the giving set, twisting until fully inserted (Fig. 4.5). Replace the bag on the infusión stand.

7. Adjust the roller clamp to the prescribed flow rate (see p. 118).

8. · Discard the used infusion bag and packaging into the clinical waste ➜ **PFP1**.

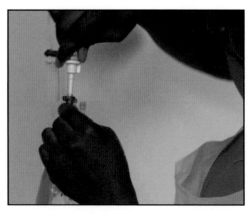

Figure 4.5 Inserting the spike of the administration set into the infusion bag.

9. Document the infusion (amount, type of fluid, time commenced, batch number and signature of the nurses) according to local policy.

10. Record the infusion on the fluid balance chart according to local policy ➡ **PFP2**.

11. Check at least hourly that the infusion is running as prescribed and the patient is not complaining of pain or discomfort at the site.

12. Observe the patient for signs of fluid overload (rising pulse and respiratory rate).

➡ Points for practice

PFP1 If discarding the administration set but retaining the bag (e.g. following blood transfusion), the spike of the set should be cut off and discarded into a sharps bin

PFP2 Most patients with an intravenous infusion will require a fluid balance chart to monitor fluid input and output (see p. 237). The new infusion and completion of the old infusion should be recorded.

4.5 Regulation of flow rate

Principles

The use of intravenous devices (pumps and syringe drivers) to regulate infusions are increasingly being used now in clinical practice. However, a large number of simple infusions will be regulated using gravity and the roller clamp only (Fig. 4.6). It is important that infusions run at a constant rate over the prescribed time.

Calculating the flow rate in 'drops per minute'

If it is a simple gravity infusion, or an infusion device that regulates the flow rate in 'drops per minute' is being used, calculation of the rate in drops per minute is necessary ➡ **PFP1**. The calculation is as follows:

$$\frac{\text{volume of infusion in ml} \times \text{number of drops per ml}}{\text{time in minutes}} = \text{flow rate in drops per minute}$$

The number of drops per ml will be determined by the administration set being used and is indicated on the packaging ➡ **PFP2**:

- Standard administration set = 20 drops per ml.
- Blood administration set =15 drops per ml.
- Paediatric set (burette) = 60 drops per ml.

Example: A patient has been prescribed 500 ml of 0.9% sodium chloride (normal saline) to be given over 6 hours using a standard administration set. The calculation is as follows:

$$\frac{\textbf{500}(\text{vol. of infusion}) \times 20(\text{No. of drops per ml})}{\textbf{360}(6 \text{ hours} \times 60 \text{ minutes})} = \frac{500 \times 20}{360} = \frac{10\ 000}{360}$$

$$= \textbf{27.77 drops per minute} \text{ (round up to 28 drops)}$$

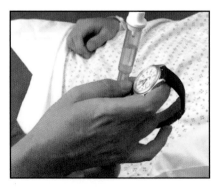

Figure 4.6 Setting the flow rate.

Example: A patient has been prescribed 420 ml of whole blood to be given over 4 hours using a blood administration set. The calculation is as follows:

$$\frac{420 \times 15}{240} = \frac{6300}{240} = \textbf{26.25 drops per minute} \text{ (round up to 27 drops)}$$

Calculating the flow rate in 'millilitres per hour'

$$\frac{\text{volume of infusion in ml}}{\text{No. of hours}} = \text{flow rate in millilitres per hour}$$

Example: A patient has been prescribed 1 litre of 5% dextrose to be given over 8 hours. The calculation is as follows: ml per hour

$$\frac{1000}{8} = \textbf{125 ml per hour}$$

➡Points for practice

PFP1 You are likely to be using a calculator for these calculations. It is important to check your answer several times to ensure that you have used the correct maths. If you are working with junior nurses, it is important to be able to demonstrate your calculation, to enable them to learn.

PFP2 The packaging of a blood administration set may state that it gives 20 drops per ml, but this relates to drops of water. Because blood is thicker than water it forms a larger drop and there are only 15 drops to each ml.

4.6 Care of peripheral cannula site

Preparation

Patient

- Inspect the cannula site to determine whether the dressing needs changing ➡ **PFP1**
- Explain the procedure, to gain consent and cooperation
- The patient must be able to cooperate by keeping the arm very still during the dressing, to prevent accidental dislodgement. If there is doubt, assistance may be required

Equipment

- The cannula site should be considered as a wound and so should not be exposed unnecessarily or during bed making, dusting, etc.
- Sterile dressing – the type will vary according to local policy, but it should be designed for intravenous cannulae ➡ **PFP2**
- If the cannula site requires cleaning, a small dressing pack will be required plus cleansing solution according to local policy

Nurse

- An apron and sterile gloves should be worn. These should be close-fitting gloves to enable manipulation of adhesive dressings and tap
- Additional protective clothing may be necessary if indicated by the patient's condition (see Ch. 1)
- Adopt a comfortable position to avoid stooping
- The hands must be washed and dried thoroughly.

Procedure

1. Ensure that all equipment is within easy reach. Protect the area under the patient's arm with a disposable dressing towel or similar, to collect any spillage.

2. Explain to the patient the importance of remaining still during the procedure, to prevent dislodgement of the cannula. Raise the bed if necessary to avoid stooping.

3. Maintaining asepsis, open the pack and new dressing and pour the cleansing solution (see Aseptic dressing technique, p. 285).

4. Put on the sterile gloves, and using the sterile disposal bag as a 'glove' (see p. 286), carefully remove the old dressing, taking care not to dislodge the cannula. Assistance may be required to secure the cannula during this procedure.

5. If necessary, clean the cannula site ➡ **PFP3**. Inspect the cannula site using a visual phlebitis score (see p. 122). If phlebitis is present this should be reported and the cannula should be removed/re-sited.

6. If the cannula site is healthy apply the new dressing, taking care not to touch the part that will be directly over the insertion site ➡ **PFP4**.

7. If an intravenous infusion is running, secure the tubing of the administration set to prevent pulling and accidental dislodgement of the cannula (Fig. 4.7).

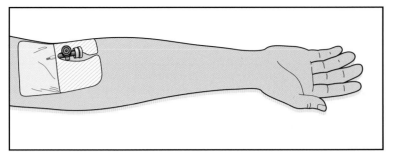

Figure 4.7 Securing the intravenous tubing.

8. Ensure the patient is comfortable and explain any restrictions to mobility and the need to protect the cannula site. Ask the patient to report any swelling, redness or pain

9. Dispose of the soiled dressing and other waste appropriately.

10. Remove gloves and apron, discard in clinical waste and wash hands.

11. Document the visual infusión phlebitis score and dressing change according to local policy. Report any abnormalities.

▶Points for practice

PFP1 The dressing will need changing if it becomes wet, blood-stained or is no longer secure (Pratt et al 2007). If it is clean, dry and secure, most local policies will state that it does not need to be changed until the cannula is removed.

PFP2 The dressing must be sterile. A moisture permeable dressing with a transparent membrane over the cannula site is ideal as they allow visual inspection of the site without removal of the dressing. The dressing is also water resistant and protects the insertion site from contamination

PFP3 The site requires cleaning if there is blood present. If pus or exudate is present, the cannula should be removed.

PFP4 If bandaging is required to protect the cannula site (e.g. a confused patient), it will need to be removed regularly to allow visual observation of the site. A light bandage that does not compress the vein should be used.

4.7 Visual infusion phlebitis (VIP) score

Principles

When a peripheral intravenous cannula (also known as a peripheral vascular access device) is inserted there are a number of local complications that can occur. These complications include:

- **Infiltration**: occurs when non-irritant fluids or medication accidently leak into the surrounding tissues

- **Extravasation**: occurs when irritant fluids or medications infiltrate the surrounding tissues, causing tissue damage and necrosis

- **Phlebitis**: occurs when the wall of the vein becomes inflamed

- **Infection**: redness or pain at the site may indicate infection.

All patients with an intravenous cannula must be assessed at least daily. It is also important to inspect the cannula site before administration of intravenous medications, before changing the intravenous administration set, and before regulating the intravenous flow rate (DH 2010). The nurse's role in assessing the cannula site is to observe for any signs of infection, ensure that the cannula and dressing is dry and secure, and inspect the site for any early signs of phlebitis. To guarantee safe and accurate practice, it is widely recognised that the visual infusion phlebitis (VIP) score helps nurses to assess and monitor the cannula site (Jackson 2008).

Procedure: using the VIP score

1. Inspect the cannulation site for signs of swelling, redness, erythema (redness and flushing of the skin), induration (abnormal hardening of the tissues), and a palpable venous cord (a hard inflamed vein is felt along the vein path with your fingertips). Ask the patient how the site feels e.g does the insertion site feel sore? Is the arm painful to touch?

2. Look at the VIP score (Fig. 4.8) and compare your findings with the descriptors to identify the condition of the site, and the score. For example: slight redness around the intravenous site indicates a score of 1 and indicates that the first signs of phlebitis may be present. Pain at the intravenous site and swelling (a score of 2) indicates signs of early phlebitis.

3. To ensure an accurate assessment, look at the next highest score to the one you have identified and compare your findings to the descriptors. If your findings do not fit those descriptors you have the correct result.

4. Refer to the VIP score to determine the required action for the score; for example, if the score is 1, the cannula will need observing. If the VIP score is 2, the cannula will need re-siting.

5. Document the VIP score, and any actions taken, according to local policy. For care of and removal of peripheral cannulae see page 124.

IV site appears healthy	0	No signs of phlebitis	OBSERVE CANNULA
One of the following is evident: • Slight pain near IV site or • Slight redness near IV site	1	Possible first signs	OBSERVE CANNULA
Two of the following are evident: • Pain at IV site • Erythema • Swelling	2	Early stages of phlebitis	RESITE CANNULA
All of the following are evident: • Pain along path of canula • Erythema • Induration	3	Mid-stage of phlebitis	RESITE CANNULA CONSIDER TREATMENT
All of the following signs are evident and extensive: • Pain along path of canula • Erythema • Induration • Palpable venous cord	4	Advanced stage of phlebitis or start of thrombophlebitis	RESITE CANNULA CONSIDER TREATMENT
All of the following signs are evident and extensive: • Pain along path of canula • Erythema • Induration • Palpable venous cord • Pyrexia	5	Advanced stage of thrombophlebitis	INITIATE TREATMENT

Figure 4.8 Example of Visual Infusion Phlebitis (VIP) score. © Andrew Jackson, Rotherham NHS Trust.

4.8 Removal of peripheral cannula

Preparation

Patient

- Explain the procedure, to gain consent and co-operation ➡ **PFP1**

Equipment/Environment

- The cannula site should be considered as a wound and so should not be exposed unnecessarily or during bed-making
- Sterile gauze squares
- Small self-adhesive dressing, or tape and sterile gauze
- Clinical waste bag
- Sharps bin

Nurse

- Raise the bed if necessary to avoid stooping
- The hands must be washed and dried thoroughly
- An apron and non sterile gloves should be worn. These should be close-fitting to enable manipulation of adhesive dressings and tape
- Additional protective clothing may be necessary if indicated by the patient's condition (see Ch. 1).

Procedure

1. Put on non-sterile gloves.
2. Carefully remove the old dressing, leaving the cannula in situ.
3. Fold a piece of gauze three or four times to create an absorbent pad.
4. Place the folded gauze over the cannula insertion site. Gently withdraw the cannula and immediately apply firm pressure over the insertion site.
5. Continue to apply pressure until the bleeding has stopped (about 3 minutes) to prevent haematoma formation.
6. Apply a small dressing, or tape and a piece of sterile gauze, over the site.
7. Discard all waste, including the plastic cannula, into the clinical waste bag.
8. Remove gloves and apron, discard in clinical waste and wash hands.
9. Ensure comfort and advise the patient to report any bleeding or discomfort at the site.
10. Document removal of cannula and report any abnormalities.

➡Points for practice

Routine replacement of peripheral cannulae every 48–72 hours is generally recommended to prevent phlebitis and catheter colonisation. However, one study found no difference when the cannula was left for 96 hours (Wilson 2006). Refer to your organisation's infection control policy.

4.9 Care of arterial line

Principles

An arterial line is most commonly inserted into the radial artery, although the femoral artery can be used. It enables invasive monitoring of blood pressure and facilitates repeated arterial blood gas sampling. It is only required for critically ill patients; its use is thus confined to critical care and high dependency areas. Any patient requiring an arterial line must be transferred to critical care or HDU. Arterial lines must be cleary labelled to prevent inadvertent drug administration. Drugs must NEVER be injected into an arterial line.

Management of an arterial line

A 500 ml infusion of 0.9% saline or heparinised saline is placed in a pressure bag and inflated to 300mgHg. This ensures a constant flow of approximately 3 ml per hour, which prevents backflow from the artery. The monitoring system will incorporate a flushing device to enable manual flushing following blood gas sampling. The aterial line is connected to a transducer by means of fine, rigid 'manometer' tubing, which transmits the pressure in the artery to the transducer. The arterial blood pressure is shown as a wave form on a bedside monitor.

Keep it visible

There is a high risk of bleeding from an arterial line and so the arterial line should be visible at all times. Because of the pressure in the artery, if the cannula should become disconnected the patient could lose large volumes of blood very quickly. Therefore it is vital that the line is always visible to allow immediate detection of any problems. Observe the site for complications in the same way as an IV cannula (see p. 120).

Use luer locks

The arterial line may be sutured in position or secured with an adhesive cannula dressing. Tubing should be secured in the usual way to prevent pulling on the catheter. Connections between the cannula and monitoring system and infusion bag must be secured with luer locks to prevent accidental disconnection. Accidental disconnection could lead to exsanguination if undetected (Scales 2010).

4.10 Intravenous pumps and syringe drivers

Principles

There are a large number of different types available from a range of manufacturers and a detailed description of each will be found in the manufacturer's user manual. To guarantee safe and accurate practice, nurses have a responsibility to ensure that they are familiar with all equipment being used. If unsure of any aspect of the pump or syringe driver, it is important to seek help from a more experienced nurse or from the department responsible for the maintenance of intravenous devices. Although intravenous devices may differ in appearance, there are a number of features that are likely to be common to all. Many hospitals have an equipment 'library' so that IV devices are purchased, stored and maintained centrally. This enables equipment to be standardized. Make sure you are familiar with the following features on the syringe driver or pump you are using:

Power supply

- Is the device powered by battery, mains electricity or both?
- If batteries, what type are they?
- If it has a rechargeable battery: how long will it run on the battery? How is the battery charged? How do you know when it needs charging?

Administration set/syringe

- Most devices can only be used with a specific administration set or type of syringe
- If it is possible to use different sizes and types, how does the device confirm recognition of the type being used?

Setting up the device

- You must be familiar with the correct procedure for setting up the device. All administration sets, cassettes and syringes are designed to be inserted easily into the device. If force is required, the correct procedure is not being followed.

Alarm systems

- Most devices have a number of alarms to alert the nurse to situations such as 'air in the line', 'infusion complete' and 'occlusion of the line'
- Most will have a mute button to allow the alarm to be silenced while dealing with the problem. It is vital that alarms are never turned off (however irritating), as dangerous situations may then go undetected
- If any alarm feature is not working properly, the device must not be used

- Some smaller devices do not have any alarms and must be checked at least once every hour to ensure safe and accurate administration of the drug or infusion.

Maintenance and repair

- All intravenous devices must be maintained regularly to ensure safe and accurate use. Most hospitals have a system of regular maintenance indicated by a sticker on the device, showing the date when maintenance is due. Pumps and syringe drivers must not be used after this date and should be returned to the relevant department for maintenance.

- Most devices that are powered by mains electricity also have a battery for short-term use when transferring a patient or during a power cut. The device should be kept plugged in to the mains at all times, even when not in use, to ensure the battery remains fully charged.

4.11 Central venous catheters: care of the site

Preparation

Patient
- Explain the procedure, to gain consent and co-operation ➡ **PFP1**
- The patient should be in a recumbent or semi-recumbent position

Equipment/Environment
- Ensure warmth, privacy and adequate light
- Dressing trolley or clean, flat surface adjacent to the patient
- Sterile dressing pack containing gloves
- Cleansing solution according to local policy (e.g. 2% chlorhexidine in 70% alcohol) ➡ **PFP2**
- Sterile dressing according to policy/protocol ➡ **PFP3**
- Alcohol hand-rub

Nurse
- The hands must be washed and dried thoroughly
- An apron should be worn
- Additional protective clothing may be necessary if indicated by the patient's condition (see Ch. 1)

Procedure

1. Assemble all equipment at the bedside.

2. Ask/assist the patient into a comfortable recumbent or semi-recumbent position and remove clothing as necessary to expose the site ➡ **PFP4**.

3. Open the pack, and using the sterile disposal bag as a 'glove', and taking great care not to dislodge the catheter, remove the old dressing and turn the bag inside out to contain it (see p. 286). Place the bag in a convenient position to allow easy access without passing used swabs across the open dressing pack.

4. Put on sterile gloves and, if necessary (i.e if there has been leakage of blood or exudate from the site ➡ **PFP1**) clean the site according to local policy and allow it to dry.

5. Apply the new dressing, making sure that insertion site is visible to allow for daily inspection ➡ **PFP1**.

6. Discard all waste and equipment appropriately. Remove gloves and wash hands.

7. Assist the patient as necessary to replace clothing and adopt a comfortable position. Instruct the patient to report any pain or discomfort at the site.

8. Document the dressing change in the nursing records and report any abnormal findings ➡ **PFP5**.

➡ Points for practice

PFP1 The central venous catheter (CVC) insertion site should be inspected at least daily (Department of Health 2011). The dressing will need changing if blood or serous fluid has collected around the catheter, as this greatly increases the infection risk

PFP2 Infusion ports and hubs should also be cleaned with chlohexidine and alcohol. Patients who are allergic to (or sensitive to) chlorhexidine should have their skin cleansed with single use povidine iodine

PFP3 Local policy or protocol will determine the type of dressing to be used. Transparent, semi-permeable dressings should be used because they are occlusive and allow easy visualisation of the site (Department of Health 2011)

PFP4 A catheter for measurement of the central venous pressure (CVP) will be inserted into the internal or external jugular vein or subclavian vein. Central venous catheters for longer term parenteral nutrition or drug administration (and, therefore, not for CVP measurement) may be inserted into the brachial vein at the antecubital fossa and then advanced until the tip rests in the subclavian vein. This is referred to as a peripherally inserted central catheter (PICC; Perry 2008)

PFP5 CVCs that are no longer required should be removed as soon as possible to reduce the risk of infection – maximum duration 1–3 weeks depending on local policy (Department of Health 2011)

4.12 Central venous pressure (CVP) measurement

In most acute hospitals, patients who require regular monitoring of their central venous pressue will be connected to a monitor via a transducer to provide a continuous central venous pressure (CVP) measurement on a monitor that is also used for cardiac monitoring (see Fig. 2.8). However in some ward settings, nurses will still use a CVP manometer to obtain readings and it is essential that this is carried out accurately.

Preparation

Patient	Equipment/Environment	Nurse
• Explain the procedure, to gain consent and cooperation	• CVP manometer with 0.9% sodium chloride infusion. CVP measurements cannot be made with any other solution	• Wash and dry hands thoroughly. Additional protective clothing may be necessary if indicated by the patient's condition (see Ch. 1)
• The patient should be lying flat or in the same position as adopted for previous CVP measurements ➡ **PFP1**		• Check previous CVP measurements and the position of the patient during these measurements (this should be indicated on the chart)

Procedure

1. With the patient lying flat or in the same position as adopted for previous measurements, level the zero point on the manometer with the patient's heart. A spirit level is incorporated into the manometer arm to ensure accurate levelling (Fig. 4.9).

2. A mark should be made at the mid-axillary line or sternal angle to indicate the level, so that all subsequent readings are made from the same point. This is in line with the right atrium and is known as the phlebostatic axis (Cole 2007).

3. If necessary, turn off any other infusions that may be running through the central venous catheter.

4. With the three-way tap in position 'A' (Fig. 4.9), allow the 0.9% sodium chloride infusion to run rapidly for a few seconds to check that the line is patent ➡ **PFP2**.

5. Stop the infusion by closing the roller clamp. Adjust the three-way tap on the manometer to position 'B', so that the fluid can flow up the manometer column. Gradually open the roller clamp to allow fluid to slowly fill the manometer column until 5–10 cm above the previous measurement. Close the roller clamp.

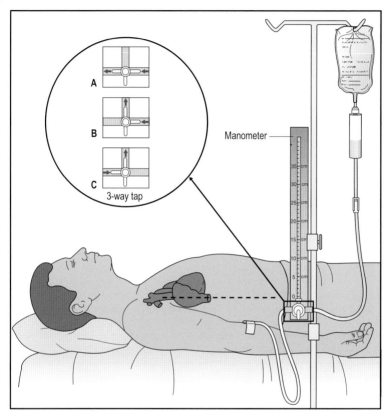

Figure 4.9 Measuring the CVP.

6. Turn the three-way tap to position 'C', so that the line to the infusion bag is closed and the other two lines (to the column and the patient) are open. The fluid in the column will now start to fall, pausing with each respiration, until it equalises with the pressure in the right atrium of the heart. The fluid should continue to rise and fall gently with respiration ➡ **PFP3**. This level, which is measured in centimetres of water (cmH$_2$O), is the CVP measurement ➡ **PFP4**.

7. Turn the three-way tap back to position 'A', so that the column of fluid is 'off', and reset the infusion to the prescribed rate. Reset any other infusions as appropriate.

8. Assist the patient into a comfortable position.

9. Ensure all equipment is secured safely and intravenous tubing does not touch the floor.
10. Record the CVP measurement on the appropriate chart. If this is the first measurement, also note the position of the patient and the reference point for readings.
11. Report any abnormalities or changes from previous measurements.

➡️Points for practice

PFP1 The patient needs to be in the same position for all readings to allow comparisons to be made and trends to be observed. If the patient's condition allows, lying flat will be the most accurate.

PFP2 If the infusion will not run freely, the CVP measurement will not be accurate. Sometimes, asking the patient to turn their head away from the CVP line can help by moving the tip of the catheter away from the wall of the blood vessel. If this makes the infusion run freely, perform the same manoeuvre when measuring the CVP.

PFP3 The fluid in the column should rise and fall gently or 'swing' with each respiration because of changes in the pressure within the chest. If the fluid falls but does not swing, it may not be an accurate measurement.

PFP4 The normal range for the CVP is 5–10 cmH$_2$O if measured at the mid axilla, and 0–7 cmH$_2$O if measured at the sternal angle. The reading should be interpreted in conjunction with other signs and the trend (i.e. whether it is rising or falling) is often more important than a single measurement.

4.13 Removal of central venous catheters (non-tunnelled)

Preparation

Patient

- Explain the procedure, to ensure understanding and cooperation
- The patient should be lying flat and slightly head-down, if possible → **PFP1**
- Ensure warmth, dignity and privacy

Equipment/Environment

Equipment to perform dressing (p. 285)

- Sterile air-occlusive dressing → **PFP2**
- Sterile scissors and sterile specimen pot (universal type)
- Cleansing solution according to local policy (e.g. chlorhexidine and alcohol or povidone iodine)
- Stitch cutter and sharps bin
- Alcohol hand-rub or hand washing facilities

Nurse

- Experienced nurses may remove non-tunnelled CVP catheters → **PFP3**. A second nurse may be required to assist during this procedure
- The hands must be washed and dried thoroughly
- An apron should be worn

Procedure

1. Ask/assist the patient to lie flat. Tilt the head of the bed down (about 15°), if the patient's condition will allow → **PFP1**. Remove clothing, bedclothes etc., as necessary, to expose the central venous catheters (CVC) site.

2. Prepare all equipment (see p. 285).

3. Turn off the infusion and loosen but do not remove the dressing covering the site.

4. Wash and dry your hands thoroughly or clean them with alcohol hand-rub.

5. Open the dressing pack, and using the waste disposal bag as a 'glove' to protect your hand, remove the dressing and turn the bag inside out to contain it (see p. 286). Place the bag in a convenient position to allow easy access.

6. Put on the sterile gloves provided in the dressing pack, and using a gauze swab and cleansing solution, clean around the insertion site → **PFP4**.

7. Use the stitch cutter to cut the stitch holding the catheter in place and make sure it is free of the skin.

8. Maintaining sterility, open the specimen pot and place it in an accessible position.

9. Fold a gauze square two or three times to create an absorbent pad. Holding this in your non-dominant hand, place it over the insertion site, ready to press immediately the catheter is withdrawn.

10. Ask the patient to hold their breath during removal of the catheter.

Withdraw the catheter by pulling in a firm, steady movement and press firmly with the gauze pad for several minutes to prevent bleeding and air embolus → **PFP1**.

11. Ask an assistant to place the tip of the catheter in the specimen pot, and using sterile scissors, cut off the tip (about 5 cm) and allow it to fall into the container. Replace the lid ➡ **PFP5**. Check that the tip is intact – a ragged broken edge may indicate that part of the tip has been left in situ which may cause a catheter embolus (Guest 2008).

12. Once the bleeding has stopped, apply the sterile air-occlusive dressing to the site.

13. Remove gloves.

14. Return the bed to the horizontal position and ask the patient to remain supine for 15–30 minutes following removal.

15. Dispose of all clinical waste and sharps appropriately.

16. Wash and dry hands thoroughly.

17. Label the specimen container, and with the appropriate request form, send for microscopy, culture and sensitivity (Guest 2008).

18. Document CVP removal and specimen request in the nursing records.

➡Points for practice

PFP1 There is a significant risk of air embolism during and after the removal of a CVC. Placing the patient in a supine, head-down position reduces this by increasing the intrathoracic pressure, making it less likely for air to be drawn in during inspiration (Guest 2008).

PFP2 An air-occlusive dressing must be used to reduce the risk of air entry leading to air embolus following removal of the catheter.

PFP3 Local policy may dictate that only nurses who have undergone additional training may remove CVCs. Tunnelled catheters must be removed by medical staff or specialist nurses and often require surgical removal.

PFP4 The site must be cleaned before removal of the catheter, to prevent contamination of the tip during withdrawal. This would lead to an inaccurate bacteriological assessment (see below).

PFP5 Trust protocol may require the tip of the catheter to be sent for bacterial examination following removal if catheter-related sepsis is suspected. If no assistance is available, place the catheter on the trolley so that the tip is resting on a corner of the sterile field, to prevent contamination. Once the dressing is securely in place, cut the tip off as described.

4.14 Care of long-term central venous catheters

Principles

Hickman and PICC lines are types of central venous catheters (CVCs) made of special hypoallergenic material that allow them to remain in situ for many months. They are often used for patients who require regular, but intermittent, intravenous therapy, such as those receiving chemotherapy or parenteral nutrition (PN; Green 2011). As with all central venous catheters asepsis is vital as there is a high risk of infection, especially with patients who are immunosuppressed and/or receiving chemotherapy. In order to reduce the risk of infection for long term PN (greater than 30 days), it is recommended that the CVC is tunnelled under the skin (Fig. 4.10) (NICE 2006). This means that the insertion site through the skin, which is very vulnerable to infection, is at some distance from the point of entry into the blood vessel, thus reducing the risk of infection (Green 2011). Most tunnelled CVCs have a Dacron® 'cuff' situated approximately 1.5 cm from the exit site (Fig. 4.10). As the patient's tissues grow around the cuff it secures the CVC in place and acts as a barrier to infection.

Another documented complication of CVC therapy is the risk of thrombi (blood clots) and fibrin plugs blocking the catheter and affecting the flow of fluid or medicine (Cummings-Winfield and Mushani-Kanji 2008). If this problem occurs, thrombolysis (medicine that 'breaks down the clot', e.g. alteplase or urokinase) may be administered. This is a high risk process and one that should be carried out under expert medical supervision.

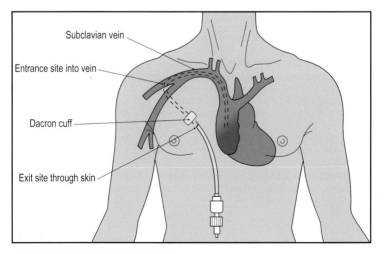

Figure 4.10 Tunnelled long-term catheter.

Care of the site

Care of long-term catheters is often undertaken at home by patients or carers or by the district nurse. The dressing over the cannula site should be changed twice weekly until the tissue around the Dacron® cuff has become fibrosed. Long-term care varies considerably from hospital to hospital, but covering the site is not usually necessary once the site has healed, except when there is a risk of it getting wet, e.g. in the shower.

Immersion of the site is not recommended, but splashing, as in the shower, is usually no problem. Bathing in a public pool and water sports are not recommended because of the risk of infection from the water. In order to remain patent, the catheter must be flushed at regular intervals to prevent clotting. Most hospitals recommend the use of saline or heparinised saline 2–3 times per week, but recommended practices vary in both frequency and the solution used.

Care of implantable ports

Implantable ports are designed for long-term intermittent venous access. They are surgically implanted under the skin of the chest wall or sometimes on the arm. It is sutured to the underlying muscle to anchor it in place. The device may have one or two ports, each of which is attached to a single lumen catheter, which is inserted into the vein. Once the wound has healed the port is accessed by insertion of a needle through the skin and through the injectable membrane of the device. Once the infusion or drug has been administered that needle is removed and the port seals off, thus reducing the risk of infection. It is almost invisible under the skin and so is more discreet that a tunnelled device, but it does require the patient to have regular needles through the skin.

Parenteral nutrition

Parenteral nutrition (PN) is most commonly administered via a central venous catheter, because of the irritant nature of the high dextrose solution. Tunnelled CVCs are recommended for PN; however, administration via a peripheral line is sometimes used for short term use. The administration set being used for PN must be changed every 24 hours with each new bag; strict asepsis is vital. Many Trusts require that nurses undergo specific training for this task. It is recommended that PN is administered via a dedicated feeding line using a volumetric pump with occlusion and air-in-line alarms (NICE 2006). The CVC being used for PN must not be used for measurement or drug administration because any interruption in the closed system increases the risk of infection. There is also a high risk of incompatibility with medicines.

The line must be flushed according to local policy before commencing and after completion of a feed. The flow rate should be continous, not intermittent, to avoid line blockages (Green 2011).

Bibliography/suggested reading

Bowden, T., 2010. Peripheral cannulation: a practical guide. British Journal of Cardiac Nursing 5 (3), 124–131.

This article provides a detailed description of the technique as well as discussion about informed consent issues, relevant anatomy, site selection and device selection. It also discusses the risks and potential complications associated with peripheral cannulation

Bowden, T., 2010. Venepuncture: a practical guide. British Journal of Cardiac Nursing 5 (2), 66–70.

This article provides a detailed description of the technique as well discussion about informed consent issues, relevant anatomy, site selection and device selection. It also shows in detail how to apply a disposable tourniquet using a quick-release knot that can be released with one hand

Bradbury, M., Cruickshank, J., 2000. Blood transfusion: crucial steps in maintaining safe practice. British Journal of Nursing 9 (3), 134–138.

This article considers nurses' responsibilities in relation to safe administration of blood and provides evidence-based guidelines using the mnemonic PACK, which stands for: Patient & Pre-transfusion checks; Asepsis & Apparatus; Checking & Clerical procedures; Keeping vigilant and Keeping accurate records.

Cole, E., 2007. Measuring central venous pressure. Nursing Standard 22 (7), 40–42.

This article describes the uses and sites of central lines, potential complications and how to record central venous pressure

Cummings-Winfield, C., Mushani-Kanji, T., 2008. Restoring patency to central venous access devices. Clinical Journal of Oncology Nurses 12 (6), 925–934. [online]. [Accessed 09.01.12] Available from: http://ons.metapress.com/content/1q1511787t16841g/fulltext.pdf.

This excellent article discusses the evidence based care needed for CVCs and the removal of thrombotic blockages. The illustrations clearly demonstrate the potential problems suffered by patients with long term CVCs. Whilst written for oncology practice, it has relelvance for all long term CVCs

Department of Health, 2010. High Impact Intervention No2. Peripheral intravenous care bundle. [online]. [Accessed 18.07.11] Available from: http://hcai.dh.gov.uk/whatdoido/high-impact-interventions.

These high impact interventions care bundles were originally published in 2007, and formed part of the saving lives campaign: reducing infection, delivering safe and clean care. They have been re-written in 2010. This particular care bundles provide a practical overview of the evidence-base principles for peripheral cannulation, including audit tools

Department of Health, 2011. High impact intervention. Central venous catheter care bundle. [online]. [Accessed 06.06.2011] Available from: http://hcai.dh.gov.uk/files/2011/03/2011–03–14-HII-Central-Venous-Catheter-Care-Bundle-FINAL.pdf.

This web page contains the Department of Health mandate on how central venous catheters should be cared for

Dougherty, L., Lamb, J., 2007. Intravenous therapy in nursing practice, second ed. Churchill Livingstone Elsevier, London.

This is a comprehensive UK text book that addresses all aspects of intravenous therapy in a variety of care settings. It also includes a chapter on intravenous therapy in children

Gabriel, J., 2009. Reducing needlestick and sharps injuries among healthcare workers. Nursing Standard 23 (22), 41–44.

Although this article focuses on the risks associated with needlestick injuries, it also addresses the different ways these injuries can be reduced to include the use of safer devices

Green, S., 2011. Nutrition and health. In: Brooker, C., Nicol, M., (Eds.), Alexanders Nursing Practice, fourth ed. Churchill Livingstone Elsevier, London.

This comprehensive chapter on nutrition and health has a section dedicated to parenteral nutrition, CVC use in nutrition, monitoring and potential complications. Using contemporary literature it provides an easily understood overview of PN

Guest, J., 2008. Specimen collection – central venous catheter tip sampling. Nursing Times 104 (22), 20–21.

This short article clearly describes how to remove a CVC and demonstrates how to obtain a catheter tip for MC&S

IV Team [online]. [Accessed 09.01.12] Available from: http://www.ivteam.com/.

An excellent web site providing links to relevant literature and advice on all aspects of IV therapy including, central venous catheters, IV pumps, arterial lines and VIP scores. It includes a short videocast by Andrew Jackson, creator of the VIP score, who explains the key problems associated with intravenous cannulation and the use of the VIP score in practice

Jackson, A., 2008. VIP score discussion from Andrew Jackson. [online]. [Accessed 18.07.11] Available from: www.youtube.com.

This short videocast by Andrew Jackson, creator of the VIP score, provides some useful information on the key problems associated with peripheral cannulation, and explains the principles for using the visual infusion phlebitis score in practice

Lavery, I., Ingram, P., 2005. Venepuncture: best practice. Nursing Standard 19 (49), 55–65.

This is a continuing professional development article that provides guidance on the theory and practice of venepuncture. It includes a useful overview of the anatomy and physiology, choice of sites and special considerations, such as venepuncture in stroke patients. Also addresses prevention of infection and other complications and the technique itself using a syringe and needle and a vacuum system

National Instituite for Health and Clinical Excellence (NICE), 2006. Nutitional support in adults – clinical guideline CG32. [online]. [Accessed 09.01.12] Available from: http://www.nice.org.uk/Guidance/CG32.

This website links to all aspects of nutrition and feeding and it makes recommendations for parenteral nutrition practice for those patients being fed via a CVC

Perry, M.C., 2008. The chemotherapy source book, frouth ed. Lippincott, Williams and Wilkins, Philadelphia.

This book discusses the various types of chemotherapy used in current practice – many of which are administered intravenously via a short- or long-term vascular device. There is a section on PICC lines and the care that patients may need in a community setting

Pratt, R.J., Pellow, C.M., Wilson, J.A., et al, 2007. epic2: National evidence based guidelines for preventing healthcare associated infections in NHS hospitals in England. Journal of Hospital Infection 65 (suppl 1), S1-S64.

Evidence-based guidelines that focus on the prevention of bloodstream infections. It includes the choice of type of CVC and the risks associated with each. The 2007 updated version has a specific focus on prevent of CVC infections

Royal College of Nursing, 2010. Standards for infusion therapy, third ed. RCN, London.

This document provides a comprehensive overview and best practice guidance on all aspects of infusion therapy including: infection control and safety, equipment, site selection, site care and complications

Scales, K., 2008. A practical guide to venepuncture and blood sampling. Nursing Standard, 22 (29), 29–36.

This article provides a good overview of relevant anatomy and physiology, consent issues, vein selection, the technique itself and sharps disposal. It also addresses the prevention and management of complications of venepuncture

Scales, K., 2010. Arterial catheters: indications, insertion and use in critical care. Nursing Standard 19 (19), IV supplement S16-S21.

An excellent article that looks at all aspects of arterial lines from indications through to arterial pressure monitoring and care and management of the arterial line, and emphasises the safety issues. It also discusses removal of an arterial line

Wilson, J., 2006. Infection control in clinical practice. third ed. Baillière Tindall Elsevier, Edinburgh.

A comprehensive text that explains basic microbiology, types of organisms and how they are spread. It then provides guidance on infection control practices, preventing wound infections and infections associated with catheters, intravenous cannulae and the respiratory and gastrointestinal systems

Chapter 5

Blood transfusion

©2012 Elsevier Ltd.

5.1 Blood transfusion

Principles of safety

- Blood transfusions are frequently administered in clinical practice, yet because there are multiple stages in the transfusion process the patient is exposed to the risk of multiple errors being made. Fatal consequences can ensue if the incorrect blood is given.

- The greatest risk to patients is that the incorrect blood component is transfused, that is, either the patient receives a blood component intended for someone else or one that is not suitable for them (SHOT, 2009). Traceability of each blood component transfused is therefore essential. There must be a clear audit trail of the collection, delivery, receipt (and return) of all blood components. Positive evidence of transfusion of each blood component must be kept for a minimum of 30 years.

- It is therefore vital that blood for transfusion is checked carefully at every stage to ensure that the correct blood is administered to the correct patient.

- The most important elements of the blood transfusion process are positive patient identification and meticulous documentation. The patient must wear an identification band that includes their first name, last name, date of birth and a unique identification number e.g. their NHS number. All documentation relating to the patient must be identical in every detail to the information on the patient's identification band.

- Whenever possible during the transfusion process, the patient should be asked to state their full name and date of birth during the checking procedures. This information must match *exactly* the information on their identification band. Patient checks should be carried out at each stage of the blood transfusion process namely: decision to transfuse, prescription; requests for transfusion; blood samples for cross matching; collection of blood and administration.

- Increasingly the use of information technology such as an electronically readable bar-code is used to improve positive identification of patients, blood samples and blood components throughout the transfusion process. Local procedure for the use of such technology, if available, should be followed.

- Guidance from the British Committee for Standards in Haematology (BCSH 2009) state that as a minimum one registered health care professional who has had their competency assessed must perform the checking procedure. If local policy requires a two person checking procedure, each person should complete all the checks independently (double independent checking). Whatever the policy it is vital that **all checking is carried out at the bedside.**

- Documentation required for all stages of the blood transfusion process should be clearly outlined in local policies.

- Adverse reactions most commonly occur within the first 30 minutes of the transfusion and so it is vital that nurses continually observe the patient during this time. For this reason it is advised that blood transfusions are not undertaken at night, unless clinically essential (Taylor et al 2010).

Storage and collection of blood

- Blood must be stored in a dedicated refrigerator at 2–6°C to prevent contaminants reproducing. It must not be kept in a ward refrigerator.

- Blood for transfusion should be collected from the blood transfusion department or dedicated refrigerator no longer than 30 minutes before it is required. This is because pathogens grow extremely quickly in blood at room temperature. Therefore, before collecting the blood component, the nurse must check that the patient is ready to start the transfusion and has patent venous access.

- If the transfusion has not commenced within 30 minutes, the blood bank must be informed and the blood may need to be discarded. If the blood is stored in a special 'blood carrier' this time may be extended (see local policy).

- It is also recommended that transfusions are completed within 4 hours of removal from a conrolled temperature environment (BCSH, 2009).

- The nurse collecting the blood must take the authorised documentation containing the patient's core identifiers and check these with the label on the blood component (Fig. 5.1). Many collection errors occur when the patient details on the laboratory produced label attached to the blood component pack (compatibility label) are not checked against the patient's identification details (BCSH, 2009).

- Unless large quantities of blood are required for rapid transfusion, only one unit of blood should be collected at a time.

- The identity of the person collecting the blood and the date and time of collection must be documented.

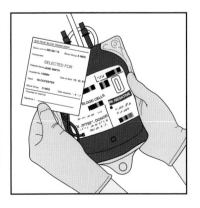

Figure 5.1 Blood bag with compatibility label.

Administration equipment

- A special blood administration set that incorporates a 170 mm filter chamber must be used. Some patients who are receiving multiple blood transfusions or who have had febrile reactions in response to previous transfusions may require an additional filter. These are fine-mesh filters that are placed between the blood bag and the administration set in order to remove microaggregates (e.g. fibrin and clots) formed during storage. The same filter can be used for up to four units of blood. If a filter is required it is usually supplied with the blood when collected from the blood transfusion department.

- When rapid transfusion or transfusion via a CVP line is necessary, blood can only be warmed by using a blood warmer during administration. Direct heat must never be used as this can cause blood to haemolyse. The design of blood warmers will vary, but most incorporate a 'zig-zag' tube or coil through which the blood passes over a heater element and is warmed before reaching the patient.

- Some infusion pumps may damage blood cells and should only be used if the manufacturer's instructions specifically state that they are safe to use with blood transfusion.

Principles of blood transfusion checking procedure

1. Check the patient's identity:
   - **all checking must take place at the bedside**
   - where possible, positively identify patients by asking them to state their full name and date of birth. Check that these match the identification band.
2. Check the patient's surname, first names, date of birth, unique identification number, blood group and rhesus factor on:
   - patient's identification band
   - blood transfusion compatibility report for.
   - compatibility label attached to the bag
   - blood bag
   - intravenous (IV) fluid/ blood prescription chart:
3. Check the expiry date of the unit of blood (and time if applicable, e.g. platelets) on:
   - compatibility label on the bag
   - blood bag.
4. Check the blood group and unique component donation number on:
   - blood bag
   - compatibility label on the bag
   - record this on the prescription chart. There is usually a peel-off section on the blood compatibility label for this.

5. Check any special requirements:
    - The unit of blood must comply with the prescription (e.g. gamma irradiated).
6. Record the date and time and signature of the nurse(s) on:
    - blood transfusion compatibility report form.
    - compatibility label.
    - intravenous (IV) fluid prescription chart.
7. Blood bag:
    - inspect the bag for any signs of leakage or damaged packaging
    - inspect blood for unusual color, turbidity or clumping of the contents.

If any discrepancies are noted, the blood must not be transfused, the blood bank must be informed, and the blood and blood transfusion compatibility form returned.

5.2 Care and management of a transfusion

Preparation

Patient
- Explain the procedure, to gain consent and cooperation ➡ **PFP1**
- The patient must be wearing an identification band.
- Advise the patient not to leave the ward during the transfusion (in many instances patients will be confined to bed)
- Unconscious patients require very close monitoring
- If an intravenous infusion is running to keep the vein open, this must be 0.9% sodium chloride

Equipment/Environment
- Blood administration set ➡ **PFP2**
- Clinical thermometer and watch
- Sphygmomanometer and stethoscope.
- Observation chart (temperature, pulse, respiration and blood pressure)
- Fluid balance chart
- Intravenous prescription chart
- Infusion stand
- Intravenous adrenaline (epinephrine) and chlorpheniramine should be available on the ward (in case of allergic reactions)

Nurse
- Wash and dry hands thoroughly.
- Gloves and an apron should be worn
- Additional protective clothing may be required according to the patient's condition (see Ch. 1)

Procedure

1. Record baseline observations of temperature, pulse, respiration and blood pressure immediately prior to commencement of the transfusion ➡ **PFP3**.

2. At the bedside, check the blood as described on p. 144 against the prescription and the patient's identification band.

3. Check the cannula site (see VIP score p. 122) .Using a non touch aseptic technique prepare the infusion as described on page 113.

4. Calculate the rate of infusion and set the infusion to the required rate (see p. 118) ➡ **PFP4**.

5. Observe the patient continuously for the first 30 minutes as this is when a reaction is most likely to occur. Record the temperature, pulse and blood pressure again 15 minutes after commencement of the transfusion. If these observations have altered significantly from baseline, the respiratory rate should be checked as well. These should be repeated during the transfusion according to local policy ➡ **PFP5** and again at the end of the transfusion.

6. Observe the urine output for volume and colour throughout the transfusion ➡ **PFP6**.

7. Observe for and encourage the patient to report any of the following ➡ **PFP7**:

   Allergic reaction/anaphylaxis (allergic reaction to 'foreign' plasma proteins):
   - wheezing and shortness of breath
   - hypotension
   - a rash on the chest or abdomen
   - oedema of the eyes or face
   - laryngeal swelling.

   Febrile reaction (reaction of the patient's antibodies to donor leucocytes):
   - pyrexia
   - feeling hot and flushed or shivering
   - rigors

   Haemolytic reaction (most serious reaction, due to transfusion of incompatible blood):
   - chest or abdominal pain, or pain in the extremities
   - lumbar or loin pain
   - oliguria
   - hypotension and shock.

   Circulatory overload (more common in elderly, especially those with heart failure):
   - rising pulse and respiration rates
   - dyspnoea or 'bubbly' respiration and frothy sputum
   - hypotension.

8. The transfusion should be stopped and medical staff informed if:
   - there is a rise in temperature of greater than 1°C
   - there is a significant rise or fall in blood pressure
   - there is a significant rise in pulse rate
   - any of the above reactions occur.

9. If a number of units of blood are transfused, the administration set should be changed every 12 hours to prevent bacterial growth.

10. The blood transfusion compatibility form must be readily available throughout the transfusion.

11. When the transfusion is complete, disconnect the infusion using a non touch technique. If an IV infusion is to follow, change the administration set.

12. Ensure the patient is comfortable and knows to report any adverse reactions as noted above.

13. Replace equipment and discard waste appropriately ➡ **PFP8**.

14. Remove gloves and apron and wash hands.

15. The time that the transfusion stopped must be documented according to local policy.

➡**Points for practice**

PFP1 Written consent is not usually required but patients must be fully informed (BCSH 2009). Some patients have a cultural and religious objection to blood transfusion, e.g. Jehovah's Witnesses, and their wishes must be respected (McInroy 2005). The nurse must be prepared to answer any questions regarding the clinical indication for the transfusion.

PFP2 A special administration set must be used for blood transfusions. This has an additional chamber above the drip chamber, which contains a filter. This filters out debris (platelets and white cells) (see Fig. 4.4b p. 114). Platelet administration requires a special administration set with no filter. Platelets must be administered rapidly (over 20–30 minutes) as soon as they are available.

PFP3 Dyspnoea and tachypnoea may both be features of serious reactions and so a baseline measurement prior to transfusion fusion is recommended.

PFP4 Electronic infusion pumps may damage blood cells and must only be used if the manufacturer's instructions specifically state that they can be used to administer blood.

PFP5 Observations during blood transfusion should be clearly dated and recorded separately from routine observations in case retrieval at a later date is necessary. Trust policies regarding the frequency of the observations required during blood transfusion may vary, but most require the temperature, pulse, respiration rate and blood pressure to be recorded before the start of the transfusion, 15 minutes after commencement, and again at the end of the transfusion. Each unit of blood should be regarded as a new transfusion.

PFP6 The urine output should be monitored for haemoglobinuria or oliguria, which are signs of an acute haemolytic transfusion reaction.

PFP7 If an adverse reaction occurs, the transfusion must be stopped immediately and the medical staff informed. The administration set should be changed and venous access maintained by an infusion of 0.9% sodium chloride. The patient's temperature, pulse, respiration rate and blood pressure, and the colour and volume of urine should be monitored. Patients who, for any reason, are unable to report adverse reactions themselves will require more frequent observation. Clearly document any adverse reactions, the action taken and the outcome.

PFP8 Ideally used blood bags are kept for at least 2 days following transfusion in case there is a delayed reaction to the blood. The procedure for storage and ultimate disposal of blood bags will vary. Local policy should be followed.

Bibliography/suggested reading

British Committee for Standards in Haematology (BCSH), 2009. Guideline on the Administration of Blood Components. [online] Available from: http://www.bcshguidelines.com/4_HAEMATOLOGY_GUIDELINES.html (accessed 10.06.11.).

This provides detailed evidence based guidelines on all aspects of blood transfusion from decision to transfuse and collection of blood samples for cross-matching to the type and frequency of observations during transfusion and completionof the transfusion episode. This is the most recent available guidance from BCSH but it is worth checking their website and the SHOT and Department of Health websites regularly for updates

Gray, A., Hart, M., Dalrymple, K., Davies, T., 2008. Promoting safe transfusion practice: right blood, right patient, right time. British Journal of Nursing 17 (13), 812–817.

This article discusses the range of national initiaves intended to support the delivery of safe and appropriate transfusion practice.It also discusses how new technologies can enhance safety in this area

McInroy, A., 2005. Blood transfusion and Jehovah's Witnesses: the legal and ethical issues. British Journal of Nursing 14 (5), 270–274.

An interesting article that examines the legal and ethical issues surrounding a patient's right to refuse blood transfusion and what type of blood products might be acceptable

National Patient Safety Agency, 2006. Right patient, right blood: advice for safer blood transfusions NPSA/2008/SPN14 [online]. Available from: http://www.nrls.npsa.nhs.uk/resources/collections/right-patient-right-blood/ (accessed 10.06.11.).

This outlines measures to improve the safety of blood transfusions, including photo identification cards for regular patients and electronic tracking systems for patients and blood. It includes competencies for staff who are involved in all stages of the process. It stipulates 3- yearly staff competency assessments

Oldham, J., Sinclair, L., Hendry, C., 2009. Right patient, right blood, right care : safe transfusion practice. British Journal of Nursing 18 (5), 312–320.

This article explores the key principles of safe transfusion practice. It focusses on the management of clinical risk in the transfusion process. It identifies legal aspects of practice and the recognition and management of transfusion reactions

Royal College of Nursing, 2004. Right blood, right patient, right time. Guidelines for the safe administration of blood and blood products. RCN, London [online]. Available from: www.rcn.org.uk (accessed 09.01.12.).

This provides comprehensive evidence-based guidance on all aspects of blood transfusion from obtaining the blood sample for cross-matching to patient monitoring during transfusion

Stevenson, T., 2007. The safe administration of blood transfusions at night. Nursing Times 103 (5), 33–34.

This paper reports an audit of blood transfusions at night in a district general hospital and found that two-thirds could have safely been delayed until morning. They suggest that, because of the greater risk of error and delayed detection of any reaction, nurses should challenge the need for transfusions at night and suggest that Trust protocols should also reflect this. They also stress that if transfusion at night is necessary greater vigilance is required to ensure patient safety

Taylor, C., Cohen, H., Mold, D., et al, on behalf of the Serious Hazards of Transfusion (SHOT) Steering Group, (Eds.), 2010. The 2009 Annual SHOT Report [online]. Available from: http://www.shotuk.org/wp-content/uploads/2010/07/SHOT2009.pdf (accessed 04.05.11.).

SHOT is the UK's professionally led haemovigilance scheme for the reporting of transfusion-related adverse events and reactions. This annual report analyses all such events and makes recommendations for improved safety standards of hospital transfusion practice. This is the most recent report available from SHOT, but it is worth checking their website and the BCHS and Department of Health websites regularly for updates

Department of Health Better Blood Transfusions [online]. Available from: www.blood.co.uk (accessed 27.01.12.).

This website has information about the history of blood transfusion, blood groups and some fun quizzes to check your knowledge

SHOT (serious hazards of transfusion) [online]. Available from: www.shotuk.org (accessed 09.01.12.).

Chapter 6

Nutrition and hydration

©2012 Elsevier Ltd.

6.1 Nutritional assessment

Principles

Good nutrition is essential not only to promote health and well-being, but also to aid recovery from trauma, surgery or disease. Yet, malnutrition is common among those who are ill whether they are in hospital or the community. People who are unwell may not eat or drink what they should or their ability to do so may be impaired due to the nature of their illness. Malnutrition is referred to as a state in which a deficiency of nutrients causes measurable adverse effects on body function and/or clinical outcome (NCCAC 2006). Although malnutrition or 'bad nutrition' associated with over-eating is also an important issue for nurses undertaking nutritional assessment, the focus of much of the literature has been on under-nutrition. Poor nutritional status is known to be associated with delayed recovery and adverse outcomes of illness and injury (NCCAC 2006). Nurses have an important role to play in the prevention of malnutrition through identifying those at risk and planning care to meet their needs (Fletcher 2009). In addition, they have a role in ensuring those who are initially well-nourished do not become malnourished whilst in hospital. Appropriate and ongoing nutritional assessment is vital.

Nutritional assessment tools

Although most hospitals have developed a tool to assist in nutritional assessment and the identification of those at risk, the NCCAC (2006) recommend use of the Malnutrition Universal Screening Tool (MUST) (Elia 2003, Todorovic et al 2003; see http://www.bapen.org.uk/pdfs/must/must_full.pdf) because it is relatively simple to use and has some validation. Its components are:

- Body mass index (BMI)
- Unplanned weight loss in the last 3–6 months
- Subjective criteria (such as those outlined below)
- Once overall risk is established, use local guidelines and/or policies to develop appropriate care plans.

Body mass index

Body mass index (BMI) is a tool for use with patients over 18 years of age and enables determination of whether the patient has a normal weight, is underweight or over-weight. However, on its own it is not a good indicator of nutritional risk; it needs to be used in conjunction with other measures. BMI is calculated by dividing the weight in kilograms (kg) by the height in metres squared (see below). If the patient's height cannot be measured the demispan of the arm, ulna height or knee height can be used to estimate height. These measurements can be converted using the guides in the MUST explanatory booklet (http://www.bapen.org.uk/pdfs/must/must_explan.pdf). If height and weight cannot be measured, BMI can be estimated using mid upper arm circumference (MUAC). If the upper arm circumference is less than 23.5 cm it is likely the BMI is less than 20 kg/m^2. If it is more than 32.0 cm the patient's BMI is likely to be more than 30 kg/m^2 (Todorovic et al 2003). A BMI of 20–24.9 indicates an average or desirable weight. A BMI of greater than 30 is classified as obese and greater than 40 as grossly obese. Patients with a BMI of less than 20 may show signs of under-nutrition. It is important to note, however, that patients who are overweight or obese can also be malnourished.

$$BMI = \frac{weight\ in\ kg}{(height\ in\ metres)^2} = \frac{60}{1.69 \times 1.69} = 20.01$$

In addition to the BMI, most nutritional assessment tools will incorporate consideration of the following factors, which are known to increase the risk of malnutrition (Dunne 2009, Holmes 2006, NCCAC 2006):

- **Age** – older adults are vulnerable to under-nutrition and its incidence rises with age irrespective of illness. A decline in lean body mass (LBM) reduces basal metabolic rate by 10–15% or more after 50 years of age. Loss of LBM enhances morbidity and mortality and impacts on cardiac, respiratory and muscle function as well as reducing body temperature (hypothermia) and increasing the risk of falls and subsequent injury.

- **Mental condition** – any deterioration in mental state or conscious level is likely to affect the patient's desire and ability to eat and drink independently and so will increase the risk of malnutrition. This includes patients who may be depressed, lethargic or apathetic.

- **Weight** – it is important to note whether there has been any recent weight loss, particularly if it is unintentional. This may be apparent from loose-fitting clothes, rings or dentures. Patients who appear thin or emaciated are at an increased risk of malnutrition. Less than 5% weight loss in 6 months is not significant. Between 5–9% is only significant if the patient is already malnourished. Between 10–20% is clinically significant and requires intervention, and more than 20% weight loss may require long-term support.

- **Appetite** – patients who are able to maintain their usual appetite and eating habits are less likely to be at risk than those who have a poor appetite or refuse meals and drinks. It is important to check whether the patient has altered their eating habits recently.

- **Functioning of the gastrointestinal tract** – the presence of diarrhoea or constipation is likely to affect the desire to eat and drink and may also lead to malabsorption. Nausea and vomiting are also likely to result in a reduced nutritional intake. Patients who are unable to take oral food or fluids following surgery involving the gastrointestinal tract or who have conditions that affect it, such as intestinal obstruction, will be at high risk.

- **Skin and pressure ulcers** – dry and scaling skin may be an indication of dehydration and possibly related malnourishment. The existence of pressure ulcers is significant and is often included on nutritional assessment tools. Pressure ulcers are regularly associated with poor nutrition and healing pressure ulcers requires increased nutritional intake.

- **Dexterity** – it is important to assess whether patients have the manual dexterity to eat and drink independently.

- **Other factors** – a number of conditions will affect the ability to eat and so will increase the risk of developing malnutrition. These include:
  - neurological conditions, especially those affecting coordination or mental state
  - difficulty swallowing (dysphagia) (e.g. after stroke) and malabsorption
  - surgery or major trauma
  - malignant disease and chronic conditions, such as chronic obstructive pulmonary disease
  - reduced mobility or confinement to bed
  - bereavement, depression or other mental ill health.

Most nutritional assessment tools involve a scoring system that allocates a score for each of the possible contributing factors. The total score will indicate whether the patient is at risk; appropriate measures can then be taken. Whether a high score indicates a high or a low risk will vary between different assessment tools. Patients identified as high risk should be referred to a dietician and nutritional support should be considered for those who are malnourished or at risk of becoming malnourished (NCCAC 2006). Patients must be assessed within 24 hours of admission. The frequency of further assessments will be determined by the result of the initial assessment. For example, if a patient is well nourished on admission then weekly reassessment is adequate. However, if the nutritional assessment score indicates at-risk then reassessment within 48 hours may be necessary.

Nutritional support

The NCCAC (2006) guidelines state that oral, enteral (e.g. nasogastric – NG – tube or percutaneous endoscopic gastrostomy – PEG) or parenteral (intravenous) nutritional support, either alone or combined, should be considered for those who are malnourished or at risk of malnourishment. They define malnourished as:
- a body mass index (BMI) of less than 18.5 kg/m^2
- unintentional weight loss greater than 10% within the last 3–6 months
- a BMI of less than 20 kg/m^2 and unintentional weight loss greater than 5% within the last 3–6 months.

Risk of malnutrition is defined as:
- having eaten little or nothing for more than 5 days and/or likely to be eating little or nothing in the next 5 days or longer
- where there is increased nutritional need, where the capacity for absorption is reduced, or where there is a high nutrient loss.

6.2 Assisting adults with eating and drinking

Preparation

Patient

- Establish what the patient would like to eat and drink and whether there are any dietary restrictions
- Ensure the patient is comfortable, i.e. has an empty bladder, clean hands, clean mouth and, if applicable, clean dentures
- Check the patient is able to swallow, to prevent choking and aspiration into the lungs
- Ask/assist the patient to sit upright if their condition allows

Equipment/environment

- Clear a space for the tray
- Remove any offensive materials from the patient's table/eating area, e.g. sputum pot, urinals, etc.
- Position a chair beside the bed for the nurse
- Napkin or paper towel, adapted cups or cutlery as required

Nurse

- Wash and dry hands thoroughly
- Put on apron (appropriate colour if applicable) ➡ **PFP1**
- Additional protective clothing may be necessary if indicated by the patient's condition (see Ch. 1)

Procedure

1. Aim to make the mealtime a pleasant experience for the patient.

2. Obtain the correct food and drink, cutlery and napkin.

3. Set the meal out in a pleasing manner to tempt the appetite.

4. Take the tray to the bedside, and if the patient is unable to see the food, describe the meal ➡ **PFP2**.

5. Cut up the food if necessary.

6. Protect the patient's clothing with a napkin or paper towel.

7. Sit down so that a more relaxed approach is conveyed. Encourage/support the patient to feed themselves if at all possible, using special cutlery if necessary ➡ **PFP3**.

8. Adjust the speed and manner in which food/drink is offered according to the patient's needs/wishes. It should not be hurried ➡ **PFP4**.

9. Allow the patient time to chew and swallow the food before presenting the next mouthful. Adjust the size of each mouthful to suit the patient.

10. Avoid asking questions while the patient is eating.

11. Respect the patient's dignity and use the napkin to remove food or drink that may run down the chin.

12. When giving a drink, tip the cup/glass very gently so that the flow is controlled. Care should be taken with hot drinks, particularly if using a polystyrene cup, as it is difficult to judge the temperature of the liquid inside.

13. Encourage the patient to eat and drink if necessary, but do not press patients once they have indicated that they have had sufficient. Small amounts taken more frequently may be more successful.

14. Assist the patient to meet hygiene needs (mouth, teeth and hands) as necessary.

15. Remove unwanted food, crockery and cutlery. Wipe up any spillages on the table or locker.

16. Replace the patient's glass of water and belongings etc. within easy reach.

17. Remove apron and wash hands.

18. Complete relevant documentation, e.g. fluid balance and/or food chart.

19. Report any abnormal occurrences, e.g. vomiting, food refusal.

Points for practice

PFP1 In some hospitals, different-coloured aprons are used for activities, such as serving meals, washing patients and doing dressings.

PFP2 If supervising the patient rather than assisting them with eating and drinking, place all food and drink within easy reach of the patient. If the patient is visually impaired, 'clock' instructions may help them locate different foods, e.g. meat is at 12 o'clock, potatoes are at 5 o'clock, etc.

PFP3 If the patient is only able to use one hand, a plate guard and non-slip mat may help. If they are unable to grip ordinary cutlery, large-handled cutlery can usually be obtained from the Occupational Therapy department.

PFP4 Always check any particular cultural practices related to eating and drinking. For example, where possible, a Muslim patient should be fed with the right hand as the left hand is considered 'unclean'.

6.3 Nausea and vomiting

Preparation

Patient	Equipment/environment	Nurse
• Respond promptly to calls for assistance	• Draw screens if time permits, to ensure privacy	• Put on apron and gloves (if time)
	• Provide vomit bowl (usually disposable)	• Additional protective clothing may be necessary if indicated by the patient's condition (see Ch. 1)
	• Provide tissues or paper towels	

Procedure

1. If possible, remove the patient's dentures (where applicable) and store them safely.

2. Ask/assist the patient to sit forward, or if lying down or semi-conscious, place in the lateral position to reduce the risk of aspiration into the lungs.

3. Support the patient's forehead.

4. Encourage the patient to breathe more deeply if possible.

5. Provide tissues and promote comfort and dignity by wiping the patient's mouth if the patient is too weak or distressed to do this unaided.

6. Never leave the patient without a vomit bowl – get a clean one before removing the used one, even if the patient feels the episode has passed.

7. Offer a mouthwash or perform mouth care if the patient is too weak.

8. Offer the patient a bowl for face and hand washing.

9. Cover the vomit bowl before removing it from the bedside.

10. Identify the type of vomit and measure the amount ➡ **PFP1**.

11. Save the vomit for inspection if necessary (e.g. haematemesis) ➡ **PFP2**.

13. Document the vomiting episode, making a note of nausea, frequency, amount and whether related to food ➡ **PFP3**. Report if vomiting is a new occurrence or if the vomiting has altered in any way.

14. Ascertain the cause of vomiting if possible, and take appropriate action.

15. If appropriate, administer anti-emetic drugs as prescribed and monitor the effect ➡ **PFP4**.

➡️ Points for practice

PFP1 The vomit may contain undigested food or be watery (gastric juices only) or a green/brown fluid (indicates presence of bile). If the vomit is brown and foul (faecal) smelling, this may indicate that there is an obstruction in the large intestine.

PFP2 The term haematemesis means blood in the vomit. If this is bright red, it indicates fresh blood from the stomach or upper gastrointestinal tract; if it is dark brown and 'coffee ground' in appearance, this is older blood that has been partially digested.

PFP3 Note the amount, frequency, whether accompanied by pain or nausea and whether associated with any medication (e.g. analgesic), surgery, type of food or other cause. Also note whether it is projectile vomit (vomit that is emitted with force).

PFP4 Nausea and vomiting causes distress and suffering for any patient who experiences it. For patients who have had surgery the prophylactic administration of prescribed anti-emetic medication can greatly reduce this (Gibson and Magowan 2011). In those who are receiving palliative care, anti-emetics are an important feature of intervention but the cause of the nausea and vomiting should also be carefully assessed (Cruickshank and Campbell 2011).

6.4 Subcutaneous fluids (hyperdermoclysis)

Preparation

Patient

- Explain the procedure, to gain consent and cooperation
- Patients receiving subcutaneous fluids are often older adults and are sometimes confused. A second nurse may be required to comfort the patient ➡ **PFP1**

Equipment/Environment

- Prescribed fluid and additive (if applicable) ➡ **PFP2**
- Standard administration set (20 drops per ml)
- Peripheral plastic cannula (e.g. Insyte-w 24G-0.7 × 19 mm) or 'butterfly'-type intravenous cannula (21G) (no longer than 20 mm) ➡ **PFP3**
- Sterile transparent occlusive dressing (approximately 10 cm × 10 cm).

Nurse

- Wash and dry hands thoroughly and put on gloves
- Only registered nurses who are competent in the use subcutaneous administration procedures may insert the cannula and subcutaneous infusions must be checked by a registered nurse

Procedure

1. Check the prescribed fluid and prime the administration set to expel all air (see p. 113) ➡ **PFP4**

2. At the bedside, ask/assist the patient to move into a suitable position to allow access to the site ➡ **PFP5**. Check the patient's name band against the prescription.

3. Clean the skin with an alcohol-impregnated swab and allow it to dry.

4. Maintaining asepsis, remove the protective cover from the cannula and hold it with the bevelled edge facing upwards. Pinch the skin up slightly and insert the needle into the subcutaneous tissue at an angle of 45° (Fig. 6.1). If

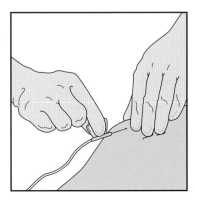

Figure 6.1 Inserting the butterfly cannula for hyperdermoclysis.

blood appears in the tubing, withdraw the cannula and repeat the process at another site using a new cannula.

5. Cover the area with the sterile transparent dressing.
6. Set the infusion to the prescribed rate (see p. 118).
7. Ensure the patient is comfortable.
8. Dispose of all clinical waste appropriately.
9. Document the subcutaneous infusion in the nursing records ➡ **PFP6**.
10. Record/monitor fluid balance according to local policy
11. Observe the cannula site for redness, swelling or discomfort.
12. Change the infusion site regularly, according to local policy ➡ **PFP7**.

➡ Points for practice

PFP1 Subcutaneous fluids are used most commonly for older adults with mild to moderate dehydration where there is no indication for intravenous fluids and where the patient requires less than 3 litres of fluid in 24 hours. It can also be used for patients who have poor venous access or where there is infected or broken skin at intravenous sites. Other palliative benefits have been reported in patients who have constipation or compromised tissue viability or those who have difficulties with oral intake, which makes them prone to dehydration. Subcutaneous administration of fluids must not be undertaken when rapid fluid replacement is needed. It is also contraindicated in those who are at risk of pulmonary congestion or pulmonary oedema, who have peripheral vascular disease of the lower extremities (Khan and Younger 2007).

PFP2 Dextrose saline or 0.9% sodium chloride are the solutions most commonly administered subcutaneously. It is not suitable for the administration of colloids, blood or total parenteral nutrition. An enzyme (hyaluronidase), which causes more rapid diffusion of the fluid by reducing normal interstitial barriers, may be prescribed. It may be injected into the site via the cannula prior to commencement of the infusion, or added to the infusion bag. However, there is conflicting evidence regarding its effectiveness and there are reported side-effects (discomfort and site irritation). Local guidelines should be followed regarding its use (Khan and Younger 2007).

PFP3 The device selected should be of the smallest gauge and shortest length necessary (RCN 2010). The choice of cannula may vary according to local policy or practice guidelines; the use of Teflon® or Vailon needles instead of steel winged infusion devices has been associated with fewer complications and reduces the need for frequent needle changes (RCN 2010).

PFP4 In most cases, all subcutaneous fluids must be checked by a registered nurse, although this may vary according to local policy. In some Trusts, two nurses are required to check intravenous and subcutaneous fluids.

PFP5 Any site with sufficient subcutaneous tissue may be used, but oedematous areas, areas with infected, broken or inflamed skin, bony prominences or sites near a joint and the patient's waistline must be avoided (RCN 2010). The nurse should consider patient comfort, mobility, ease of access and skin condition when choosing the site. The abdomen and thighs are commonly used, although the areas over the scapula and anterior chest wall are ideal.

PFP6 Line labels that indicate the time and date of insertion should be used. Documentation in the patient's notes should include an outline of the need for subcutaneous infusion, the insertion site and device used, any directions for monitoring of the infusion and the patient's response to treatment (Khan and Younger 2007, RCN 2010).

PFP7 Ideally the infusion site should be changed after 2 litres of fluid (Khan and Younger 2007) or rotated at least every 3 days (RCN 2010). The administration set should be changed at least every 72 hours (RCN 2010).

6.5 Nasogastric tube insertion

Preparation

Patient

- Explain the procedure, to gain consent and cooperation
- Draw screens to ensure privacy.
- Ensure the patient is comfortable – sitting upright if possible, with the head neither tilted backwards nor forwards ➡ **PFP1**
- Protect the patient's clothing with a towel. A glass of water and a straw will aid swallowing during insertion.

Equipment/Environment

- Prepare space at the bedside
- Nasogastric tube of appropriate size and type (e.g. Ryle's type, fine bore) ➡ **PFP2**
- Lubricant (water-soluble jelly or sterile water).
- pH strips
- Receiver or vomit bowl
- A 20/50 ml syringe ➡ **PFP3**
- Two small gallipots
- Adhesive tape, tissues, clinical waste bag

Nurse

- Wash and dry hands thoroughly
- Put on apron and gloves
- Additional protective clothing may be necessary if indicated by the patient's condition (see Ch. 1).

Procedure

1. Take the equipment to the bedside.
2. Agree with the patient a signal (e.g. hand signal) that can be used should he/she want the nurse to stop.
3. Estimate the length of tube to be inserted by measuring the distance from the patient's nose to the tip of the earlobe and then to the xiphisternum, and make a note of where this is on the tube (Fig. 6.2) ➡ **PFP4**.

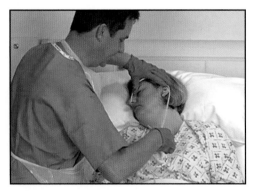

Figure 6.2 Measuring the length of the tube to be inserted.

4. Ask/assist the patient to remove dentures and to clear nasal passages by blowing the nose. Select the best nostril (not tender, no deviated septum, etc.).

5. Encourage the patient to relax as much as possible and to breathe steadily.

6. Prepare the tube as per manufacturer's instructions (e.g. lubricating the tip of the tube and injecting sterile water down the tube to activate coating).

7. Pass the tube gently into the nostril and pass backwards (not upwards) along the floor of the nose to the nasopharynx. (If a blockage is felt, change to the other nostril.)

8. Pause to allow the patient to draw breath and recover.

9. Ask the patient to breathe through their mouth and swallow. As the patient swallows, and while keeping the head level, gently advance the tube. A glass of water with a straw will help the patient to 'swallow' the tube without moving their head.

10. When the tube has reached the measured distance, check it is in the stomach by one or more of the following methods:

    • Aspirate a small amount of stomach contents (0.5–1 ml) from the tube. Apply aspirate to a pH strip, leave for 1 minute and then compare with the colour bars to get a reading. A pH of 5.5 or less confirms gastric placement ➡ **PFP5**.

    • If unable to obtain any aspirate or the pH is greater than 5.5, injecting 10–20 ml of air using a 50 ml syringe will dispel any residual fluid. Advance the tube by 10–20 cm, turn the patient onto their side, leave for 15–30 min and try aspirating again. If the pH is still greater than 5.5 the position of the tube should be confirmed by X-ray. An X-ray should be used to confirm the position of the tube in all unconscious patients ➡ **PFP6** and Figure 6.3.

11. Secure the tube with tape ensuring that friction or pressure on the tip of the nose is avoided and the patient's vision is not obstructed.

12. If a fine-bore tube has been used, remove the guide wire using gentle traction ➡ **PFP7**.

13. Ensure the patient is comfortable.

14. Clear away the equipment and dispose of waste appropriately.

15. Remove gloves and apron and wash hands.

16. Document nasogastric tube insertion ➡ **PFP8**.

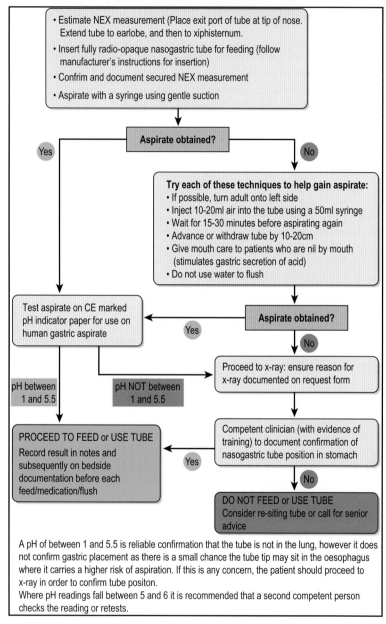

- Estimate NEX measurement (Place exit port of tube at tip of nose. Extend tube to earlobe, and then to xiphisternum.
- Insert fully radio-opaque nasogastric tube for feeding (follow manufacturer's instructions for insertion)
- Confirm and document secured NEX measurement
- Aspirate with a syringe using gentle suction

Aspirate obtained?

Yes

No

Try each of these techniques to help gain aspirate:
- If possible, turn adult onto left side
- Inject 10-20ml air into the tube using a 50ml syringe
- Wait for 15-30 minutes before aspirating again
- Advance or withdraw tube by 10-20cm
- Give mouth care to patients who are nil by mouth (stimulates gastric secretion of acid)
- Do not use water to flush

Test aspirate on CE marked pH indicator paper for use on human gastric aspirate

Aspirate obtained?

Yes

No

Proceed to x-ray: ensure reason for x-ray documented on request form

pH between 1 and 5.5

pH NOT between 1 and 5.5

Competent clinician (with evidence of training) to document confirmation of nasogastric tube position in stomach

Yes

No

PROCEED TO FEED or USE TUBE
Record result in notes and subsequently on bedside documentation before each feed/medication/flush

DO NOT FEED or USE TUBE
Consider re-siting tube or call for senior advice

A pH of between 1 and 5.5 is reliable confirmation that the tube is not in the lung, however it does not confirm gastric placement as there is a small chance the tube tip may sit in the oesophagus where it carries a higher risk of aspiration. If this is any concern, the patient should proceed to x-ray in order to confirm tube positon.

Where pH readings fall between 5 and 6 it is recommended that a second competent person checks the reading or retests.

Figure 6.3 Decision Tree for nasogastric tube placement in Adults (from NPSA 2011, with permission).

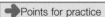Points for practice

PFP1 Insertion of the nasogastric tube may be for feeding or for gastric aspiration. The upright position is best for nasogastric tube insertion; if this is not possible, the patient should be lying on one side.

PFP2 If the nasogastric tube is being inserted for the purpose of enteral feeding, a fine- or small-bore tube must be used. They are radio-opaque throughout their length and have externally visible length markings (NPSA 2011). They reduce patient discomfort and provide a decreased risk of aspiration. They are also less likely to cause complications such as gastritis, oesophageal and nasal irritation. The wide bore (Ryles's tube) should only be used for gastric drainage, medication administration, gastric lavage and diagnostic testing.

PFP3 Using a larger syringe allows gentle pressure and suction. A smaller syringe may produce too much pressure and split the tube. Only appropriate oral/ enteral syringes should be used (NPSA 2007)

PFP4 The measurement from the tip of the nose, to the earlobe and the xiphisternum is known as the NEX measurement (NPSA 2011). Having undertaken the measurement the amount that will remain outside the nose must be recorded. The tube may have markings on it to facilitate this. It is important to measure the tube to ensure that it does not pass through the stomach and into the duodenum. Once the tube is inserted the amount of tube outside the nose must be recorded and confirmed before each feed (NPSA 2011).

PFP5 A pH between 1 and 5.5 is considered safe when determining if the tube is in the stomach. See Figure 6.3.

PFP6 Advancing or withdrawing the tube may assist the tube locate in the stomach. Flushing the tube with 10/20 ml of air will dispel any residual fluid (nasopharyngeal secretions/water) and may also dislodge the tip of the tube from the gastric mucosa. Turning the patient on their side will enable the tube to enter the gastric fluid pool. Changes to the pH strip may not occur in some clinical conditions (e.g. pernicious anaemia or previous gastrectomy) or if the patient is receiving H_2-receptor antagonists (which decrease the secretion of gastric acid) or if the tube has passed through the pylorus. X-ray is only the second line method for testing the position of the nasogastric tube when no aspirate has been obtained or the pH indicator has failed to confirm the location (NSPA 2011; Fig. 6.3) However, it is the method of choice in patients who are unconscious with no gag reflex. **The following methods are never used to test the position of the tube:** auscultation, litmus paper tests, the 'whoosh test' (injecting air and listening for a bubbling sound) and absence of respiratory distress in the patient (NPSA 2011).

PFP7 If an X-ray is required when a fine-bore tube has been inserted, the guide wire should not be removed until confirmation of its position in the stomach has been established. The guide wire is then removed by holding the tube at the nose with one hand and pulling the wire out with the other. If it is difficult to remove, then the tube should be removed as well. Do not reinsert the guide wire after removal, as there is a risk of perforation of the oesophageal or stomach wall.

PFP8 In order to reduce the risk of adverse events or outcomes, the NPSA (2011) has indicated that the following must be documented in the patient's medical records:

- The person who passed the tube must record the tube type, size and external length once secured.

- The result of pH testing including the pH if aspirate was obtained, the person who checked the pH and a confirmation as to the safety of commencing feed and/or medication.

- The position of the tube must be checked and recorded at least once daily and before each feed, before administration of medicine, in the event of new or unexplained respiratory symptoms and following any incidences that may have affected the tube placement (coughing, vomiting, retching). Testing should not be undertaken within 1 hour of feeding or medication administration as it may affect the pH result.

6.6 Nasogastric feeding

Preparation

Patient

- Explain the procedure, to gain consent and cooperation
- Ensure the patient is comfortable and sitting upright if condition permits

Equipment

- Nasogastric feeding pump, or reservoir bottle or bag if a gravity method is being used
- Prescribed nasogastric feed plus enteral administration set
- 20/50 ml oral/enteral syringe and water/sterile water ➡ **PFP1**
- 50 ml oral/enteral syringe, gallipot and pH strips to check tube position ➡ **PFP2**

Nurse

- Wash and dry hands thoroughly
- Put on apron. Additional protective clothing may be necessary if indicated by the patient's condition (see Ch. 1)

Procedure

1. Take the equipment to the bedside.

2. Check the nasogastric tube is in the stomach by aspirating a small amount of stomach contents (0.5–1 ml) from the tube. Apply aspirate to a pH strip and then compare to colour bars to get a reading. A pH of 5.5 indicates gastric placement (see p. 163 and Fig. 6.3).

3. Flush the tube with at least 30 ml of water before commencing the feed.

4. Check the expiry date of the feed.

5. Remove the cap of the feed bottle and attach the administration set according to manufacturer's instructions. If a separate reservoir is being used, pour the feed into the bag/reservoir and attach the administration set. (Sterile water may be given via this method.)

4. Allow the feed to run through the tubing to expel all air and then close the roller clamp.

5. Connect the administration set to the nasogastric tube securely.

6. If using a pump, insert the administration set according to the manufacturer's instructions and open the roller clamp. Switch the pump on (Fig. 6.4), set it to the prescribed rate and press 'start'. If no pump is being used, adjust the roller clamp until the prescribed flow rate is achieved.

7. Clear away the equipment and wipe up any spillages.

8. Remove apron and wash hands.

9. Record the feed on the fluid balance chart and other relevant documentation.

10. Ensure the patient is comfortable and observe for signs of abdominal discomfort, nausea, gastric reflux or dyspnoea while the feed is being administered.

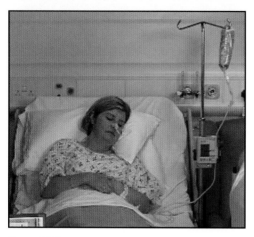

Figure 6.4 Nasogastric feeding via a pump.

11. Ensure throughout that the feed is being administered at the correct rate. Check for signs of a blocked tube ➡ **PFP3**. Report any complications.

12. Attend to the patient's hygiene (mouth, lips and nostrils) as necessary.

13. Observe for diarrhoea or constipation.

14. When the feed has finished, detach the bottle from the administration set and flush the nasogastric tube with at least 30 ml of sterile water to prevent stasis of feed and maintain patency of the tube ➡ **PFP4**.

15. Change the administration set every 24 hours. Attach label indicating date and time commenced.

➡ Points for practice

PFP1 Sterile water should be used for patients who are immunosuppressed.

PFP2 It is vital to check the position of the tube prior to each feed (see p. 163).

PFP3 As the feeding solution can be 'sticky', the tube can become blocked if it has not been adequately flushed.

PFP4 If a second bottle of feed is due to commence, ensure that the first does not empty completely, allowing air to enter the administration set. If this does happen, the set will need to be disconnected and primed again before the second feed can commence.

6.7 Care of gastrostomy site

Principles

- A gastrostomy is a tube is placed directly into the stomach and is the most common type of enteral, long-term feeding device. It is introduced either endoscopically (percutaneous endoscopic gastrostomy – PEG) or radiologically (radiologically inserted gastrostomy – RIG). A RIG is used for patients for whom an endoscopy is contraindicated, for example, those whose airway would be compromised by an endoscope or patients who have an obstruction (e.g. tumour) that would make passing an endoscope difficult.

- There are different types of gastrostomy tubes, some of which lie flush with the skin and others that protrude. There are those that have a one-way valve to prevent reflux and a silicone dome that acts as an internal anchoring device. Most have both internal and external fixators although low-profile balloon gastrostomy devices do not (Roberts 2007). A RIG has stitches known as T-Fasteners, which help secure the stomach to the abdominal wall and facilitate the stoma tract to form. These stay in place for 10–14 days following insertion.

- The tube should be secure but not too tight. If the internal or external part of the tube is too tight against the abdominal wall it can cause severe discomfort and cellulitis and bleeding. The external fixation device should be placed 2–3 mm from the abdominal skin surface to facilitate the normal extension and deflation of the abdomen that takes place during breathing, laughing, coughing etc. (Best 2009).

- The main disadvantage of percutaneous endoscopic gastrostomy (PEG) is the risk of wound infection due to contamination by oral flora during insertion. Therefore, the site should be treated as a wound and prophylactic antibiotics may be prescribed. The patient's temperature and pulse rate should be monitored for the first 7 days post-insertion of the gastrostomy tube.

- In the first 24 hours, the incision site should be monitored closely for redness, leakage of feed or swelling (Slater 2009). Should any of these occur feeding should be stopped and medical advice sought.

- Some serosanguinous drainage can be expected initially but excessive bleeding or oozing is not normal (Slater 2009). In this instance a pressure bandage should be applied and medical assistance sought.

- The patient should also be assessed regularly for pain at the insertion site. Some pain is to be expected initially but it should decrease (Slater 2009).

- Until the site has granulated and healed, cleaning and dressing changes should be undertaken aseptically. Patients who have a RIG inserted should have their dressing changed aseptically until the T-Fasteners are removed.

- Although local practices vary, most policies recommend that around the stoma site and under the retention device should be cleaned daily with sterile 0.9% sodium chloride or sterile water and lint-free gauze and a dry dressing applied. When the area has healed, no dressing is necessary.

- The PEG tube should not be taped to the abdomen for the first two weeks to ensure a straight stoma formation (Best 2008). However, a RIG may be lightly taped to avoid traction on the tube (Fogg 2007).

- The sides of the external fixation device should be lifted gently to check the skin around the stoma but the device itself should not be disturbed for the first 14–21 days to facilitate the formation of a stoma tract (Roberts 2007). After this time, the stoma should be cleaned daily with lint-free gauze or a flannel and mild soapy water.

- The external fixation device should be released regularly to clean the skin around the stoma. Manufacturer guidelines should be referred to when releasing the tube from the external fixation device as the procedure differs for each tube.

- Before replacing the external fixation device, the tube should advanced (2–3 cm) and rotated completely (360°). The tube should then be pulled back to rest against the internal gastric wall. Care should be taken that it is not pulled back too tight as to do so may cause ulceration of the gastric mucosa. This procedure is thought to prevent 'buried bumper syndrome' where the internal fixator becomes embedded in the gastric mucosa. Advancing and rotating the tube should be undertaken at least twice a week (Best 2009).

- RIG tubes have an increased risk of displacement due to the type of internal device (pigtail device with a string running through it). Therefore, it is important that traction on the tube is avoided and they must not be rotated or advanced (Fogg 2007).

- For patients with a RIG, the external length of the tube should be recorded. If, on assessment, it appears to be moving too much or appears longer and the external fixator is in the correct position, medical assistance must be sought as the internal fixator may have broken (Best 2008).

- If a patient is showering or bathing the gastrostomy tube should be closed and the site dried thoroughly afterwards. Showering is preferred to bathing as the stoma site should not be immersed in water until site is healed. Creams and talcum powder should not be used around the site. Cream can impact on the grip of the fixation device and talcum powder, when moist, can contribute to skin breakdown or infection (Best 2009).

- Once the wound is healed, ongoing care of the site involves ensuring it remains clean and dry. If infection becomes evident, careful cleaning with soap and water or antibacterial solutions and the application of a topical antibiotic is necessary (NCCAC 2006).

- Feeding via a PEG can be commenced 4 hours after insertion when it is safe and well tolerated (NCCAC 2006), although this may be longer if the patient has had a general anaesthetic as gastric function may be disrupted. The presence or absence of bowel sounds to initiate feeding is debated. Patients with a RIG may not have feeding commenced for 24 hours.

- The most common cause of blockage of the tube is inadequate flushing. The tube should be flushed with 30–50 ml of water (Fig. 6.5) at least twice daily if the feeds are continuous, before and after feeds and the administration of

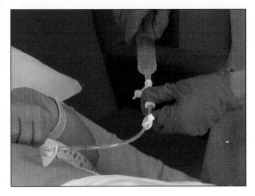

Figure 6.5 Flushing the gastrostomy tube.

drugs. The type of water used will vary according to local policy but for patients who are not immunocompromised, fresh water from a drinking source or cooled boiled water is sufficient. Sterile water must be used for immunocompromised patients.

• In some instances patients have a tube placed into the jejunum because they have had upper gastrointestinal surgery or they have difficulties associated with gastric emptying. The care of a jejunostomy tube is similar to that of a PEG with some notable exceptions. The lumen of the tube for a jejunostomy is much narrower than a gastrostomy and particular care must be taken to maintain patency. Therefore, 4-hourly flushing of the tube with sterile water is recommended (British Association for Parenteral and Enteral Nutrition – BAPEN– 2003). Also, a jejunostomy tube must not be rotated only advanced, as the jejunal extension may become dislodged (Best 2008).

6.8 Feeding via percutaneous endoscopic gastrostomy (PEG)/radiologically inserted gastrostomy (RIG)

Preparation

Patient

- Explain the procedure, to gain consent and co-operation ➡ **PFP1**
- It is advisable for the patient to be sitting up (unless the feed is given very slowly) ➡ **PFP2**
- Bowel sounds should be present ➡ **PFP3**

Equipment/Environment

- Prescription chart and prescribed feed ➡ **PFP4**
- Enteral feed administration set.
- Enteral syringe and 30–50 ml of sterile water (to flush tube)
- 20 ml oral/enteral syringe, receiver and pH strips to check tube position
- Enteral feed pump
- Infusion stand
- Fluid balance chart

Nurse

- Wash and dry hands thoroughly
- Put on apron. Additional protective clothing may be necessary if indicated by the patient's condition (see Ch.1)

Procedure

1. Take the equipment and the feed to the bedside and check the patient's name band.

2. Check the gastrostomy tube is in the stomach, aspirating a small amount of stomach contents with a 20 ml oral/enteral syringe. Apply aspirate to a pH strip and then compare to the colour bars to get a reading. A pH of 5.5 indicates gastric placement (see p. 163 and Fig. 6.3).

3. Draw up 30–50 ml (depending on local policy) of sterile water and flush the tube using the 50 ml enteral syringe ➡ **PFP5**.

4. Remove the cap of the feed bottle.

5. Maintaining asepsis, open the enteral feed administration set, attach it to the bottle according to the manufacturer's instructions, and close the flow control roller clamp ➡ **PFP6**.

6. Attach the hanger to the feed container and hang the feed container on the infusion stand.

7. Open the roller clamp on the administration set, allow the feed to run through to expel all air and then close the clamp. The plastic cap on the end of the administration set should remain in place so that the tube remains sterile.

8. Insert the administration set into the pump according to the manufacturer's instructions, remove the plastic cap at the distal end of it and attach it to the PEG tube.

9. Open the roller clamp and turn on the pump.

10. Set the flow rate as prescribed (e.g. 125 ml per hour) and start the pump.
11. Check that the feed is running, it is not leaking at the connection with the PEG tube, and that the tube is not kinked or blocked.
12. Ensure the patient is comfortable. Observe PEG site regularly ➡ **PFP7**.
13. Clear away equipment and wipe up any spillages, especially on the pump.
14. Remove apron and wash hands.
15. Document the type of feed, time started, rate of flow and volume of water used to flush the tube.
16. Return regularly, to check the feed is running as prescribed. The pump usually has alarms to indicate when the feed has finished or if the tube has become blocked or kinked. If there are no alarms, extra checking is required.
16. Observe the patient for nausea, vomiting or diarrhoea.
17. On completion of the feed, disconnect the administration set and flush the tube with sterile water according to local policy ➡ **PFP8**.

➡ Points for practice

PFP1 As eating and drinking are social activities as well as physical necessities, it is important to try and make gastrostomy feeds as pleasant and 'normal' as possible, e.g. if the feed is not continuous, by administering the feed when others are eating their meals.

PFP2 Ideally, patients receiving enteral feeding should be semi-upright or upright during the administration of the feed and should remain in this position for at least 30 minutes after the feed has finished. This is thought to reduce the risk of reflux and aspiration (Roberts 2007). This is particularly important for patients who are receiving bolus feeds.

PFP3 The presence or absence of bowel sounds to initiate feeding is a matter of debate (Slater 2009)

PFP4 Feeding via a PEG tube may be intermittent or continuous. Pump feeding can be administered continuously 24 hours or over a shorter 16–18 period. The NCCAC (2006) concluded that there is no clinical benefit to using the shorter period although it may be more acceptable to patients. For patients in intensive care continuous feeding may be of benefit in preventing a high level of gastric residue and stabilising blood glucose levels.

PFP5 Avoid adding anything to the feed. If drugs are to be administered via the PEG tube, they must be soluble in water and the tube should be flushed with 30–50 ml of sterile water before and after their administration to prevent blockage (BAPEN 2003).

PFP6 When flushing the PEG tube, care should be taken when attaching the syringe, to avoid damaging the connection. A 50 ml enteral syringe should be used to flush the tube, as the pressure exerted by smaller syringes is too great. If the PEG tube is not being used for feeding for a period of time, it should be flushed twice a day to maintain patency (Best 2009: Fig. 6.5)

PFP7 The site should be inspected daily for signs of leakage, swelling, skin irritation or breakdown, soreness or excessive movement of the tube (Green 2011)

PFP8 The administration set must be changed every 24 hours and should be labelled to indicate the date that the change is due.

Bibliography/Suggested reading

Best, C., 2008. Nutrition: a handbook for nurses. Wiley, Chichester.

This book explores all aspects of nutrition for nurses as well as guidance to caring for patients with specific nutritional needs

Best, C., 2009. Percutaneous endoscopic gastrostomy feeding in the adult patient. British Journal of Nursing 18 (12), 724–729.

This article explores the insertion of a PEG tube, the care required and the complications associated with PEG feeding and the steps that can be taken to minimize their occurrence

British Association for Parenteral and Enteral Nutrition, 2003. Administering drugs via enteral feeding tubes. [online]. Available from: www.bapen.org.uk (accessed 18.01.12.).

This is a useful website for exploring multiple aspects of parenteral and enteral nutrition

Cruickshank, S., Campbell, K., 2011. Nursing the patient with cancer. In: Brooker, C., Nicol, M. (Eds.), Alexander's Nursing Practice, fourth ed. Churchill Livingstone, Edinburgh.

This chapter addresses aspects of the care of the patient with cancer and includes oncology as a speciality, medical intervention and nursing management

Department of Health, 2003. The essence of care. DoH, London.

The Essence of Care launched in February 2001 provides a tool to help practitioners take a patient-focused and structured approach to sharing and comparing practice. It enabled healthcare personnel to work with patients to identify best practice and to develop action plans to improve care. Food and nutrition is one of the eight benchmarks of care

Dunne, A., 2009. Management of malnutrition in older people within the hospital setting. British Journal of Nursing 18 (17), 1030–1035.

This article discusses the prevalence of malnutrition among older people in the UK. It discusses the role of screening and outlines practical steps that can be taken to improve the nutritional management of older people within the hospital environment

Elia, M., 2003. The 'MUST' report: nutritional screening of adults: a multidisciplinary responsibility. Development and use of the 'Malnutrition Universal Screening Tool' ('MUST') for adults. A report by the Malnutrition Advisory Group of the British Association for Patenteral and Enteral Nutrition. British Association for Parenteral and Enteral Nutrition (BAPEN), Redditch.

Fletcher, J., 2009. Identifying patients at risk of malnutrition: nutrition screening and assessment. Gastrointestinal Nursing 7 (5), 12–17.

This article identifies ways in which nurses can identify patients at overall risk of malnutrition. The article is beneficial as it provides a clear overview of nutritional screening and assessment as part of the overall holistic nursing assessment

Fogg, L., 2007. Home enteral feeding part 1: an overview. British Journal of Community Nursing 12 (6), 246–252.

This article is the first of two that examine key aspects of management of patients in the community who are being fed enterally

Gibson, C.E., Magowan, R., 2011. Nursing the patient undergoing surgery. In: Brooker, C., Nicol, M. (Eds.), Alexander's Nursing practice, fourth ed. Churchill Livingstone, Edinburgh.

This chapter addresses all aspects of the care of patients undergoing surgery and includes pre-surgical care, informed decision making, pre-operative preparation, peri-operative safety, postoperative care, discharge planning and rehabilitation

Green, 2011. Nutrition and health. In: Brooker, C., Nicol, M. (Eds.), Alexander's Nursing practice, fourth ed. Churchill Livingstone, Edinburgh.

This chapter addresses the principles of nutritional science, public health nutrition, nutrition screening and assessment, nutritional intervention, enhancing nutritional intake, enteral and parenteral nutrition

Holmes, S., 2006. Barriers to effective nutritional care for older adults. Nursing Standard 21 (3), 50–54.

Although this article focuses on the older person, the issues identified are pertinent for the majority of hospitalised patients. The barriers to achieving nutritional adequacy once patients have been admitted to hospital are considered and suggestions for overcoming them are made

Khan, M., Younger, G., 2007. Promoting safe administration of subcutaneous infusion. Nursing Standard 21 (31), 50–56.

This articles discusses safe practice for the administration of subcutaneous infusion including the anatomical sites, guidelines for insertion and the patient care required

National Collaborating Centre for Acute Care (NCCAC), 2006. Nutrition support in adults: oral nutrition support, enteral tube feeding and parenteral nutrition. Methods, evidence and guidance. NCCAC, London.

This guideline is essential reading as it addresses all aspects of nutritional support using the best available evidence www.nice.org.uk/nicemedia/pdf/cg032fullguideline.pdf

National Patient Safety Agency, 2007. Promoting safer measurement and administration of liquid medicines via oral and other enteral routes.[online]. Available from: www.nrls. npsa.nhs.uk (accessed 18.01.12.).

This site is useful for keeping updated on many safety issues

National Patient Safety Agency, 2011. Reducing the harm caused by misplaced nasogastric feeding tubes in adults, children and infants. [online]. Available from: www.npsa.nhs.uk/ advice (accessed 18.01.12.).

This site is useful for keeping updated on many safety issues. In this instance there are clear guidelines about assessing the position of the nasogastric tube

Roberts, E., 2007. Nutritional support via enteral tube feeding in hospital patients. British Journal of Nursing 17 (16), 1058–1062.

This article provides a practical overview of enteral feeding solutions and their administration that facilitates nurses understanding of the possible prescribed regimens

Royal College of Nursing, 2010. Standards for infusion therapy, third ed. RCN, London.

This document provides a comprehensive overview and best practice guidance on all aspects of intravenous and subcutaneous infusion therapy including: infection control and safety, equipment, site selection, site care and complications

Slater, R., 2009. Percutaneous endoscopic gastrostomy feeding: indications and management. British Journal of Nursing 18 (17), 1036–1043.

The article looks specifically at PEG as a form of enteral nutrition delivery, how it is undertaken, and the care needs of the patient post-insertion of a PEG tube

Thompson, I., 2004. The management of nausea and vomiting in palliative care. Nursing Standard 19 (8), 46–53.

This article discusses safe practice for subcutaneous infusions including the most appropriate sites for administration, guidelines for insertion and patient care

Todorovic, V., Russell, C., Stratton, R., Ward, J., Elia, M., 2003. The 'MUST' explanatory booklet: a guide to the 'Malnutrition Universal Screening Tool' ('MUST') for adults. British Association for Parenteral and Enteral Nutrition (BAPEN), Redditch [online]. Available from http://www.bapen.org.uk/pdfs/must/must_explan.pdf (accessed 18.01.12.).

Medicines management

©2012 Elsevier Ltd.

7.1 Storage of medicines

Principles

In line with legal requirements and local policies, it is part of the nurse's role to ensure that medicines are safely stored. The following principles apply to all situations involving the storage and administration of medicines:

- All medicines, lotions and reagents (except intravenous fluids and drugs for use in emergency situations) must be stored in locked cupboards. Drugs for emergency use (e.g. cardiac arrest) may be kept with the emergency equipment, but must be in a sealed container, which is then replenished and resealed after use.

- All medicines, including emergency drugs and intravenous fluids, must be stored in an environment that meets the manufacturers' recommendations, e.g. minimum or maximum temperature.

- Contents of boxes of dose units e.g. intravenous fluids, sterile topical fluids and ampoules should not be emptied out of their original containers and stored loose as this has been identified as a contributory factor in medication incidents.

- Medicine cupboards must be kept locked at all times; drug trolleys must be locked and secured to the wall when not in use, and individual medicines cabinets (sometimes called 'patient's own dispensary') must be locked when not in use.

- Controlled drugs must be kept separate from other medicines, and the keys to the controlled drugs cupboard kept separately from other drug keys. A controlled drugs register must also be kept. There are requirements for regular auditing in relation to ensuring the safety and security of controlled drugs.

- All stock must be rotated so that medicines are used before their expiry date. Regular checks of stored medication must be made to ensure that stock rotation is effective. The stock list of medicines kept in the clinical area is agreed by pharmacy staff and the senior nurse.

- The security of medicines is the responsibility of the nurse in charge of the clinical area. No unauthorised person must be allowed access to the keys (refer to local policy regarding who has authorised access to the keys).

7.2 Self-administration of medicines

Principles

- In some hospitals and care homes patients/residents (hereafter called patients) are given responsibility for taking their own prescribed medicines. This may be in preparation for their discharge home or to maintain their independence. It is also thought that encouraging patients to take responsibility for taking their own medicines will improve concordance.

- Local policies will differ, but the principles for self-administration of medicines are based upon the availability of suitable storage (usually locked cupboards attached to the patient's locker or in their room), a medicines regimen that is not subject to frequent change and individually dispensed medicines from the pharmacy.

- The medicines may be dispensed in separate packs or in compliance aids such as a monitored dose container or a daily/weekly dosing aid.

- The nurse's role in self-administration of medicines is to support and educate the patient in the safe administration of their medicines and in the use of any compliance aids that may be used. In some instances it may be the nurse's role to support and educate carers or support workers in this role rather than the patient themselves.

- Collaborative working between all members of the healthcare team is imperative if the individual's suitability for self-administration is to be assessed and appropriate education and support provided.

- The nurse must assess the patient's ability to self-administer their medicines prior to entering them into the programme. Most policies for self-administration of medicines include obtaining written consent from the patient before entering them into the programme. Patients have the right to withdraw their consent at any time.

- Most programmes also have varying levels of supervision according to the patient's ability and the level of support and education required. The level should be documented in the notes and reviewed regularly.

- The Nursing and Midwifery Council (NMC 2007) identify three levels of self-administration:

  Level 1: the nurse may administer the patient's medicines whilst implementing a planned programme of education. The education programme should include detailed information (both verbal and written) about the medicines, their dosage and times for administration, intended effects and any possible side-effects. The written information should include patient information leaflets and also an individualised card indicating the times and dosages for each medicine. During this period the nurse can assess the need for any compliance aids that may be required, such as bottle-top openers or large print on labels.

Level 2: the nurse remains responsable for the safe storage of medicines, but the patient is encouraged to call the nurse when medicines are due. The nurse checks the prescription, opens the locker and asks the patient to identify which medicine is due. The nurse will then observe the patient taking the medicine, offer additional supervisión or information as required.

Level 3: the patient administers their own medicines and is given responsibility for the key to their cabinet. It is important that sufficient time is allocated to the programme, so that patients have time to fully understand their medicines prior to discharge home or the implementation of the programme in a residential home.

- It is important to reassess the patient's ability to self-administer medications at frequent intervals or if the patient's condition changes.

- Nurses may find that, in some instances, they have to take responsibility for repackaging dispensed medicines into compliance aids for patients. This must be undertaken with care and the nurse must be aware of the risk of error in this procedure (NMC 2007). The procedure must be documented and all medicines must be accounted for.

7.3 Drug calculations

It is sometimes necessary to perform drug calculations in order to administer prescribed medicines correctly, for example, when the medicines are not available in the exact dosage that has been prescribed.

Converting from one unit of measurement to another

It is sometimes necessary to convert from one unit of measurement to another in order to be able to administer the correct amount of medicine. To convert units you need to know the following:

1 kilogram (kg) = 1000 grams (g)

1 gram (g) = 1000 milligrams (mg)

1 milligram = 1000 micrograms (mcg)

To convert grams (g) to milligrams (mg) or milligrams (mg) to micrograms (mcg) you need to multiply by 1000. This is achieved by moving the decimal point three places to the right, e.g. 6.5 mg × 1000 = 6500 mcg

To convert micrograms (mcg) into milligrams (mg) or milligrams (mg) to grams (g), you need to divide by 1000. This is achieved by moving the decimal point three places to the left, e.g.: 2500 mcg = 2.5 mg

Percentage concentration and ratios

Sometimes drug concentration may be measured as a percentage (%) weight to volume (w/v). The percentage equates to the number of grams (weight) per 100 millilitres (volume) and the percentage remains constant, irrespective of the size of the container.

1% lignocaine means 1 g of lignocaine dissolved in every 100 ml (i.e.1000 mg per 100 ml or 10 mg per ml)

5% glucose means 5 g of glucose dissolved in every 100 ml (i.e. 5000 mg per 100 ml or 50 mg per ml)

Occasionally drug concentrations are written as ratios. The ratio 1 : 1000 equates to 1 g per 1000 ml and the ratio: 1 : 10 000 equates to 1 g per 10 000 ml. e.g. adrenaline (epinephrine) 1 : 1000 (1 g per 1000 ml):

= 1000 mg per 1000 ml

= 1 mg per ml

e.g. adrenaline (epinephrine) 1 : 10 000 (1 g per 10,000 ml)

= 1000 mg per 10,000 ml

= 1 mg per 10 ml

= 0.1 mg per ml

Calculating the number of tablets required

In order to calculate the correct number of tablets, use the following formula:

$$\text{number of measures required (i.e. tablets)} = \frac{\text{dose prescribed}}{\text{dose per measure}}$$

Firstly you need to convert the amount required into the same units of measurement as the tablets, then use the formula.

For example, 1 g of paracetamol is prescribed. Paracetamol is dispensed in 500 mg tablets:

$$1\,g = 1000\,mg$$

$$\text{Number of tablets} = \frac{100\,mg}{500\,mg}$$

$$= 2 \text{ tablets to be given}$$

Calculating the volume to give or draw up

In order to calculate the correct volume, use the following formula:

$$\text{volume to give} = \frac{\text{dose required}}{\text{dose available}} \times \text{volume available}$$

For example, 75 mg of pethidine is prescribed. Pethidine is dispensed in ampoules containing 100 mg in 2 ml

$$\text{volume to give} = \frac{75}{100} \times 2 = 1.5\,ml$$

Calculating infusion rates

See 'Intravenous therapy', 'Regulation of flow rate'.

7.4 Principles of administration of medicines

Principles

Safety is of paramount importance when administering medication by any route and emphasis has been placed on organisational responsibility for ensuring medicines safety (Department of Health 2011, National Patient Safety Agency 2009). In order to ensure that administration of medication is safe it is imperative that the nurse remembers the '6 rights' (O'Brien et al. 2011):

1. Right patient: the patient's identity should be checked against their identification (ID) band and the prescription chart. In primary care, where patients will not have an ID band, alternative means of identification should be used such as a photograph of the patient.

2. Right medicine: check that the prescription is legible, signed by an authorised prescriber and that it matches the the label on the medication. It is also important to ensure that you understand the reasons why the medication is prescribed and that the patient does not have any allergies to the medication. If a patient has a known allergy they should wear a red allergy band. Some Trusts have instigated 'traffic light' systems to alert staff to preparations that contain penicillin. The prescriber should use the generic name, rather than a trade name on the prescription.

3. Right dose: check that the correct dosage has been prescribed and carry out any calculations required to ensure the correct amount is administered. Check that the maximum daily dose has not been exceeded.

4. Right route: check that the prescribed route is appropriate for the patient and that a suitable preparation for that route is available.

5. Right time: check that the medication is given at the prescribed time. It is also important to check if the medication has to be given at a particular time such as before or after food.

6. Right documentation: it is imperative that the prescription chart is signed to state that the medication has been given. If for any reason the medication is not able to be administered, this must also be documented with the reason for non administration clearly identified. Documentation of the effects of the medication is also required e.g. whether anti-emetics have been effective or if any unwanted side-effects have been reported by the patient.

The following procedure applies to the administration of all medicines, regardless of route. Additional route specific guidelines will follow.

Preparation

Patient

- Check the location of the patient before dispensing the medication. Do not leave medicines unattended for administration at a later time
- Check the patient understands the reasons for the medication being administered and any special instructions, e.g. swallow whole or after food, etc. Ensure that they have consented to receiving the medicine ➡ **PFP1**
- Ascertain whether the patient has any drug allergies ➡ **PFP2**
- The patient should be wearing an identification wrist band

Equipment/Environment

- Medicines to be administered and equipment appropriate to the route of administration.
- Patient's prescription chart
- Drug reference book, e.g. British National Formulary

Nurse

- **Medicines may only be administered by a registered nurse ➡ PFP3**
- The nurse must have knowledge of the action, usual dose and side-effects of the drugs being administered and knowledge of legislation and local policies relating to the administration of medicines (NMC 2007)
- Local policy may require that two nurses check certain medicines before administration
- Wash hands or use alcohol hand rub

Procedure

1. Check the prescription chart has the patient's full name and hospital number and read the prescription to ascertain which medicines require administration ➡ **PFP4**.

2. Check by which route each medicine is to be given.

3. Check the prescription is dated and is legible and signed by an authorised prescriber ➡ **PFP5**.

4. Check it is the correct time to administer the medicine and that the patient has not already received it. Check any special observations (e.g. blood pressure or pulse rate) or requirements relating to the medication (e.g. before or after food).

5. Identify the correct medication by checking the medicine container against the prescription chart.

6. Check the expiry date of the medicine.

7. Calculate how much is needed to achieve the prescribed dose (e.g. how many tablets or how much of the ampoule is to be drawn up) ➡ **PFP6**.

8. Repeat steps 2–7 for all medicines due at this time.

9. Check the patient's identity – using the patient's nameband, a photograph or verbally, against the prescription chart, according to local policy ➡ **PFP7**.

10. Administer the medicine as prescribed. **Medicines must not be left at the bedside unattended.** The patient may forget to take them or another patient may take them by mistake.

11. Dispose of any packaging and other waste.

12. Ensure the patient is comfortable and knows how to report any unwanted side-effects of the medication.

13. Sign/initial the prescription chart according to local policy, to indicate that the medicine has been administered. If the medication cannot be administered for any reason, this must also be documented and reported.

14. Monitor the effects of the medication and document in the nursing records. Report any abnormal effects/side-effects immediately.

⬤ Points for practice

PFP1 Except in exceptional circumstances, medicines for patients who refuse to take them should not be given covertly by disguising them in food (NMC 2007).

PFP2 If the allergy section of the prescription chart has not been completed, check with the patient and/or the medical notes before administering any medicines. If the patient has no known allergies, this should be indicated in the allergy box; it should not be left blank.

PFP3 Student nurses may only participate in the administration of medicines under the direct supervision of a registered nurse. A registered nurse must countersign all student signatures.

PFP4 Patient Group Directions (PGDs) are sometimes used in lieu of an individual prescription. These are written instructions for the supply or administration of medicines to groups of patients. They must be approved by a doctor or dentist AND a pharmacist who have been involved in developing them AND they must be approved by the appropriate healthcare body, e.g. an Acute Healthcare Trust or Primary Care Trust. Some employers require specific training for those who use PGDs and so local policy must be followed (NMC 2007). Student nurses may **not** administer medication under a PGD even under direct supervision of a registered nurse (NMC 2007).

PFP5 Instruction by telephone to administer a previously unprescribed substance is not acceptable. In exceptional circumstances, where the authorised prescriber is unable to issue a new prescription for an altered dose of an existing prescription, fax or e-mail may be used. This must be followed up with a new prescription confirming the new prescription. The NMC (2007) suggest that this should be within 24 hours.

PFP6 If the dosage of medication is related to weight, the patient's weight should be recorded on the prescription chart.

PFP7 To reduce the risk of error all patients should wear an identification wrist band. If checking their identity verbally it is important to ask them to state their name and date of birth.

7.5 Oral route

Preparation

Patient	**Equipment**	**Nurse**
• Ask/assist the patient to assume a position that allows easy swallowing	• Medicines to be administered plus medicine pots, tablet cutter, tissues, jug of water and/or milk if appropriate	• **Only registered nurses may administer medicines** ➡ **PFP1**
• Ensure the patient has plenty of appropriate fluid with which to take the medicine	• Prescription chart	• Clean hands thoroughly
	• Drug reference book, e.g. British National Formulary	• Additional protective clothing may be necessary if indicated by the patient's condition (see Ch. 1)

Procedure

1. Check the '6 rights' and follow the principles of administration as described on pages 183–185.

2. Calculate the volume of liquid or number of tablets or capsules required to achieve the prescribed dose (see p. 181). Do not break tablets unless they are scored across the middle. Scored tablets may be broken with a file, tablet cutter or using a tissue, to avoid handling ➡ **PFP2**.

3. Dispense the prescribed amount into a medicine pot. If not in a blister pack, shake the tablets/capsules into the top of the container before transferring to the medicine pot, to avoid handling them (Figure 7.1). Liquid preparations may be drawn up in an oral syringe for accuracy of measurement and then transferred into a medicines pot or the liquid can be squirted from the syringe directly into the patient's mouth ➡ **PFP3**

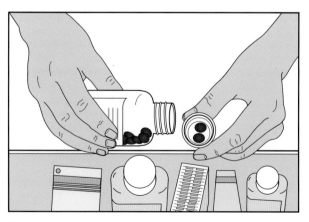

Figure 7.1 Non-touch technique for oral medicines.

4. Repeat this procedure for all oral medicines due at this time.

5. Check the patient's identity – using the patient's nameband or verbally, according to local policy – against the prescription chart.

6. Make sure the patient is in an appropriate position to swallow the medicine and has sufficient fluid.

7. Watch or assist the patient to take the medicines and ensure they have swallowed them all. **Do not leave medicines unattended at the bedside** for later administration ➡ **PFP4**

8. Dispose of any packaging, disposable medicine pots, etc., in the clinical waste

9. Document drugs admnistered according to local policy

10. Clean used equipment as appropriate and according to local policy.

➡ Points for practice

PFP1 Student nurses may only participate in the administration of medicines under the direct supervision of a registered nurse. A registered nurse must countersign all student signatures.

PFP2 Only soluble or dispersible preparations may be dissolved in water. If the patient is unable to swallow whole tablets, the pharmacist should be consulted to identify an alternative preparation, e.g. suspension or elixir. Tablets should not be crushed as this may alter the chemical properties of the medication. Additionally, crushing a tablet usually renders it 'unlicensed' and as such the manufacturer will not assume any liability (NMC 2007). Medication must only be crushed with the permission of the authorised prescriber and pharmacist and with the patient's consent. The reasons for crushing the medication must also be clearly documented.

PFP3 Oral syringes are a different colour from other syringes (often a purple colour) to ensure that oral medications could never be inadvertently given intravenously.

PFP4 Except in exceptional circumstances, medicines for patients who refuse to take them should not be given covertly by disguising them in food (NMC 2007).

7.6 Nasogastric route

Some patients are unable to take nourishment and medicines orally. If they have a nasogastric tube, medicines may be administered via this route. It is imperative that the pharmacist is consulted to determine whether tablets may be crushed and mixed with water or whether alternative solutions, such as suspensions and elixirs, are available (see ➡ **PFP2** on p. 187 regarding crushing tablets). You should also consider whether any interaction with the feed may occur and the possibility of blockage of the tube. See nasogastric feeding (p. 167) for technique.

7.7 Controlled drugs

Preparation

Patient

- Explain the procedure, to gain consent and cooperation
- Check the patient understands the reasons for having the medication

Equipment/Environment

- Patient's prescription chart
- Controlled drugs register

Nurse

- Ensure knowledge of legislation and local policies relating to the administration of controlled drugs
  ➡ **PFP1 & 2**
- Two nurses are usually required, one of whom must be a registered nurse (check local policy)
- Wash hands or use alcohol hand rub
- Additional protective clothing may be necessary if indicated by the patient's condition (see Ch. 1)

Procedure

If local policy stipulates two nurses, they must both be involved in **all** stages of this procedure:

1. Read the prescription to ascertain which drugs require administration and by which route.

2. Check that the prescription has the patient's full name and hospital number and is legible, dated and signed by the authorised prescriber.

3. Check that it is the correct time to administer the drug and that the patient has not already received it. You may also need to check that the appropriate time has elapsed since the previous dose and any special considerations, such as the maximum dosage allowed in 24 hours.

4. Open the controlled drugs cupboard and select the appropriate drug, checking that the quantity corresponds with that indicated in the controlled drugs register. Check the expiry date.

5. Remove the drug from its container and check it against the prescription.

6. Check the quantity remaining and replace in the cupboard. Lock the cupboard.

7. Check the amount required, route, time and patient's identity again with the prescription.

8. Select/draw up the correct amount/volume of the drug, performing any calculation as required. Any unused drug should be discarded into a sharps bin ➡ **PFP3**.

9. In the controlled drugs register, record the patient's full name, the dose to be administered (any wastage must also be recorded), the time and the stock number remaining.

10. At the bedside, check that the information on the patient's nameband corresponds with that on the prescription. Check again the drug, dose, route and time against the prescription.

11. Administer the drug by the prescribed route and discard all waste appropriately.

12. Ensure the patient is comfortable and is aware of the effects and side-effects of the drug.

13. Both nurses must sign the prescription chart and the controlled drugs register. Ensure the Controlled Drugs register is returned to the appropriate place ➡ **PFP4**

14. Monitor the effects of the drug and report any side-effects immediately.

➡Points for practice

PFP1 The keys to the controlled drugs cupboard must be kept separately from other keys and must be carried by the registered nurse in charge of the ward. No unauthorised personnel must have access to these keys.

PFP2 Some drugs are controlled drugs in certain preparations only. For example, intramuscular dihydrocodeine (DF118) is a controlled drug but the oral preparation is not.

PFP3 It is important to ensure that any unused drug is discarded safely and cannot be used by unauthorised persons. It is recommended that unused/wasted drugs should be discarded into a sharps bin. Unused fluids should be either emptied onto an absorbant pad which is then put in the sharps bin or the ampoule emptied directly in the sharps bin. When the bin is sent for destruction it should be labelled 'contains mixed pharmaceuticals waste and sharps – for incineration' (DoH 2007). Wasted/discarded drugs should be witnessed and accounted for in the Controlled Drugs register.

PFP4 Controlled-drug registers must not be thrown away when full, but must be retained in storage for at least 2 years. Check local policy for details.

7.8 Subcutaneous injection

Preparation

Patient

- Explain the procedure and ensure, to gain consent and cooperation
- Ask/assist the patient to choose the site of injection
- The patient should be wearing an identification wrist band

Equipment

- Patient's prescription chart
- Prescribed medication (this is often a pre-filled syringe with needle)
- Cardboard tray or receiver
- Syringe of appropriate size (0.5–2 ml) if necessary
  ➡ **PFP1**
- Orange (25G) sterile needle if necessary
- Draw curtains/ blinds to ensure privacy, dignity
- Small clinical wipe/tissue
- Sharps bin

Nurse

- **Only registered nurses may administer medicines**
  ➡ **PFP2**.
- Knowledge of local drug administration polic.
- Wash hands / use alcohol hand rub
- An apron and non-sterile gloves should be worn
  ➡ **PFP3**
- Protective clothing may be necessary if indicated by the patient's condition (see Ch. 1).

Procedure

1. Check the '6 rights' and follow the principles of administration as described on pages 183–185. Check the medication against the prescription chart.

2. If using a pre-filled syringe it is not necessary to expel the air bubble ➡ **PFP4**. If it is not a pre-filled syringe, prepare the medication as for intramuscular injection (see p. 195)

3. Raise the bed to a safe working height to avoid stooping.

4. Select the site of administration (Figure 7.2) ➡ **PFP5**. Ask/assist the patient to adopt a suitable position, if necessary and expose the chosen injection site.

5. It is not necessary to clean the skin ➡ **PFP6**. Pinch up the skin using the thumb and first finger of your non-dominant hand and insert the short needle into the subcutaneous tissue at an angle of 90° (Figure 7.3) ➡ **PFP7** and ➡ **PFP8**.

6. It is not necessary to withdraw the piston as it is unlikely that a blood vessel of any size will be punctured.

7. Keeping the skin pinched, inject the solution slowly. On completion, pause briefly before withdrawing the needle as this helps to prevent backtracking.

8. Do not massage the site ➡ **PFP9**. If necessary, use the tissue to wipe away any blood.

9. Dispose of the syringe and needle into the sharps bin immediately (see p. 14). **Do not resheath the needle.**

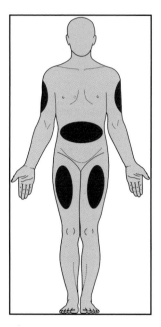

Figure 7.2 Sites commonly used for subcutaneous injection.

10. Lower the bed. Ensure the patient is comfortable and is aware of the effects and side-effects of the medication. Some local irritation may occur at the injection site.

11. Dispose of any waste, gloves and apron in the clinical waste.

12. Wash hands/use alcohol hand rub.

13. Sign the prescription chart as per local policy to indicate that the medication has been administered. Document any abnormalities or complications with the procedure.

14. Store medications according to the manufacture's guidance. Some medications (e.g. insulin) have to be kept in the refrigerator.

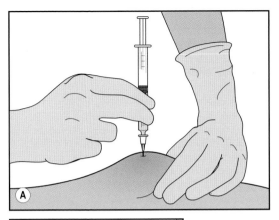

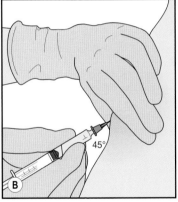

Figure 7.3 Subcutaneous injection technique.

➡ Points for practice

PFP1 No more that 2 ml should be given by the subcutaneous route.

PFP2 Only registered nurses may administer medications. Student nurses may only participate in the administration of medicines under the direct supervision of a registered nurse. A registered nurse must countersign student signatures.

PFP3 Gloves must be worn for all invasive procedures (Pratt et al. 2007)

PFP4 Some drugs (e.g. heparin) are manufactured in pre-filled syringes. Unlike all other injections, the air in a heparin syringe is not expelled, but is designed to remain in the syringe, next to the piston. When the small amount of drug is given, the air fills the needle hub/nozzle of the syringe and needle ensuring that all fluid has been expelled from the syringe. This prevents the drug tracking back to the surface as the needle is withdrawn, which can cause skin irritation.

PFP5 Patients receiving regular subcutaneous injections (e.g. insulin) should rotate the injection site; repeated injections into the same area causes hardening of the subcutaneous tissues, which will interfere with absorption (King 2003). Possible sites are: the upper arms, the anterior aspect of the thighs, and the abdomen (see Figure 7.2). Heparin is usually given into the subcutaneous tissue of the abdominal wall.

PFP6 The skin is not cleaned because, with repeated use, alcohol causes the skin to harden and many patients will be having subcutaneous injections over a long period of time, possibly for the rest of their life.

PFP7 Pinching the skin into a fold lifts the adipose tissue away from the underlying muscle to ensure the medication reaches the subcutaneous tissue (King 2003).

PFP8 If not using a pre-filled syringe or insulin 'pen', the needle will be longer than 5–8 mm; longer needles should be inserted at an angle of 45° (see Figure 7.3).

PFP9 Massaging the skin affects the absorption of the drug

7.9 Intramuscular injection

Preparation

Patient

- Explain the procedure, to gain consent and cooperation
- Check the patient's understanding of the reason for the injection
- Patient should be wearing an identification wrist band

Equipment/environment

- Patient's prescription chart
- Prescribed medicine and diluent, if required
- Cardboard tray or receiver
- Sterile syringe of appropriate size (2–5 ml)
- Sterile needle-usually green (21G) for adult patients ➡ **PFP1**
- Alcohol-impregnated swab
- Small clinical wipe/tissue
- Sharps bin

Nurse

- **Only registered nurses may administer medicines.** A second nurse may be required depending on the local drug administration policy ➡ **PFP2**
- Wash and dry hands thoroughly
- An apron and non-sterile gloves should be worn

Procedure

1. Check the '6 rights' and follow the principles of administration as described on pages 183–185. Check the medicine and any diluent against the prescription chart and check expiry dates.

2. Open the syringe packaging at the plunger end and remove the syringe. Check that the plunger will move freely inside the barrel.

3. Taking care not to touch the nozzle end, hold the syringe in one hand and open the needle packaging at the hilt (coloured) end. Attach the needle firmly to the syringe and loosen, but do not remove, the needle cover (sheath). Place in the tray/receiver.

4. If a glass ampoule of liquid is being used, ensure that all the contents are in the bottom of the ampoule, then break off the top using a clinical wipe or tissue to protect your fingers. If a plastic ampoule is being used, break off the top, taking care not to touch the top of the ampoule with your fingers.

5. Pick up the syringe and needle and allow the needle cover to slide off into the tray or receiver.

6. Carefully insert the needle through the neck of the ampoule and into the solution, taking care not to allow it to scrape against the bottom of the ampoule, as this blunts the needle.

7. Draw back on the plunger, using your thumb and middle finger on the plunger with your first finger against the flange of the syringe until the required amount is in the syringe (Figure 7.4).

8. If the medicine is in powder form, draw up the diluent, clean the rubber stopper of the ampoule/vial with an alcohol-impregnated swab and allow it to dry. Inject the appropriate amount of diluent (see manufacturer's instructions; usually 1.5–2 ml) into the ampoule/vial. Mix thoroughly by

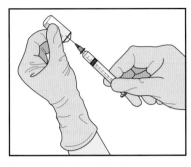

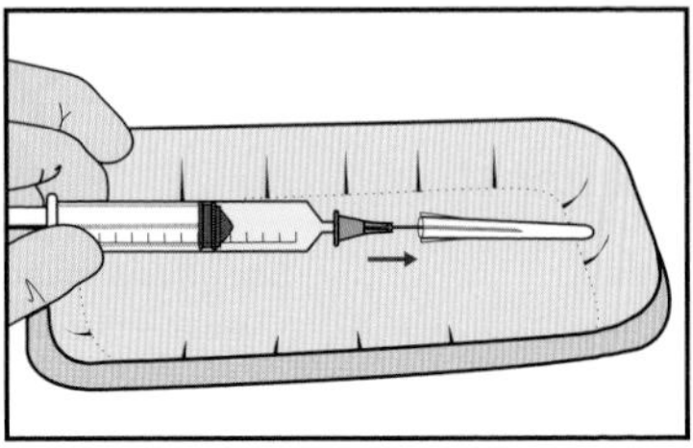

Figure 7.5 Safe re-sheathing technique.

Figure 7.4 Drawing up injection.

gently agitating or rolling the ampoule/vial until all the powder has dissolved ➡ **PFP3**.

9. Holding the ampoule/vial upside down at eye level, pull back the plunger to draw the liquid into the syringe. Make sure that the needle remains below the surface of the liquid to prevent air being drawn into the syringe (Figure 7.4).

10. Replace the ampoule in tray/receiver. Taking care not to touch the needle with your hand, carefully resheathe the needle using the non-touch method (Figure 7.5) ➡ **PFP4**.

11. Hold the syringe upright at eye level and encourage any air to rise to the top of the syringe. Gently tap the barrel of the syringe if necessary to make air bubbles rise to the top. Expel the air by gently pressing the plunger until droplets of liquid are seen at the top of the needle (Figure 7.6). If necessary, attach a new needle ➡ **PFP5**.

12. Take the tray/receiver containing the syringe, ampoule and alcohol-impregnated swab plus the sharps bin to the patient. Check the medicine and prescription again and the patient's nameband.

13. Ensure privacy. Raise the bed to a safe working height to avoid stooping.

14. Select the site. Ask/assist the patient to adopt a suitable position and pull back the bedclothes to exposure the injection site (Figure 7.7) ➡ **PFP6**.

15. Clean the skin with the alcohol-impregnated swab allow it to dry ➡ **PFP7**.

16. Stretch the skin slightly with your non-dominant hand ➡ **PFP8**.

17. Holding the syringe like a dart in your dominant hand, warn the patient, then insert the needle swiftly and firmly at an angle of 90° to the skin (Figure 7.8). Leave 0.5–1 cm of the needle showing ➡ **PFP9**.

18. With the ulnar border of your hand against the skin, hold the coloured part of the needle (hilt) to prevent movement.

19. Withdraw the plunger slightly to check the needle has not inadvertently entered a blood vessel ➡ **PFP10**.

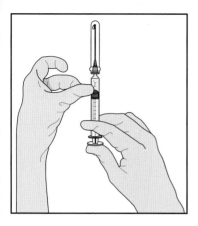

Figure 7.6 Expelling the air.

20. Depress the plunger steadily, not too quickly, until the syringe is empty.

21. Quickly and smoothly withdraw the needle from the skin and press firmly on the site with the swab or a tissue until any bleeding stops.

22. **Do not resheathe the needle.** Discard it, still attached to the syringe, into the sharps bin ➡ **PFP11**.

23. Assist the patient into a comfortable position and replace the bedclothes. Lower the bed to a safe height.

24. Dispose of any waste, gloves and aprons in the clinical waste.

25. Wash and dry hands.

26. Document administration according to local policy.

27. Intramuscular medicines will usually take effect within 20 minutes. Check for the desired effect and for any side-effects, especially if administering an analgesic or anti-emetic. Document and report any complications or adverse reactions.

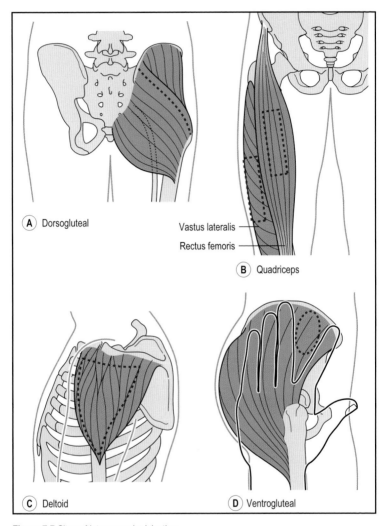

(A) Dorsogluteal

Vastus lateralis
Rectus femoris

(B) Quadriceps

(C) Deltoid

(D) Ventrogluteal

Figure 7.7 Sites of intramuscular injection.

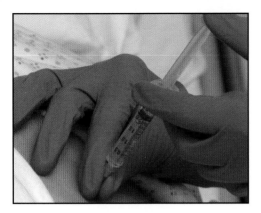

Figure 7.8 Intramuscular injection technique.

➡ Points for practice

PFP1 If the patient is very thin or cachexic, the same gauge needle is used but it is not inserted so deeply. Using a smaller gauge needle requires more pressure to inject the liquid, which causes more discomfort, not less (King 2003).

PFP2 Each institution will have its own drug administration policy, which will indicate whether two nurses are required to check certain drugs. It will also indicate the role of the student nurse in drug administration.

PFP3 When mixing the medicine, keep the needle inside the ampoule so that it remains sterile. If there is pressure within the vial, you may need to keep your thumb on the plunger. Mix gently as vigorous shaking will make it frothy and difficult to withdraw into the syringe.

PFP4 Resheathing the needle before administration to the patient using the non-touch technique shown is perfectly safe and ensures that droplets of the drug are not inhaled or sprayed onto the skin as air is expelled from the syringe.

PFP5 To avoid patient discomfort, a new sterile needle may be required if the tip of the needle has become blunt or bent whilst mixing and drawing up the medication.

PFP6 The recommended sites for intramuscular injection are the ventrogluteal (gluteus medius) and the lateral aspect of the vastus lateralis, which is one of the quadriceps (Nisbet 2006, Cocoman and Murray 2010). The dorsogluteal (gluteus maximus) site is potentially associated with more risks due to the presence of major blood vessels and nerves. Also, the drug absorption rate is much lower in gluteal muscles. If the patient is obese (i.e. has large amounts of adipose tissue) it is harder to be confident that the injection will reach the gluteus maximus so the vastus lateralis may be a better site (Greenway 2004, Nisbet 2006). Smaller intramuscular injections, such as vaccinations, are usually given into the deltoid area (see Figure 7.7).

PFP7 The skin should be washed if visibly dirty. Some local policies no longer recommend skin cleansing prior to intramuscular injection because they regard it as unnecessary if the skin is clean (Wynaden et al. 2005) and the nurse prepares the injection using the required handwashing and asepsis (O'Brien et al. 2011). However, when using an alcohol impregnated swab allow the skin to dry; otherwise skin cleansing is ineffective.

PFP8 An alternative technique is the Z-track method. This involves pulling the skin sideways or downwards from the injection site to displace the skin and subcutaneous tissue from the underlying muscle. Once the medication is given, release the tension on the skin to seal off the needle pathway and puncture site. This prevents the drug from seeping out through the injection site or into the subcutaneous tissues (Cocoman and Murray 2010).

PFP9 Leaving a little of the needle exposed means that it will be possible to remove the needle in the event of needle breakage.

PFP10 If blood appears in the syringe at step 19, stop, withdraw the needle and start the procedure again with a new syringe and drug (Wynaden et al. 2005). This happens only very rarely.

PFP11 If you are unable to take the sharps bin to the patient, the needle and syringe should be placed in a cardboard tray or receiver and then tipped into the sharps bin without further handling (see p. 14).

7.10 Intravenous drug administration

Preparation

Patient

- Explain the procedure, to gain consent and cooperation
- The patient should be resting in a chair or in bed
- If the cannula site is covered by a bandage, this must be removed to allow inspection of the site

Equipment/environment

- Prescription chart and prescribed medicines
- 'Needle free' system or orange needle if an injectable bung is used
- 0.9% sodium chloride to flush the cannula
  ➡ **PFP1**
- Alcohol and chlorehexidine swab
- Sharps bin

Nurse

- Only registered nurses who have undergone the appropriate training may administer intravenous medicines in accordance with local policies
  ➡ **PFP2**
- Clean hands thoroughly and put on non-sterile gloves. Additional protective clothing may be necessary if indicated by the patient's condition (see Ch. 1)
- Goggles may be necessary with certain medicines, e.g. cytotoxic drugs

Procedure

1. Check the '6 rights' and follow the principles of administration as described on pages 183–185 Whether you need to check IV medicines with another nurse will depend on the local intravenous drug administration policy ➡ **PFP2**.

2. Prepare the medicine for administration, as described for intramuscular injections (see p. 195). Prepare 10 ml of 0.9% sodium chloride flush (more if several medicines are to be administered) ➡ **PFP1**.

3. At the bedside, check the medicine and the patient's nameband against the prescription again.

4. Adopt a comfortable posture (sitting is probably best) in a position that allows easy access to the cannula. Face the patient so that any adverse reaction may be observed, and if the patient is undergoing cardiac monitoring, this should also be in view.

5. Inspect the cannula site using a visual infusion phlebitis score (see p. 122). Do not continue with administration if phlebitis is noted.

6. If cannula site is healthy, thoroughly disinfect the rubber membrane of the injection port or injectable bung on the extension set according to local policy and allow to dry. If there is an infusion running, the intravenous bolus may be administered via the giving set side port which is situated approximately 10 cm from the cannula ➡ **PFP3** and ➡ **PFP4**.

7. If the cannula has no infusion in progress, open the the clamp on the extension tubing and insert the nozzle of the syringe to the needle free injection port or insert a small needle (25 guage) into the intermittent injection bung ➡ **PFP5** (Figure 7.9).

8. Before administering the medicine, administer a small amount (1–2 ml) of the 0.9% sodium chloride flush to confirm the patency of the cannula. If

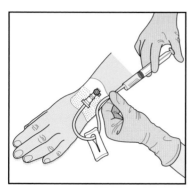

Figure 7.9 Intravenous injection technique.

resistance is felt, do not continue as this may dislodge a clot at the end of the cannula ➡ **PFP6**.

9. After administering the flush remove the syringe and insert the nozzle into the top of the 0.9% sodium chloride ampoule to keep it sterile. Next, connect the syringe of the medicine to be given and slowly administer the medicine according to the prescription, the manufacturer's instructions, and/or local policies and procedures,

10. Administer the remaining flush or, if a number of medicines are being given, flush between each one to prevent mixing in the cannula.

11. Close the clamp on the extension tubing and remove the syringe.

12. If a needle was used, do not resheathe the needle. Discard it immediately, still attached to the syringe, into the sharps bin.

13. Remove your gloves.

14. Ensure the patient is comfortable and advise them to report any side-effects.

15. Document the medicines administered according to local policy and observe the patient for the desired effect and any adverse side-effects.

16. Discard any waste appropriately and wash your hands.

➡ Points for practice

PFP1 0.9% sodium chloride is used for flushing purposes except in a few instances when the drug being administered is incompatible with sodium chloride. In these cases (e.g. amphotericin), 5% glucose should be used instead. In many NHS Trusts, the 0.9% sodium chloride or 5% glucose flush may be administered without prescription.

PFP2 Although single-nurse administration is common for other routes of administration, some local policies require two nurses to administer intravenous drugs. It is vital that both nurses check thoroughly – you should never rely on the other nurse to check that it is correct.

PFP3 If an infusion in progress is prescribed to run at a very slow rate (e.g. dobutamine or insulin) it is advisable to use a separate cannula for bolus intravenous medications. If this is not possible, administer the flush and the bolus at a slower rate than the infusion to ensure that the infusion is not given faster than the prescribed rate.

PFP4 Although some cannulae have an integral injection port on the top of the cannula, this should not be used for drug administration as it is difficult to keep the port clean and provides a reservoir for bacterial contamination.

PFP5 There are a number of 'needle-free' injection caps available. These allow the syringe to be fitted directly into the injection cap without the need for a needle, thus reducing the risk of a needle-stick injury.

PFP6 If the patient complains of pain at the site, this may be due to infiltration or extravasation. If a small amount of flush solution is administered before the medicine to test patency, it will only be 0.9% sodium chloride rather than some potentially more damaging substance that is administered into the surrounding tissues.

7.11 Instillation of nose drops/ nasal spray

Preparation

Patient
- Explain the procedure, to gain consent and co-operation ➡ **PFP1**
- For nose drops ask the patient to lie down or sit in a chair where they are able to hyperextend their neck. A pillow under the shoulders is beneficial
- For nasal sprays the patient should be sitting upright with the head slightly forward

Equipment
- Prescription chart
- Nose drops/ nasal spray as prescribed
- Clean tissues

Nurse
- Only registered nurses may administer medicines ➡ **PFP2**
- Wash hands and dry thoroughly
- Additional protective clothing may be necessary if indicated by the patient's condition (see Ch. 1)

Procedure

1. Check the '6 rights' and follow the principles of administration as described on pages 183–185. Note whether the drops/spray are to be instilled into one or both nostrils.

2. If required ask the patient to clear their nosrils by either blowing their nose or wiping the inside of the nostrils with a moistened tissue.

For nose drops:

1. Ask the patient to hyperextend their neck.

2. Remove the cap from the nose drops container and place it on end to avoid contamination.

3. Using the dropper, administer the correct number of drops into each nostril, taking care not to touch the nose with the dropper. Replace cap.

4. Ask the patient to remain in this position for at least 2 minutes to allow absorption of the medication.

5. Wipe away any excess medication with a tissue.

For nasal spray:

1. Remove the cap from the spray and place it on end to avoid contamination.

2. Prime the spray if necessary.

3. Insert the spray into the nostril whilst occluding the other nostril with a tissue.

4. Ask the patient to inhale at the same time as activating the spray.

5. Repeat in other nostril if prescribed. Replace cap.

6. Ask the patient to refrain from blowing their nose for about 20 minutes and instruct them not to sniff too vigorously following admnistration ➡ **PFP3**.

7. Ensure the patient is comfortable.

8. Discard any used tissues into clinical waste.

9. Return the nose drops/ nasal spray to the appropriate storage area.

10. Wash hands or use alcohol hand rub.

11. Document administration on the prescription chart accordin to local policy.

12. Evaluate the effect of the nose drops/spray in the nursing records and report any abnormalities.

➡ Points for practice

PFP1 Patients may be able to administer nose drops/ nasal sprays themselves. Nurses should ensure that they are using the correct procedure (see self-administration of medicines, p. 179)

PFP2 Only registered nurses may administer medications. Student nurses may only participate in the administration of nose drops/nasal sprays under the direct supervision of a registered nurse. A registered nurse must countersign all student signatures.

PFP3 The nurse should explain that nose drops may run into the back of the throat, causing the patient to experience an unusual taste.

7.12 Instillation of ear drops

Preparation

Patient

- Explain the procedure, to gain consent and cooperation
- Explain the action of the ear drops and the expected outcome
- Ask the patient to sit upright with their head tilted slightly away from the affected ear or to lie on their side with the affected ear uppermost ➡ **PFP1**

Equipment/environment

- Prescription chart
- Ear drops as prescribed
  ➡ **PFP2**
- Clean tissues

Nurse

- Only registered nurses may administer medicines ➡ **PFP3**
- Clean hands thoroughly
- Additional protective clothing may be necessary if indicated by the patient's condition (see Ch. 1)

Procedure

1. Check the '6 rights' and follow the principles of administration as described on pages 183–185. Check the ear drops against the prescription chart, noting which ear is to have the drops instilled.

2. Remove the cap from the ear drops container and and place on end to avoid contamination.

3. Gently pull the pinna of the ear upwards and backwards.

4. Squeeze the bottle or dropper to dispense the prescribed number of drops into the ear taking care not to touch the skin with the dropper (Figure 7.10).

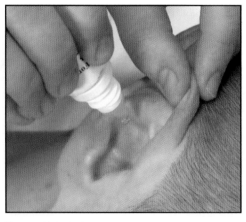

Figure 7.10 Instillation of ear drops.

5. Release the pinna.

6. Provide the patient with a tissue to cover their ear, but ask them not to push it into the ear as this may absorb the ear drop.

7. Replace the cap.

8. Instruct the patient to remain in this position for 1–2 minutes to allow the drops to reach the eardrum.

9. When the patient is sitting upright, use the tissue to wipe away any excess fluid from the outer ear.

10. If prescribed, repeat the process in the other ear after 5–10 minutes.

11. Ensure the patient is comfortable.

12. Dispose of used tissues in clinical waste. Return the nose drops/ nasal spray to the appropriate storage area.

13. Wash hands or use alcohol hand rub

14. Record administration on the prescription chart.

15. Evaluate the effect of the ear drops in the nursing records and report any abnormalities.

⇨Points for practice

PFP1 Patients may be able to administer ear drops themselves. Nurses should ensure that they are using the correct procedure (see Self-administration of medicines, p. 179).

PFP2 If drops are prescribed for both ears there may be a separate bottle for each ear.

PFP3 Only registered nurses may administer medications. Student nurses may only participate in the administration of ear drops under the direct supervision of a registered nurse. A registered nurse must countersign student signatures.

7.13 Instillation of eye drops or ointment

Preparation

Patient
- Explain the procedure, to gain consent and cooperation
- Instruct the patient to tilt their head backwards and look up
  ➡ **PFP1**
- Explain that vision maybe blurred for a short while after administration of the drops/ointment

Equipment/Environment
- Prescription chart
- Eye drops and/or ointment as prescribed
  ➡ **PFP2**
- Clean tissues

Nurse
- Only registered nurses may administer medicines
  ➡ **PFP3**
- Clean hands thoroughly
- Additional protective clothing may be necessary if indicated by the patient's condition (see Ch. 1)

Procedure

1. Check the '6 rights' and follow the principles of administration as described on pages 183–185. Check the eye drops against the prescription, noting which eye is to have the drops/ointment instilled ➡ **PFP4**.

Eye drops

1. Take a clean tissue and fold it several times to make a small pad.
2. Shake the bottle and remove the cap from the container and place it on end to avoid contamination.
3. Using the tissue pad, gently pull the lower lid downwards to form a small pocket for the drops/ointment.
4. Rest the edge of your hand on the patient's forehead.
5. Hold the dispenser between your thumb and middle finger about 2–3 cm from the patient's eye.
6. Press the bottom of the bottle with your forefinger to dispense the prescribed number of drops (Figure 7.11).
7. Ask the patient to close (but not squeeze) the eye for about 60 seconds to disperse the medication.
8. Repeat for other eye if prescribed.

Eye ointment

1. Remove the cap from the container and place it on end to avoid contamination.
2. Using a tissue, gently pull the lower lid downwards.

3. Squeeze the tube gently until a small amount (about 1–2 cm) of ointment forms a 'ribbon'. Apply the ribbon inside the lid margin, from the inner to outer aspect of the eye (Figure 7.12). Do not touch any part of the eye with the tube.

4. Ask the patient to close (but not squeeze) their eyes to disperse the medication. They should keep their eyes closed for approximately 60 seconds.

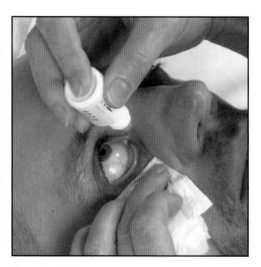

Figure 7.11 Instillation of eye drops.

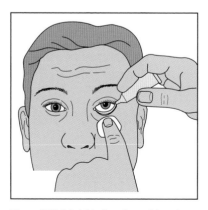

Figure 7.12 Administration of eye ointment.

5. Wipe away any excess medication that runs down the cheek with a clean tissue.

6. Repeat for other eye if required.

7. Replace the cap of eye drops/ointment.

8. If more than one medication is required, repeat the process after 2–3 minutes.

9. Ensure the patient is comfortable and that visión has returned to normal.

10. Dispose of used tissues in clinical waste. Return the eye drops/ointment to the appropriate storage area.

11. Wash hands or use alcohol hand rub.

12. Document administration on the prescription chart.

13. Evaluate the effect of the drops/ointment in the nursing records and report any abnormalities.

▶Points for practice

PFP1 Patients may be able to administer eye drops themselves. Nurses should ensure that they are using the correct procedure (see Self-administration of medicines, page 179). They may find it easier to self-administer the drops if they balance the bottle across the bridge of their nose and then squeeze the bottle to administer the drops. Specialist compliance aids are also available for patients who have difficulty with fine movement of the fingers or hands.

PFP2 If both eyes are being treated, there may be a separate bottle/tube for each eye. If one eye has obvious infection, treat the uninfected eye first. For patients who wear contact lenses, check with the prescriber if the lenses should be removed prior to instillation of eyedrops/ointment.

PFP3 Only registered nurses may administer medications. Student nurses may only participate in the administration of eye drops/ointment under the direct supervision of a registered nurse. A registered nurse must countersign all student signatures.

PFP4 If both eye drops and ointment are to be administered, administer the eye drops first as the grease base of the ointment can inhibit the absorption of drops.

7.14 Topical application

Preparation

Patient
- Explain the procedure, to gain cooperation and consent
- If possible patients should apply the cream or ointment themselves. The nurse should ensure they are applying it correctly (see Self-administration of medicines, p. 179)

Equipment
- Ensure the screens are pulled round to promote dignity and comfort
- Prescription chart
- Cream, ointment, lotion or topical patch as prescribed
- Non sterile gloves and sterile gauze to apply cream/lotion/ointment

Nurse
- Only registered nurses may administer medicines ➡ **PFP1**
- Clean hands thoroughly
- Put on apron. Additional protective clothing may be necessary if indicated by the patient's condition (see Ch. 1)

Procedure

1. Check the '6 rights' and follow the principles of administration as described on pages 183–185. Check the lotion/ointment/patch against the prescription.
2. Locate the appropriate part of the body and assess the skin.
   - If a topical patch is prescribed, remove backing and apply the patch to clean, dry skin PFP.
   - If cream, ointment or lotion, put on gloves and rub in with a piece of sterile gauze. Your gloves will protect you from absorption of the active ingredients.
3. Ensure the patient is comfortable.
4. Remove apron and gloves and discard, with the used gauze, in clinical waste.
5. Wash hands thoroughly.
6. Document administration and the condition of the skin according to local policy.

➡ Points for practice

PFP1 Only registered nurses may administer medications. Student nurses may only participate in the administration of topical applications under the direct supervision of a registered nurse. A registered nurse must countersign all student signatures.

PFP2 If the medicine comes in the form of a topical patch, the site of application should be varied according to the manufacturer's instructions, i.e. the same site should not be used on consecutive applications and the patch may need to be removed after a certain time period.

7.15 Vaginal preparations

Preparation

Patient

- Explain the procedure, to gain cooperation and consent
- Wherever possible the woman should be assisted as necessary to administer the cream or pessary herself. If this is not possible, ask/assist her to lie on her back with her heels together, knees bent and legs apart

Equipment

- Ensure the screens are pulled round to promote privacy, dignity and comfort
- Prescription chart
- Cream or pessary as prescribed
- Vaginal applicator
- Gauze swabs or tissues
- Receiver/tray
- Protective pad or panty liner
- Disposable clinical waste bag

Nurse

- Only registered nurses may administer medicines ➡ **PFP1**
- Clean hands thoroughly
- Put on gloves and apron. Additional protective clothing may be necessary if indicated by the patient's condition (see Ch. 1).

Procedure

1. Check the '6 rights' and follow the principles of administration as described on p. 183–185. Check the pessary/cream against the prescription chart.

2. Remove the pessary from the packaging and insert into the applicator. If using a vaginal cream, this is usually pre-loaded in the applicator. Place in tray.

3. Raise bed to a safe working height to avoid stooping.

4. Place an absorbent pad under the patient's buttocks.

5. Expose the genital area and retract the labia to expose the vagina. Warn the patient and gently insert the applicator into the vagina as far as is comfortable.

6. Holding the applicator, press the plunger to release the pessary or cream high in the vagina (Figure 7.13).

7. Remove the applicator and place in the tray. Wipe away any traces of cream and remove the absorbent pad. Discard all waste into the clinical waste bag.

8. Offer the patient a panty liner or pad to protect underwear. Replace bedclothes.

9. Remove gloves and place in clinical waste bag.

10. Ensure the patient is comfortable and lower the bed to a safe height. Ask the patient to remain recumbent for as long as possible ➡ **PFP2**.

11. Remove apron and wash hands.

12. Document administration according to local policy.

13. Evaluate effect of medication in nursing records.

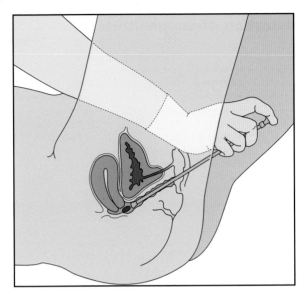

Figure 7.13 Insertion of a vaginal pessary.

➡ Points for practice

PFP1 Only registered nurses may administer medications. Student nurses may only participate in the administration of vaginal preparations under the direct supervision of a registered nurse. A registered nurse must countersign student signatures. A male nurse will require a female chaperone to carry out this procedure.

PFP2 Vaginal preparations are best administered last thing at night, when the patient will be recumbent for several hours, to allow absorption of the medication.

7.16 Administration of suppositories

Preparation

Patient

- Explain the procedure, to gain consent and cooperation
  ➡ **PFP1**
- If the suppository is for drug administration (e.g. paracetamol) the bowels should be opened prior to administration if possible
- A rectal examination to assess whether faecal matter is present may be performed prior to administration of suppositories designed to relieve constipation
- Ask/assist patient to remove clothing below the waist, and lie in the left lateral position
  ➡ **PFP2**
- Place an absorbent pad under the buttocks

Equipment

- Draw the curtains/screen to ensure dignity, privacy and comfort
- Prescription chart
- Suppositories as prescribed
- Cardboard tray or receiver
- Sachet or tube of lubricant
- Small clinical waste bag
- Gauze swabs or tissues

Nurse

- Only registered nurses may administer medicines
  ➡ **PFP3**
- Clean hands thoroughly
- Put on apron and gloves
- Additional protective clothing may be necessary if indicated by the patient's condition (see Ch. 1)

Procedure

1. Check the '6 rights' and follow the principles of administration as described on pages 183–185. Check the suppository against the prescription chart.
2. Remove all packaging around suppository.
3. Squeeze some lubricant onto a piece of gauze and lubricate the blunt end of the suppository ➡ **PFP4**.
4. Raise the bed to a safe working height to avoid stooping.
5. Pull back the bedclothes and ask the patient to draw up their knees.
6. With your left hand, part the patient's buttocks and visualise the anus, noting any haemorrhoids or skin tags that may make insertion difficult.
7. Warn the patient that he/she will feel suppository being inserted into the rectum.
8. Ask patient to relax; encouraging deep breathing may help
9. Gently insert the suppository into the anal canal blunt end first, using the index finger of your right hand (Figure 7.14) ➡ **PFP4**.
10. Repeat the process if more than one suppository is required.

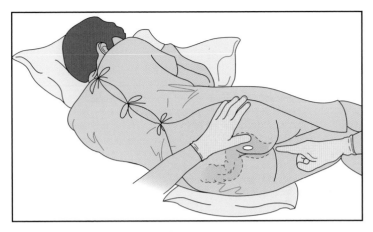

Figure 7.14 Administration of suppositories.

11. Wipe away excess traces of lubricant from the anal area and remove gloves.

12. If it is an evacuant suppository (e.g. glycerine or bisacodyl) leave the patient in a comfortable position with a call bell at hand. To be effective, the suppositories need to remain in position for at least 15 minutes and patients should be discouraged from opening their bowels before this time.

13. Replace bedclothes and lower the bed.

14. Place all used equipment, gloves and apron in clinical waste and wash hands

15. Document administration of the suppository as per local policy.

16. Document the effect of the suppository and report as appropriate.

Points for practice

PFP1 If a suppository may be required whilst a patient is in the operating theatre, consent should be obtained prior to surgery.

PFP2 It is necessary for the patient to be in the left lateral position because of the position of the rectum. This means that for effective insertion, even left-handed nurses must use their right hand to insert the suppository.

PFP3 Only registered nurses may administer medications. Student nurses may only participate in the administration of suppositories under the direct supervision of a registered nurse. A registered nurse must countersign all student signatures.

PFP4 There is some evidence to suggest that if the suppository is inserted blunt end first, insertion and retention of the suppository is easier, however, more research is required to confirm this (Kyle, 2009).

7.17 Respiratory route – metered dose inhaler

Preparation

Patient

- Explain the procedure, to gain cooperation and consent

Equipment/Environment

- Metered dose inhaler and any adjuncts such as a volumatic spacer ➡ **PFP1**
- Prescription chart
- Patients should use inhalers themselves, the nurse's role is to ensure they utilise the correct technique (see self administration of medicines p. 179)

Nurse

- Only registered nurses may administer medicines ➡ **PFP2**
- Clean hands thoroughly.

Procedure

Check the '6 rights' and follow the principles of administration as described on pages 183–185. Check the inhaler against the prescription chart.

Using inhaler only. Instruct the patient to:

- Remove the cap and shake inhaler.
- Breathe out gently and make a seal around the mouthpiece (Figure 7.15). As they start to inhale, press the top of the canister to actuate the inhaler and hold their breath for a minimum of 10 seconds and then exhale gently.
- Wait 30 seconds before taking another inhalation.

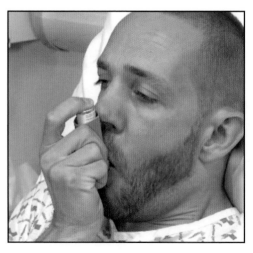

Figure 7.15 Inhaler technique.

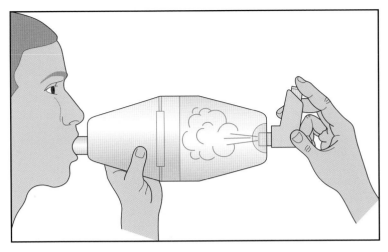

Figure 7.16 Volumetric spacer device.

Using inhaler with volumatic spacer. Instruct the patient to:
- Shake the inhaler and insert it into the end of the spacer (Figure 7.16).
- Place their mouth around the mouthpiece of the spacer and press the canister once to release the drug into the spacer.
- Breathe in and out slowly five times and then remove the spacer from the mouth. The valve of the mouthpiece will move in and out as the patient breathes.
- Wait 30 seconds before administering a second dose.
  1. Replace the cap on the patient's inhaler and return it to usual storage area.
  2. If the inhaler contains steroids advise/assist the patient to rinse their mouth following administration ➡ **PFP3**.
  3. Ensure the patient is comfortable.
  4. Spacers should be washed with clean water once a month or if visibly soiled. They should be left to air dry ➡ **PFP4**.
  5. Document that the inhaler has been administered as per local policy and evaluate its effectiveness.

➡️Points for practice

PFP1 Adjuncts such as a volumatic spacer device can be used for patients who are very breathless or find it difficult to coordinate pressing the canister and breathing (see Figure 7.16). It also helps to reduce deposition of the powder in the throat. Specialist respiratory nurses will be able to advise on other suitable inhaler devices should the patient have difficulty using a metered dose inhaler.

PFP2 Only registered nurses may administer medications. Student nurses may only participate in the administration of inhaled medications under the direct supervision of a registered nurse. A registered nurse must countersign student signatures.

PFP3 Rinsing the mouth after inhalation of steroids reduces deposition of the powder in the mouth, which can lead to candida (thrush) infections.

PFP4 Spacers should be replaced every 6–12 months as the volumatic valve wears out.

7.18 Variable dose intravenous infusions

Some patients are prescribed variable dose (commonly known as 'sliding scale') intravenous infusions that require variable rates each hour according to physiological parameters. These are prescribed for medications that need to respond to changes in the patient's condition. For example, the rate of an insulin infusion may need to be adjusted according to the blood glucose levels or glyceryl tri-nitrate adjusted in response to chest pain scores and blood pressure.

In these cases the prescription must state clearly the parameters for titration by the nurse. For example, sliding scale insulin regimens will specify the number of units of insulin per hour to be administered acording to the blood glucose level that hour. Only registered nurses who have undertaken additional training relating to intravenous therapy may change the settings on intravenous pumps or syringe drivers with such regimes. Students may not change the hourly rate (even under direct supervision). See Chapter 4 for more information about intravenous infusions.

Bibliography/Suggested reading

British National Formulary (BNF). London: Royal Pharmaceutical Society of Great Britain and RCPCH Publications,BMJ Publishing Group.

This is published twice a year and so the most recent edition should be used. This publication lists all medications and their classification. It identifies indications, cautions, contraindications and dose for each medication.(Available at www.bnf.org – in order to access the latest edition, registration is necessary at this website, but there is no charge for this.)

Care Quality Commission, 2010. The safer management of controlled drugs. Annual Report 2009. CQC, London [online]. Available from: http://www.cqc.org.uk/_db/_documents/20100802_CDAR_2009_FINAL_201008104818.pdf (accessed 30.05.11.).

This report describes how the arrangements for safer management of controlled drugs have continued to develop and reports on the progress with the recommendations made in the 2008 report. It identifies examples of good practice which are useful for all practitioners involved in the administration of controlled drugs

Cocoman, A., Murray, J., 2010. Recognizing the evidence and changing practice on injection sites. British Journal of Nursing 19 (18), 1170–1174.

This paper presents a comprehensive review of the evidence-base for using the ventrogluteal injection site for intramuscular injections in place of the more commonly used dorsogluteal site (upper outer quadrant). Despite the agreement that the ventrogluteal site is preferable there is a reluctance to use this site in practice. The paper sets out to discuss the reasons for this and presents some solutions to help change practice

Department of Health, 2007. Safer management of controlled drugs: a guide to good practice in secondary care (England). DoH, London.

This sets out systems for procuring, storing, supplying, transporting, prescribing, administering, recording and safely disposing of CDs whilst ensuring that patients who require CDs have appropriate and convenient access. The document is organised in chapters dealing with legislative requirements and guiding principles

Department of Health, 2011. The 'never events' list 2011/12 [online]. Available from: http://www.dh.gov.uk/prod_consum_dh/groups/dh_digitalassets/documents/digitalasset/dh_124580.pdf last accessed 6/6/2011.

This guidance sets out the policy for reporting on the 25 'never events' which the DH states are serious and largely preventable. 9 of the 25 'never events' relate to medicines. The report identifies national guidlines available to reduce errors and promote good practice in relation to each 'never event'

Greenway, K., 2004. Using the ventrogluteal site for intramuscular injection. Nursing Standard 18 (25), 39–42.

This article discusses the use of the ventrogluteal site for intramuscular injection in place of the dorsogluteal (upper, out quadrant of the buttock) that was traditionally used. Includes the rationale for use of this site, clear diagrams to locate the ventrogluteal site and discusses potential complications when using the dorsogluteal site

Hunter, J., 2008. Subcutaneous injection technique. Nursing Standard 22 (21), 41–44.

This article provides a step-by-step approach to administering a subcutaneous injection with underpinning rationale for the key principles

Hunter, J., 2008. Intramuscular injection techniques. Nursing Standard 22 (24), 35–40.

This paper describes the technique for intramuscular injection with rationale for the key principles

King, L., 2003. Subcutaneous insulin injection technique. Nursing Standard 17 (34), 45–52.

This article discusses the injection technique required to ensure insulin is not inadvertently injected into muscle. It discusses the rationale for the 'pinch up' method, which reduces the risk of inadvertent intramuscular injection by lifting the subcutaneous tissue away from the muscle.

Kyle, G., 2009. Practice Questions: solving your clinical dilemmas. Nursing Times 105 (2), 16.

This article tries to answer whether suppositories should be inserted blunt end or pointed end first, based on the evidence available

Jevon, P., Payne, E., Higgins, D., Endacott, R., 2010. Medicines management s guide for nurses. Wiley-Blackwell, Chichester.

This book covers legal and safety issues, prescribing and different systems of administration. It also covers errors and pharmacology of common medications

Lawson, E., Hennefer, D., 2010. medicines management in adult nursing. Learning Matters, Exeter.

This covers a wide range of medicines management issues such as legislation; ethical frameworks; drug calculations, pharmacology and partnership working

National Asthma Council Australia, 2010. Using your inhaler. [online]. Available from: http://www.nationalasthma.org.au/content/view/548/984/ (accessed 30.05.11.).

This website has a series of short video clips demonstrating how to use a variety of inhalers

National Institute for Health and Clinical Excellence, 2009. Medicines adherence. NICE Clinical Guideline 76 NICE, London.

This guideline makes recommendations about how practitioners can enable patients to make informed decisions about their medication

National Patient Safety Agency, 2009. Safety in doses: improving the use of medicines in the NHS. [online]. Available from: http://www.nrls.npsa.nhs.uk/resources/?entryid45=61625 (accessed 06.06.11.).

This reports analyses reported medicines safety incidents from 2007 and identifies lessons learned from these. It identifies good practice in risk management and promotes initiatives to reduce medicines errors

NHS Education for Scotland Toolkit for the self administration of medicines (SAM) in hospital. [online]. Available from: www.nes.scot.nhs.uk/media/6798/samsbrochure.pdf (accessed 30.05.11.).

A useful toolkit identifying best practice when implementing a self administration policy in hospital. It includes useful forms and information for staff and patients

Nisbet, A.C., 2006. Intramuscular gluteal injections in the increasingly obese population: retrospective study. BMJ 332, 637–638.

A study to measure ventrogluteal depth in 100 patients. It concluded that standard green and blue needles do not reach the gluteal muscle in a considerable number of patients, which results in the injection being given subcutaneously instead of intramuscularly. It recommends that the vastus lateralis muscle may be a better choice in obese patients.

Nursing and Midwifery Council, 2007. Standards for medicines management. NMC, London.

These standards give an overview of the principles of medicines management that should be followed. They were reviewed in 2010 – although numbers were added to each section for ease of reference, the content has not been changed

O'Brien, M., Spires, A., Andrews, K., 2011. Introduction to medicines management in nursing. Learning Matters, Exeter.

A good introductory text that covers principles of administration; basic pharmacology, legal and professional issues and drug calculations. It has relevant student actvities and worked examples/answers in each chapter

Olsen, J., Giangrasso, A., Shrimpton, D., Dillon, M., Cunningham, S., 2010. Dosage calculations for nurses. Pearson, Harlow.

One of the numerous books available to help with drug calculations. This text has numerous examples, exercises and think points. It has the added bonus of a companion website with additional drug calculations exercises and study skills tips

Pratt, R.J., Hoffman, P.N., Robb, F.F., 2005. The need for skin preparation prior to injection: point-counterpoint. British Journal of Infection Control 6 (4), 8–20.

An interesting debate about the need or otherwise for skin preparation prior to injection. Both sides of the argument are presented with rationale/evidence. It concludes that skin preparation is probably not necessary in healthy individuals with visibly clean skin but is recommended for injections in the thigh, for elderly and immunocompromised hospital patients and when injections are close to colonised wounds/lesions

Pratt, R.J., Pellowe, C.M., Wilson, J.A., et al, 2007. Epic2: national evidence-based guidelines for preventing healthcare-associated infections in NHS hospitals in England. Journal of Hospital Infection 65 (1) suppl 1: S1–S64.

These national evidenced-based guidelines set out the broad principles of best practice for preventing HCAI in NHS hospitals in England. The document describes key principles for preventing infections and the required interventions

Ware 2 Care, 2008. Medication administration for nurses:adult, second ed. CD.

This CD is interactive and provides the opportunity for students to undertake drug calculations and pharmacology quizzes and engage in simulated drug rounds. Whilst feedback on specific errors is not given, the activities certainly help to provide some structured and fairly realistic exercises relating to medication administration

Watkinson, S., Seewoodhary, R., 2008. Adminsitering eye medications. Nursing Standard 22 (18), 42–48.

This article has a good section about types of medication and model of action for ophthalmic conditions.

Wynaden, D., Landsborough, I., Chapman, R., McGowan, S., Lapsley, J., Finn, M., 2005. Establishing best practice guidelines for administration of intramuscular injections in the adult: a systematic review of the literature. Contemporary Nurse 20, 267–277.

This Australian paper presents a comprehensive review of approximately 150 articles in order to produce these best practice guidelines. The guidelines address all aspects of intramuscular injection including; choice of site, needle size, volume of medication, techniques to reduce discomfort, skin cleansing and angle, and speed of injection

Chapter 8

Elimination

©2012 Elsevier Ltd.

8.1 Observation of faeces

Principles

Normal faeces (also known as 'stool') is brown, soft and formed; it has an odour, but should not be offensive smelling. When observing faeces, the following should be noted and any abnormality reported. the classifications of the bristol stool chart (Figure 8.1) are used in many clinical areas.

- Amount – particularly if diarrhoea, as patients may lose a lot of fluid this way.

- Frequency – the 'normal' frequency will vary from patient to patient.

- Consistency – the normal consistency is soft and formed. The following should be noted: hard faeces (constipation); liquid (diarrhoea); mucus evident (ulcerative colitis or Crohn's disease); fatty, offensive smelling and floats (steatorrhoea, seen in biliary disease); whether parasites are present.

- Colour – a pale, putty colour suggests the absence of bile pigments. The presence of bright-red blood may indicate bleeding from haemorrhoids or rectal bleeding. If the stool appears black and tarry in consistency (melaena), this indicates digested blood from the stomach or small intestine. If the stool is black and hard in consistency, this may be the result of iron medication.

- Pain/discomfort associated with a bowel action.

- Flatus – the presence of this indicates gut motility and is an important observation following abdominal surgery.

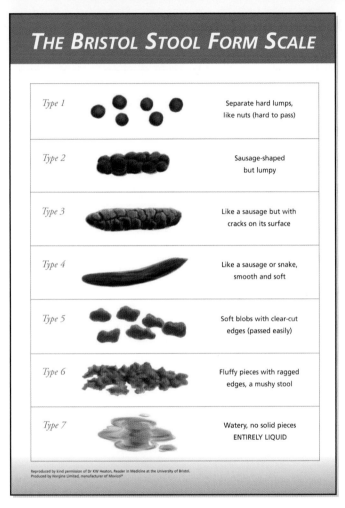

Figure 8.1 Bristol Stool Chart. Reproduced by kind permission of Dr K. W. Heaton, Reader in Medicine at the University of Bristol. © 2000 Norgine Pharmaceuticals Ltd

8.2 Obtaining a specimen of faeces

Preparation

Patient	Equipment	Nurse
• Explain the procedure, to gain consent and cooperation.	• Sterile specimen container with spoon-shaped spatula • Specimen bag • Pathology request form or computer print out • Patient detail label	• Put on apron and gloves • Additional protective clothing may be necessary if indicated by the patient's condition (see Ch. 1).

Procedure

1. Ask/assist the patient to use a bedpan or commode (see pp 231–234). Offer/ assist with hand washing.

2. Open the sterile specimen container with atached spoon-shaped spatula (usually attached to the lid) ➡ **PFP1**.

3. Use the spatula to remove a small quantity of faeces from the bedpan. Place the faeces and the spatula into the container and secure the lid. See Figure 8.2.

4. Complete the patient's details on the label of the container ➡ **PFP2**.

5. Place the specimen container in the specimen bag, seal it and insert the pathology request form into the pocket.

6. Dispose of faeces and place bedpan in the washer or disposal system as appropriate. If used, clean the commode according to local policy.

7. Remove gloves and apron and wash hands.

8. Place specimen in the designated area to await transport to the laboratory.

9. Document that specimen has been collected.

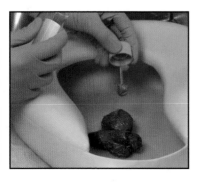

Figure 8.2 Specimen of faeces

➡ Points for practice

PFP1 If no spoon-shaped spatlua is provided, use a disposable wooden tongue depressor.

PFP2 If a series of specimens is being collected, ensure the correct sequence is identified. This may be requested in order to detect bleeding from the gastrointestinal tract.

8.3 Administration of an enema

Preparation

Patient
- Explain the procedure, to gain consent and cooperation
- Ask/assist the patient to remove clothing below the waist and lie in the left lateral position ➡ **PFP1**
- Cover the patient with a blanket
- Place an absorbent pad under the buttocks

Equipment
- Prescription chart ➡ **PFP2**
- Enema as prescribed ➡ **PFP3**
- Cardboard tray/receiver
- Gauze swabs/tissues
- Lubricant
- Bedpan or commode, plus toilet paper.

Nurse
- Put on apron and gloves
- Draw screens to ensure privacy
- Additional protective clothing may be necessary if indicated by the patient's condition (see Ch. 1)

Procedure

1. Check the anal area for soreness, haemorrhoids or skin tags. If present seek advice before proceeding.
2. Remove the cover or removable tip from the nozzle and lubricate the tip.
3. Ask the patient to relax and take deep breaths.
4. Part the buttocks with the left hand. With the right hand, hold the nozzle of the enema and *gently* insert it through the anus and into the anal canal ➡ **PFP4** (Figure 8.3).
5. Squeeze the bag/pack until all the contents have been deposited – some packs may be rolled (like a tube of toothpaste) to expel the last of the contents.

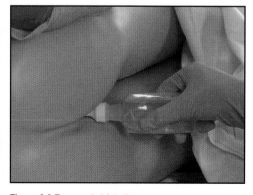

Figure 8.3 Enema administration

6. While still squeezing gently withdraw the nozzle ➡ **PFP5**.

7. Wipe away any residual lubricant and leave the patient dry. Cover the patient. Be aware that the patient may feel faint and/or nauseous.

8. **Evacuant enema:** ask the patient to hold the enema for as long as possible but the effect is likely to be rapid. Assist the patient onto the bedpan or commode as necessary (see pp 231–234).

9. **Retention enema** (drug administration): the patient should be instructed to stay in the left lateral position for at least 30 minutes to aid retention and absorption of the fluid. Raising the foot of the bed may also help.

10. After the patient has opened their bowels, observe the nature of the faeces (see p. 225).

11. Dispose of faeces and place bedpan in the washer or disposal system as appropriate. If used, clean the commode according to local policy. Offer/assit with hand washing.

12. Remove gloves and apron and wash hands.

13. Document/report the result of the enema.

➡Points for practice

PFP1 It is necessary for the patient to be in the left lateral position because of the position of the rectum.

PFP2 If the enema is for drug administration (retention enema), this must be prescribed and checked as described on pp. 183–185.

PFP3 Some enemas may need to be warmed before administration. Do this by placing it in a bowl of warm water. Test a little on your forearm before administration to check it is not too hot.

PFP4 Because the patient needs to be in the left lateral position even left-handed nurses must use their right hand to insert the nozzle of the enema.

PFP5 Keeping the bag rolled/squeezed while removing the nozzle prevents fluid running back into the bag.

8.4 Assisting with a bedpan

Preparation

Patient
- Assess the patient to determine whether a standard or slipper bedpan is required ➡ **PFP1**
- Ensure privacy and dignity are maintained throughout

Equipment
- Bedpan and cover
- Toilet paper

Nurse
- An apron should be worn. Gloves must be worn when handling the bedpan and assisting with toileting
- Additional protective clothing may be necessary if indicated by the patient's condition (see Ch. 1)

Procedure

1. Take the covered bedpan and toilet paper to the bedside.
2. Ensure the screens are completely drawn.
3. Raise the bed to a safe working height (see Ch. 12).
4. Ask/assist the patient to raise their buttocks and place the bedpan underneath the patient's pelvis – wide rim of bedpan under the buttocks, and narrow area between legs ➡ **PFP2**
5. When using a slipper bedpan (Figure 8.4B), if the patient cannot raise their buttocks assist the patient to roll to one side and slip the bedpan underneath from the side; talcum powder applied to the bedpan will assist this process. The handle end should be positioned between the legs.
6. For female patients, make sure that the legs are slightly apart, otherwise urine may trickle down the legs onto the sheet. For male patients, ensure that the penis is positioned over the bedpan ➡ **PFP3**.
7. Preserve the patient's privacy and dignity by covering the patient with the bedclothes.

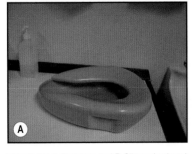
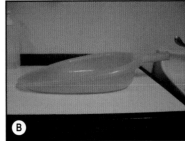

Figure 8.4 A Bed pan and B Slipper bed pad

8. Ensure the call bell is within easy reach and leave the patient but remain within earshot.

9. When the patient has finished, provide assistance with wiping/cleansing as necessary. Remove the bedpan and make the patient comfortable ➡ **PFP4**

10. Dispose of excreta safely and measure the urine if patient is on a fluid balance chart

11. Place the bedpan in the washer or disposal system as appropriate.

12. Remove gloves and apron and wash hands.

13. Offer a the patient bowl of water to wash their hands. Return the bedside table and belongings to within easy reach of patient.

14. Document urine output and bowel action (see p. 225 – observation of faeces skill).

➡ Points for practice

PFP1 The slipper bedpan (Figure 8.4B) is used for patients who are unable to sit on a standard bedpan. Its wedge shape makes it easier to insert and more comfortable to use. It is inserted with the handle between the patient's legs and the smooth, flat part underneath the buttocks.

PFP2 Dependent patients will require two nurses for this procedure.

PFP3 When using a slipper bedpan male patients may find it easier to use a urinal as well (see p. 235).

PFP4 After a bowel action the perianal area should be washed and dried thoroughly.

8.5 Assisting with a commode

Preparation

Patient

- Explain the procedure, to gain consent and cooperation
- Clear the bed area and draw the screens to ensure privacy
- Assess the patient's level of mobility and ability to assist with the procedure

Equipment

- Commode containing clean bedpan.
- Toilet paper.

Nurse

- An apron should be worn. Gloves should be worn when assisting with toileting and removing the commode
- Additional protective clothing may be necessary if indicated by the patient's condition (see Ch. 1).

Procedure

1. Take the commode (with seat in place, covering bedpan) and toilet paper to the bedside ➡ **PFP1**.

2. Ensure the screens are completely drawn.

3. Check the bed brakes are on.

4. Position the commode so that the patient has sufficient room to get out of bed without banging their legs, and apply the brakes.

5. Assist the patient to a sitting position on the edge of the bed.

6. Offer slippers and dressing gown and djust the bed to enable the patient to stand easily.

7. Assist the patient as necessary to transfer to the commode.

8. If the patient is frail, position the commode so that the patient is close to and facing the bed. Apply the brakes and place a pillow at the edge of the bed for the patient to lean on (Figure 8.5).

9. Ensure the patient has access to a call bell. Provide privacy by leaving but remain within earshot.

10. When the patient has finished, assist with cleaning/washing as necessary and help the patient back to bed. Re-arrange the pillows, bed clothes and bed table as necessary.

11. If appropriate measure the volume of urine and note the bowel action. Dispose of excreta and place the bedpan in the washer or disposal system.

12. Clean the commode and indicate that it has been cleaned, according to local policy ➡ **PFP2**.

13. Remove gloves and apron and wash your hands.

14. Take the patient a bowl of water to wash for hand washing.

15. Document urine output and bowel action according to local policy.

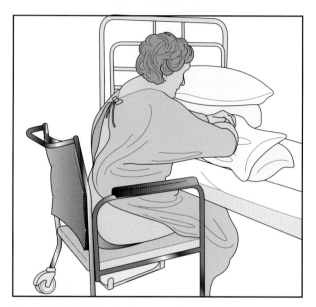

Figure 8.5 Frail patient using the commode

➡ Points for practice

PFP1 If there is no toilet roll holder, placing it in a bowl or receiver will prevent it rolling off the commode when being wheeled to the bedside.

PFP2 Local policy for cleaning the commode may vary but usually involves cleaning with hot water with detergent followed by thorough drying. The use of detergent is important as it breaks up grease and improves the ability of water to remove it so that approximately 80% of micro-organisms are removed (Wilson 2006). Local policy may require you to place a strip of coloured tape on equipment after cleaning to indicate that it is clean. This is dated and signed by the person who cleaned it.

8.6 Assisting with a urinal

Preparation

Patient
- Explain the procedure, to gain consent and cooperation
- Assess the patient's level of mobility/dexterity and ability to assist with the procedure
- Ensure privacy and dignity are maintained

Equipment
- Urinal ➡ **PFP1**
- Cover/paper hand towel to cover the urinal

Nurse
- An apron and gloves should be worn
- Additional protective clothing may be necessary if indicated by the patient's condition (see Ch. 1).

Procedure

1. Ask/assist the patient to adopt an appropriate position. Standing is often best if this is possible ➡ **PFP2**.

2. If necessary, assist the patient to hold the urinal and position the penis inside.

3. When the patient has finished urinating, assist as necessary with clothing and returning to bed/chair.

4. Cover the urinal and take to the sluice/dirty utility room. Measure urine if the patient is on a fluid balance chart.

5. Dispose of the urine (unless it is being collected, e.g. 24-hour urine collection – see p. 248) and discard the urinal or clean it as per local policy.

6. Remove gloves and apron and wash hands. Record amount on fluid balance chart (where applicable) (see p. 237).

7. Offer the patient hand washing.

➡ Points for practice

PFP1 Many patients prefer to keep a urinal at the bedside. This should be kept in a holder attached to the bed, not on the bedside locker or bed table.

PFP2 If the patient is sitting on the edge of the bed, make sure the brakes are on and the bed is at a suitable height for their feet to touch the floor.

8.7 Monitoring fluid balance

Preparation

Patient
- Explain why fluid balance monitoring is required and the need to measure urine
  ➡ **PFP1**

Equipment
- Fluid balance chart
- Measuring jug

Nurse
- Apron and gloves should be worn if handling body fluids
- Additional protective clothing may be necessary if indicated by the patient's condition (see Ch. 1)

Procedure

1. All oral, intravenous and nasogastric intake should be recorded on the fluid intake side of the fluid balance chart (Figure 8.6). If continuous bladder irrigation (see p. 265) is in progress it is usually recorded on a separate chart. The urine output must be transposed to the fluid balance chart.

2. In the **output section** record: all urine output, diarrhoea or stoma output, nasogastric aspiration and vomit. Any other output that can be measured or weighed (e.g. wound drainage) should also be recorded.

3. The sections labelled **'Other'** should be annotated according to individual patient requirements (see Figure 8.6).

4. Patients who are independent in meeting their oral needs should be asked to note the nature and quantity of their oral fluid intake. If the patient is not independent, the nurse must do this.

5. Patients who are independent will often be able to measure and chart their own urine output. If they are unable to do this themselves, provide them with a clearly labelled jug to leave in the sluice/toilet area for the nurse to measure.

6. Assess individual needs and monitor and record input and output at regular intervals ➡ **PFP2**

7. A new chart will be needed for each 24-hour period. The fluid intake and output for the previous day is then totalled and the balance is calculated ➡ **PFP3**

			Fluid balance chart				

Hospital/Ward: ST. SWITHINS **Date:** 21.09.2012

Hospital number: 1928374

Surname: PATEL **Forenames:** RASHID

Date of birth: 13.12.1951 **Sex:** FEMALE

	Fluid intake			Fluid output			
Time(hrs)	Oral	IV	Other (specify route)	Urine	Vomit	Other (specify)	
01.00						Diarrhoea	
02.00	200						
03.00							
04.00							
05.00							
06.00							
07.00	180			300	250		
08.00							
09.00	100				800		
10.00		125	N/Saline				
11.00		125					
12.00		125					
13.00	180	125		25			
14.00		125	Cannula tissued				
15.00	180						
16.00						450	
17.00		250	Glucose Saline				
18.00		250		35	650		
19.00		250			NG tube inserted		
20.00		250					
21.00		125	Glucose Saline +KCl				
22.00		125					
23.00		125				225	
24.00		125			450		
TOTAL	840	2,125		360	2150	675	

KEY:
NBM = NIL BY MOUTH
B/F = BROUGHT FORWARD

ALL MEASURMENTS IN MILLILITRES (ML.)
TOTAL INPUT = 2965
TOTAL OUTPUT = 3185
Balance = –220 ML.

Figure 8.6 Fluid balance chart

➡Points for practice

PFP1 If the patient is on a fluid restriction (e.g. in renal failure), all oral fluid, including jelly, yoghurt and milk taken with cereal, has to be recorded.

PFP2 Accurate recording of intake and output is vital to be able to calculate the fluid balance. Gaps in recording (e.g. if the patient has been to theatre or for a test) make the balance inaccurate. In acute situations it may be necessary to measure the urine output every hour.

PFP3 If there is more intake than output, the patient is in a positive fluid balance. If there is more output than intake, the patient is in a negative fluid balance. In some patients, especially renal patients who do not pass urine, changes in weight will be used to calculate fluid loss or gain.

8.8 Observation of urine

Preparation

Patient
- Explain the procedure to gain cooperation and consent

Equipment
- Clean container/jug for the urine

Nurse
- An apron and gloves should be worn
- Additional protective clothing may be necessary if indicated by the patient's condition (see Ch. 1)

Procedure

1. Ask the patient to provide a urine sample.
2. If necessary, transfer the specimen to a clear container or jug ➡ **PFP1**.
3. Observe the urine for colour, concentration, odour and the presence of particles ➡ **PFP2**.
4. Dispose of urine safely. Clean or dispose of the container/jug according to local policy.
5. Remove gloves and apron and wash hands.
6. Document findings and report abnormalities.

➡ Points for practice

PFP1 A clear container or jug should be used if possible to enable the colour and clarity of the urine (e.g. presence of particles) to be assessed.

PFP2 Normal urine is straw-coloured and clear. Dark-yellow urine indicates that it is more concentrated than normal. The smell of ammonia will develop if the urine specimen is left standing. A malodorous or 'fishy' smell and/or particles in the urine may indicate a urine infection. Any blood in the urine should always be reported, although in female patients menstruation may be the cause.

8.9 Application of a penile sheath

Preparation

Patient

- Explain the procedure to gain consent and cooperation
- Ensure complete privacy and dignity

Equipment/environment

- Sheath sizing tool and correctly sized penile sheath ➡ **PFP1**
- Card or paper with a hole cut ➡ **PFP2**
- Catheter drainage bag or leg bag as appropriate
- Warm water, soap, disposable washcloth and towel

Nurse

- Hands must be clean and an apron and non sterile gloves should be worn
- Additional protective clothing may be necessary if indicated by the patient's condition (see Ch. 1).

Procedure

1. Assist the patient into a supine position.

2. Prepare the catheter drainage bag.

3. Expose the patient's genitalia and place the penis gently on a towel. Measure the penis and select the correct size sheath ➡ **PFP3**.

4. Gently grasp the shaft of the penis. If the patient has not been circumcised, retract the foreskin.

5. Wash the tip of the penis at the urethral meatus and work outwards.

6. Wash the shaft of the penis in a downward stroke.

7. Repeat until the penis is clean, then rinse and dry gently. Leave to air dry for a few minutes.

8. If using a skin protection wipe, allow to dry according to manufacturer's instructions before applying the sheath. Do not use powders or creams as this will affect adhesion.

9. Ensure the foreskin is returned to its normal position.

10. Clip hair at the base of the penis as this is likely to prevent adhesion ➡ **PFP4**.

11. Place the penis through the hole cut in the card or paper ➡ **PFP2**. Gently press on the pubic hairs to keep them away from the adhesive during application.

12. Apply the sheath according to the manufacturer's guidelines. Application technique will depend on whether you are using a one-piece or two-piece sheath ➡ **PFP5**.

13. If using a leg bag, attach it to the leg first to avoid sheath twisting.

14. Readjust bedclothes and ensure the patient is comfortable

15. Dispose of clinical waste appropriately. Remove gloves and apron and wash hands thoroughly.

16. Observe for leakage from the bag/tubing.

17. Document application of sheath, noting the condition of the penile skin, size and type of penile sheath, and any difficulties during the procedure.

18. Continue to check and document skin integrity at least once daily when attending to patient hygiene ➡ **PFP6**. Advise the patient to wear loose clothing and underwear.

➡Points for practice

PFP1 The correct sizing of a penile sheath is important as if it is too small there may be difficulties with fitting and it may restrict urinary flow and blood to the penis. If it is too loose, it will crease and leakages will occur.

PFP2 A card or tissue paper with a hole for the penis acts as pubic hair protector. Some companies provide sheath packages, which include a pubic hair shield (Robinson 2006).

PFP3 Sizing tools for correct selection of penile sheath come as either a tape measure or a card with cut-out sections in various sizes. If using a cut-out it must be measured with the cut-out section on the upper surface of the penis and not underneath. Always use the sizing tool supplied by the same company as the penile sheath as companies use different measuring scales (Robinson 2006). Measurement should be taken from the shaft of a flaccid penis, just behind the glans. It the penis is erect then the circumference should be measured and the penile sheath also fitted in this state. Penile retraction (penis retracted into pelvic cavity), is not uncommon in older men and its extent must be determined before attempting to attach a sheath. If partial, a shorter sheath may be appropriate, but if there is complete retraction a penile sheath is not appropriate as it is likely to roll off as the penis retracts, causing disconnection and leakage.

PFP4 It is important that hair is clipped as shaving could make the skin sore. Clipping prevents pubic hair from around the base of the penis adhering to the adhesive strip, which will cause discomfort if pulled.

PFP5 Penile sheaths are available in latex and non-latex (silicone) materials, can be one-piece or two-piece, are available in short and standard lengths, have various penile shaft fittings and have anti-kinking devices (Booth and Lee 2005). Sheaths in silicone materials are recommended because of the risk of latex allergy. One-piece sheaths have adhesive already applied to the inside of the sheath. Fitting instructions vary; therefore, it is important to carefully follow the manufacturer's instructions.

Two-piece sheaths come with a double-sided hydrocolloid strip. One side of the strip adheres to the penis shaft and the other to the sheath. The adhesive strip should be gently stretched and then attached to the shaft of the penis beginning from behind the glans in a spiral direction. Ensure the sides meet. The sheath is then rolled over the shaft of the penis adhering to the outer side of the strip (Robinson 2006).

PFP6 Skin soreness or breakdown on the shaft of the penis can be caused by poor hygiene, latex allergies and pulling or rough handling of the sheath. If the skin on or around the penis becomes damaged, use of a sheath should be discontinued until healing has occurred.

8.10 Urinalysis

Preparation

Patient
- Ask/assist the patient to provide a urine specimen
- If catheterised, obtain a catheter specimen (see p. 246).

Equipment/Environment
- Fresh urine specimen in clean container/jug
  ➡ **PFP1**
- Urine reagent sticks
- Watch with a secondhand

Nurse
- An apron and gloves should be worn
- Additional protective clothing may be necessary if indicated by the patient's condition (see Ch. 1)

Procedure

1. Check the expiry date of the reagent sticks and make sure that you are familiar with the manufacturer's instructions for use.

2. Remove a stick, making sure that you do not touch the coloured reagent pads with your hands. Replace the lid ➡ **PFP2**.

3. Dip the stick into the urine so that the reagent pads are completely covered. Remove straight away and slowly draw the edge of the stick across the top of the container/jug to remove excess urine ➡ **PFP3**.

4. Note the time on your watch. Accurate timing according to the manufacturer's instructions is crucial.

5. When the correct period of time has elapsed, read off the results by holding the stick alongside (but not touching) the pot and comparing the colour of each reagent pad with those displayed on the side (Figure 8.7). Make a mental note of the results ➡ **PFP4**.

Urine reagent sticks commonly test for the following:
- **Specific gravity** (SG: normal range 1001–1035). A raised SG may indicate concentrated urine due to dehydration; a low SG may indicate renal disease or diabetes insipidus (Rigby and Gray 2006).

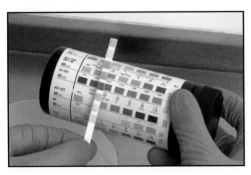

Figure 8.7 Matching the reagent pads in urinalysis

- **pH** (normal range 4.5–8.0). Normal urine is slightly acidic; a low pH may indicate respiratory or metabolic acidosis and a high pH may indicate respiratory or metabolic alkalosis. Some drugs can affect the urinary pH: ascorbic acid can make the urine more acidic and sodium bicarbonate, potassium citrate and sodium citrate can make the urine more alkaline (Skinner 2005).

- **Protein, glucose, ketones, blood and bilirubin**. All of these are negative in normal urine. The presence of these abnormalities might indicate the following (Rigby and Gray 2006):
  - Protein (proteinuria) – urinary tract infection, pyelonephritis, pre-eclampsia, congestive cardiac failure.
  - Glucose (glycosuria) – diabetes mellitus, acute pancreatitis, Cushing's syndrome or sometimes in pregnancy.
  - Ketones (ketonuria) – excessive fat metabolism due to diabetic ketoacidosis, vomiting or severe dieting/starvation.
  - Blood (haematuria) – kidney disorders (e.g. glomerulonephritis), disorders of the urinary tract (e.g. kidney stones, tumours, infection), trauma or menstruation.
  - Bilirubin – liver disease (e.g. hepatitis) or biliary tract obstruction (e.g. gall stones, carcinoma of the head of pancreas).

- **Nitrite and leucocytes.** These are both negative in normal urine. Urinary tract infection causes a rise in measured nitrite and leucocytes (Skinner 2005).

- Discard the used stick in the clinical waste and clean or dispose of the container/jug according to local policy.

- Remove gloves and apron and wash hands.

- Document urinalysis and report any abnormalities. Discuss the results with the patient as appropriate.

➡Points for practice

PFP1 The urine sample should be less than 2 hours old as urine left to stand will become alkaline (Skiner 2005).

PFP2 The lid of the reagent-sticks pot must always be replaced immediately after use to prevent moisture getting in.

PFP3 Removing excess urine from the testing stick will prevent it dripping and prevent the coloured reagent pads running into each other, which could give inaccurate readings.

PFP4 Make a mental note of the results or if necessary jot them down on a piece of paper. Do not take the patient's charts into the sluice/dirty utility room to prevent contamination or splashing with water.

8.11 Midstream specimen of urine

Preparation

Patient

- Explain the procedure, to gain consent and cooperation
- Ensure privacy and dignity are maintained
- MSU specimen specimen pot
  ➡ **PFP1**
- Gauze swabs, soap and water

Equipment/Environment

- Toilet, urinal or bedpan

Nurse

- Apron and gloves should be worn
- Paper towels
- If assisting the patient, additional protective clothing may be necessary if indicated by the patient's condition (see Ch. 1)

Procedure

Male patient

1. Instruct/assist the patient to retract the foreskin and clean the skin surrounding the urethral meatus with soap and water, using each gauze swab only once. Dry with paper towels.
2. Ask the patient to start urinating into the urinal/toilet then stop, pass the middle part of the stream into the specimen pot (10 ml is sufficient) and then finish urinating into the urinal/toilet.
3. Remove the funnel part of the pot and close the lid securely.

Female patient

1. Instruct/assist the patient to clean the urethral meatus with soap and water, using each gauze swab only once. Swab from front to back. Dry with paper towels.
2. Ask the patient to start urinating into the bed pan/toilet then stop, pass the middle part of the stream into the specimen pot (10 ml is sufficient) and then finish urinating into the urinal/toilet.
3. Remove the funnel part of the pot and close the lid securely.

Male and female patients

1. Discard all clincal waste safely and offer the patient hand washing facilities.
2. Remove gloves and apron and wash hands.
3. Complete patient details on the label ➡ **PFP2**. Place in a plastic specimen bag with the pathology request form (Figure 8.8) ➡ **PFP3**.
4. Place the specimen in the refrigerator for dispatch to the laboratory as soon as possible ➡ **PFP4**.
5. Document the date and time of the MSU according to local policy.

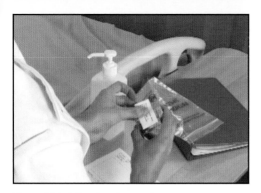

Figure 8.8 Labelling the urine specimen

➡️Points for practice

PFP1 Most specimen pots for midstream urine sample have a funnel attached to facilitate collection. This is removed and discarded in the clinical waste before the specimen is sent to the laboratory.

PFP2 The patient's details should include: surname, first name, date of birth, hospital number, ward (these are often on a computer generated label) and the type of specimen (i.e. MSU).

PFP3 If the test is ordered by computer, the request form should be printed off to accompany the sample.

PFP4 The specimen should be placed in a refrigerator because urine readily supports growth of bacteria. The multiplication of bacteria in specimens stored at room temperature can give misleading results (Wilson 2006).

8.12 Catheter specimen of urine

Preparation

Patient

- Explain the procedure, to gain consent and cooperation
- Maintain dignity and privacy throughout the procedure

Equipment/Environment

- Alcohol-impregnated swab
- Non-toothed clamp
  ➡ **PFP1**
- Orange (25 G) needle and sharps bin ➡ **PFP2**
- A 20 ml syringe
- Sterile universal specimen container

Nurse

- Hands must be washed and dried thoroughly
- An apron and gloves should be worn
- Additional protective clothing may be necessary if indicated by the patient's condition (see Ch. 1)

Procedure

1. If there is no urine present in the catheter tubing, apply a non-toothed clamp below the sampling port for 15–20 minutes to allow urine to collect.

2. Clean the sampling port on the tubing with the alcohol-impregnated swab and allow it to dry.

3. Insert the needle or syringe into the sampling port and aspirate the required amount of urine ➡ **PFP3**. If a needle is being used, take care not to go right through the tubing and out the other side (Figure 8.9).

4. Remove the needle and discard into the sharps bin ➡ **PFP4**. Transfer the urine to the specimen pot and replace the lid securely.

5. Remove the clamp, if used, to allow free drainage.

6. Discard clinical waste safely. Remove gloves and apron and wash hands.

7. Label the specimen ➡ **PFP5** and place it in a plastic specimen bag with the laboratory request form ➡ **PFP6**.

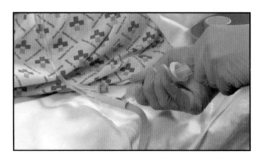

Figure 8.9 Obtaining a catheter specimen of urine

8. Place the specimen in the refrigerator for dispatch to the laboratory as soon as possible ➡ **PFP7**.

9. Document the date and time of specimen according to local policy

---

➡ Points for practice

PFP1 It is important that a non-toothed clamp is used to prevent damage to the tubing.

PFP2 Some catheter bags have a 'needle-free' sampling port as part of the tubing, which allows the syringe to be connected without a needle. If a needle is required, an orange needle (25 G) should be used.

PFP3 A 10 ml sample of urine is usually sufficient.

PFP4 If a needle has been used, remove it from the syringe before transferring the specimen, in case it falls into the pot and contaminates the specimen.

PFP5 The patient's details should include: surname; first name; date of birth; hospital number; ward; and date, time and type of specimen (i.e. CSU).

PFP6 If the test is ordered by computer, the request form should be printed off to accompany the sample.

PFP7 The specimen should be placed in a refrigerator because urine readily supports growth of bacteria. The multiplication of bacteria in specimens stored at room temperature can give misleading results (Wilson 2006).

8.13 24-hour urine collection

Preparation

Patient
- Explain the procedure, and assess the patient's ability to participate in obtaining the collection.

Equipment/Environment
- Urinal/bedpan as required and jug
- Bed/door sign indicating 24-hour urine collection is in progress, time started and completion time
- A 24-hour urine collection container (more than one may be required) ➡ **PFP1**

Nurse
- Apron and gloves should be worn
- Additional protective clothing may be necessary if indicated by the patient's condition (see Ch. 1)

Procedure

1. Label the container clearly with the patient's name, hospital number and ward.
2. When urine is passed, discard it. The 24-hour period begins at this point; write this time on the container.
3. Every time the patient passes urine, it is collected and placed in the container, which is stored in the sluice/dirty utility room ➡ **PFP2**.
4. If the patient is undertaking collection independently, check compliance and continued understanding.
5. Ask/assist the patient to empty their bladder at the end of the 24-hour collection period and write the time on the container.
6. Transfer the 24-hour urine collection and laboratory request form to the laboratory as soon as possible ➡ **PFP3**.
7. Clean or discard the jug according to local policy and remove sign from the bed/door.
8. Document the 24-hour urine collection according to local policy.

➡ Points for practice

PFP1 Bottles containing hydrochloric acid or nitric acid may be required if the collection is to test for: catecholamines (VMA), creatinine, calcium, phosphate, oxalate, citrate and magnesium. Plain bottles are usually required for: sodium, potassium, urea, creatinine, urate, albumin, Bence Jones Protein, and urine free cortisol. histamine. The volume of acid will need to be deducted from the total volume – check local policy.

PFP2 Should a sample of urine become contaminated or accidentally be discarded, the collection must be terminated and restarted.

PFP3 If the test is ordered by computer, the request form should be printed off to accompany the sample.

8.14 Early morning urine specimen

Preparation

Patient

- Explain the collection procedure and the need for three consecutive early morning specimens ➜ **PFP1**
- Ensure privacy and dignity are maintained
- The urine specimen should be collected as soon as possible after waking

Equipment/Environment

- Sterile universal specimen pot
- Gauze swabs, soap and water
- Paper towels
- Toilet, urinal or bedpan

Nurse

- Apron and gloves should be worn if the patient requires assistance
- Additional protective clothing may be necessary if indicated by the patient's condition (see Ch. 1).

Procedure

Ask/assist female patients to clean and dry the vulval area around the urinary meatus, using wet gauze swabs and paper towels. Ask male patients to retract the foreskin and clean and dry the end of the penis.

For cytology

Ask/assist the patient to hold the specimen pot in a gloved hand and pass the beginning and the end of the stream of urine into the pot ➜ **PFP2**. The middle of the stream should be passed into the toilet, bedpan or urinal ➜ **PFP3**. Repeat the procedure on the next two consecutive days if required.

For other test (e.g.TB, pregnancy)

1. Ask/assist the patient to hold the specimen pot in a gloved hand and pass the first part of the stream into the pot. The remainder of the stream should be passed into the toilet, urinal or bedpan.

2. Ensure the specimen pot is securely closed. Label the pot ➜ **PFP4** and place in a plastic specimen bag with the laboratory request form. Refrigerate until dispatch to the laboratory ➜ **PFP5**.

3. Document the date and time of specimen collection according to local policy.

4. The patient may be unaware of the possible diagnosis; deal with the patient's questions with sensitivity.

➡ Points for practice

PFP1 A urine specimen for cytology is requested when a malignancy is suspected. The patient may not be aware of this at this point and care must be taken to avoid unnecessary alarm.

PFP2 The first part and end of the stream of urine are collected as these are most likely to contain malignant cells if present in the bladder.

PFP3 If the patient is unable to stop and start the stream of urine, the bladder should be emptied completely into a sterile container and a small portion (10–20 ml) of that amount put into the specimen pot.

PFP4 The patient's details should include: surname; first name; date of birth; hospital number and ward. Each specimen must also be clearly labelled with the date and time, and numbered to ensure the correct sequence is known in the laboratory.

PFP5 The specimen should be placed in a refrigerator because urine readily supports growth of bacteria. The multiplication of bacteria in specimens stored at room temperature can give misleading results (Wilson 2006).

8.15 Female catheterisation

Preparation

Patient
- Explain the procedure, to gain consent and cooperation
- Ensure the patient's privacy and dignity are maintained throughout
- Ask/assist the patient to wash the perineal area and dry thoroughly

Equipment/Environment
- Clean trolley or other appropriate surface
- Sterile catheterisation pack ➡ **PFP1**
- Two urinary catheters of appropriate size ➡ **PFP2**
- Sachet of sterile 0.9% sodium chloride
- Catheter bag with stand/holder
- A 10 ml syringe and 10 ml ampoule of sterile water for injection
- Disposable waterproof absorbent pad
- Alcohol hand-rub or hand washing facilities
- Good light source
- Single use sterile anaesthetic gel
- Sterile universal specimen container

Nurse
- Wash and dry hands thoroughly
- An apron should be worn. Additional protective clothing may be necessary if indicated by the patient's condition (see Ch. 1)
- Two nurses may be necessary if the patient needs assistance to adopt the required position

Procedure

1. Take the prepared trolley to the patient's bedside and position it on the right or left depending on the nurse's dominant hand.

2. Raise the bed to a safe working height and ensure a good light source.

3. Ask/assist the patient to adopt a supine position with knees flexed and thighs relaxed to externally rotate the hip joints. If the patient is unable to adopt this position, assist her onto her side with her upper leg flexed at the hip and knee.

4. Arrange the bedclothes to expose the genital area, and place the disposable pad beneath the buttocks.

5. Wash your hands or clean them with alcohol hand-rub.

6. Maintaining asepsis, open the catheterisation pack and any additional packs and equipment.

7. Open the catheter, but do not remove it from its internal wrapping, and place it in the sterile receiver on the trolley. Expose the tip of the catheter by pulling off the top of the wrapper at the serrated edge.

8. Pour the sachet of 0.9% sodium chloride into the gallipot.

9. Open the catheter bag and arrange it at the side of the bed, ensuring that the catheter connection is easily accessible and remains sterile.

10. Draw up the amount of sterile water required to inflate the balloon ➡ **PFP3**.

11. Attach the nozzle to the anaesthetic lubricating gel.

12. Wash your hands or clean them with alcohol-based rub, and put on the sterile gloves ➡ **PFP4**.

13. Place sterile dressing towels onto the bed area between the patient's legs and over the patient's thighs.
14. Using a gauze swab and your non-dominant hand, retract the labia minora to expose the urethral meatus (Figure 8.10). This hand should be used to maintain labial separation until catheterisation has been completed.
15. Clean the perineal area with 0.9% sodium chloride, using a new gauze swab for each stroke and cleaning from the front towards the anus.
16. Gently insert the nozzle of the anaesthetic gel into the urethra. Squeeze the gel into the urethra, remove and discard the tube. Leave for approximately 5 minutes ➡ **PFP5**.
17. Place the receiver holding the catheter on the sterile towel between the patient's legs.
18. Holding the catheter so that the distal end remains in the receiver and gradually advancing it out of its wrapper, introduce the catheter into the urethra in an upward and backward direction for approximately 5–7 cm or until urine flows out of the catheter end. Advance the catheter a further 5 cm. Do not force the catheter ➡ **PFP6**.
19. Attach the syringe of water to the balloon port and inflate the balloon with the correct amount of water (see Figure 8.13 – in male catheterisation).

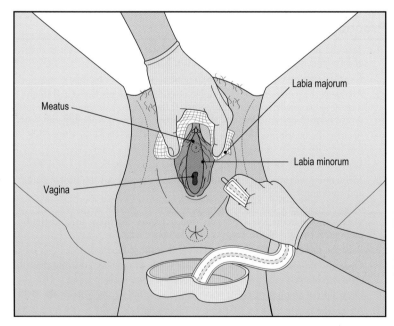

Figure 8.10 Female catheterisation

20. Gently withdraw the catheter until resistance is felt; the inflated balloon will hold it in place in the bladder

21. Maintaining asepsis, attach the catheter drainage bag and position it so that there is no pulling on the catheter ➡ **PFP7**. The catheter can be secured by using a securement device or by taping it to the patient's leg ➡ **PFP8**

22. Remove the sterile towel by tearing it on one side.

23. Ensure the catheter drainage bag is positioned below the patient's bladder ➡ **PFP9**.

24. Cover the patient and replace the bedclothes. Make sure the patient is dry and comfortable.

25. Place a small amount of urine (10–20 ml) into the specimen pot ➡ **PFP10**.

26. Dispose of equipment and clinical waste appropriately.

27. Measure and record the amount of urine contained in the receiver.

28. Remove gloves and apron and wash hands.

29. Document catheterisation in the patient's records ➡ **PFP11**

30. Send the specimen, with the request form, to the laboratory as soon as possible, for culture and sensitivity

31. If the patient's condition allows, encourage oral fluids ➡ **PFP12**. Document urine output on a fluid balance chart.

➡ Points for practice

PFP1 A catheterisation pack usually contains the following sterile items: kidney dish/receiver, dressing towels, gloves, gallipot and gauze swabs. If a catheterisation pack is not available, a sterile dressing pack containing gloves can be used and the other items added as required.

PFP2 When choosing the size of catheter to be inserted, choose the smallest size possible. The external diameter of the catheter shaft is measured in Charrière (ch) also known as French gauge (Fg) units. For most women a 12 ch/Fg or 14 ch/Fg will be adequate, although a larger size may be necessary if there is blood or sediment in the urine. A second catheter is useful in case catheterisation is unsuccessful with the first. Female length catheters are 23–26 cm. They reduce the risk of kinking and looping, and so allow more efficient drainage, and can also be more easily concealed if being used with a leg bag (Robinson 2006). However, they are not suitable for all women and male standard length catheters are recommended for women postoperatively, in those who are critically ill, immobile or clinically obese (RCN 2008). Moreover, the National Patient Safety Agency (2009) recommend that female catheters should only be available in specialist units meaning that females in general ward settings may have standard length (male) catheters inserted.

PFP3 The volume of water required will be indicated on the catheter. A balloon size of 10 ml is recommended for the routine drainage of clear urine, as this is usually sufficient to retain the catheter. Larger balloon sizes may irritate the bladder and cause bladder spasm and bypassing of urine (Nazarko 2010). 30–80 ml balloons are used in specialised catheters in urology units and should not be used for routine catheterisation. It is important to use the exact amount of water as indicated on the catheter.

PFP4 Concerns about contamination of the hands during urethral cleansing and instillation of gel can be overcome by using two pairs of sterile gloves (one on top of the other) at the start of the procedure. The outer pair can then be removed after cleansing, prior to catheter insertion.

PFP5 Anaesthetic gel is recommended for use in female catheterisation to prevent urethral trauma and to reduce discomfort for the patient (Head 2006).

PFP6 If the catheter is accidentally inserted into the vagina, leave it in place to prevent it happening again, and use a new catheter. Once this is successfully in place, remove the first catheter.

PFP7 In some instances a patient may have a catheter valve fitted instead of a drainage bag. This allows the bladder to fill up and is emptied intermittently (e.g. 4-hourly). They are most suitable for patients requiring long-term catheterisation who have good bladder capacity, good cognitive function and the dexterity to manage the valve. They should not be used for patients who have poor bladder sensation, urgency or who are cognitively impaired.

PFP8 Securing the urinary catheter was identified by the RCN (2008) as being a key competency in its catheter care guidelines. There are a number of devices on the market that can be classified broadly as adhesive and non-adhesive. There are advantages and limitations to both types but what is important is that the catheter is secured sufficiently to enable the patient to move without discomfort, reduce the risk of urethral traction or catheter dislodgement and encourage good urine flow (Fisher 2010).

PFP9 Positioning the catheter drainage bag below the level of the patient's bladder aids gravity flow and prevents reflux of urine. Ensure the bag is not touching the floor as this is an infection risk (Head 2006).

PFP10 Urine from the sterile receiver or contained within the plastic wrapper can be tipped into the specimen pot.

PFP11 Record of the catheterisation should include: the reason for catheterisation, the date and time of catheterisation, the type of catheter (size, length, gauge), the batch number and manufacturer of the catheter (an adhesive label showing the batch number is often provided with the catheter), the size of balloon and the amount of water used to inflate it. A plan of care including review/assessment date should be documented.

PFP12 Traditionally people with an in-dwelling urinary catheter were encouraged to have a high fluid intake, which was thought to reduce the incidence of catheter-associated urinary-tract infections (CAUTI). This has now been discredited, but good fluid intake will result in more dilute urine, which in turn enables smaller diameter catheters to be used and so reduce the risk of urethritis (Pomfret 2006). Most acute patients will have a fluid balance chart.

8.16 Male catheterisation

Preparation

Patient

- Explain the procedure, to gain consent and cooperation
- Ensure the patient's privacy and dignity are maintained throughout
- Ask/assist the patient to wash the penis and perineal area and dry thoroughly

Equipment/Environment

- Clean trolley or other appropriate surface
- Sterile catheterisation pack ➡ **PFP1**
- Two urinary catheters of an appropriate size ➡ **PFP2**
- Single use sterile anaesthetic lubricating gel
- Sachet of sterile 0.9% sodium chloride
- A 10 ml syringe and 10 ml ampoule of sterile water for injection
- Catheter drainage bag and stand/holder
- Sterile universal specimen container
- Alcohol hand-rub or hand washing facilities
- Waterproof absorbent pad
- Good light source

Nurse

- Wash and dry hands thoroughly
- An apron should be worn. Additional protective clothing may be necessary if indicated by the patient's condition (see Ch. 1)
- Two nurses may be necessary if the patient needs assistance to adopt the required position ➡ **PFP3**

Procedure

1. Take the prepared trolley to the patient's bedside and position it on the right or left depending on the nurse's dominant hand.

2. Raise the bed to a safe working height and ensure a good light source.

3. Wash your hands or clean them with alcohol hand-rub.

4. Maintaining asepsis, open the catheterisation pack and any additional packs and equipment.

5. Open the catheter, but do not remove it from its inner wrapper, and place it in the sterile receiver on the trolley. Expose the tip of the catheter by pulling off the top of the wrapper at the serrated edge. Replace it in the sterile receiver.

6. Draw up the amount of sterile water required to inflate the balloon ➡ **PFP4**.

7. Pour the sachet of 0.9% sodium chloride into the gallipot.

8. Open the catheter drainage bag and arrange it at the side of the bed, ensuring the attachment tip is easily accessible and remains sterile.

9. Arrange the bedclothes to expose the genital area, and place the absorbent pad underneath the buttocks.

10. Ask/assist the patient to adopt a supine position with the legs extended.

11. Wash your hands or clean them with alcohol hand-rub. Put on a one or two pairs of sterile gloves ➡ **PFP5**.

12. Tear a hole in the centre of the sterile towel. Cover the patient's abdomen and thighs with the towel, with the penis protruding through the hole.

13. Attach the nozzle to the anaesthetic lubricating gel.

14. With your non-dominant hand and using sterile gauze, grasp the shaft of the penis and retract the foreskin.

15. Clean the glans penis with the sterile 0.9% sodium chloride, ensuring the tips of the fingers remain sterile (Figure 8.11A).

16. Still holding the penis, gently insert the nozzle of the anaesthetic lubricating gel into the urethra and instill the gel into the urethra (Figure 8.11B).

17. Massage the gel along the urethra and wait 5 minutes for it to act.

18. Put on a new pair of sterile gloves or remove the top pair revealing the second pair underneath

19. Place the receiver containing the catheter between the patient's thighs.

20. Grasp the shaft of the penis with your non-dominant hand and hold the penis upwards, to extend the peno-scrotal flexure ➡ **PFP6**.

21. With your dominant hand holding and gradually withdrawing the wrapper, insert the catheter 15–25 cm into the urethra until urine flows (Figure 8.12). If resistance is met at the external sphincter, extend the penis further towards the abdomen. Ask the patient to cough or strain gently as if passing urine. If resistance continues, do not force the catheter: stop the procedure and seek medical advice.

22. When urine is flowing, advance the catheter further, to ensure the catheter is in the bladder.

23. Inflate the balloon with the correct amount of sterile water (Figure 8.13).

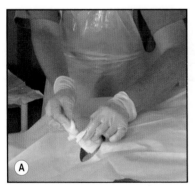
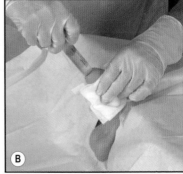

Figure 8.11 (A & B) Cleaning the glans penis and instilling anaesthetic gel

24. Gently withdraw the catheter until resistance is felt; the inflated balloon will hold it in place in the bladder

25. Maintaining asepsis, attach the catheter drainage bag and position it so that there is no pulling on the catheter ➡ **PFP7**. The catheter can be secured by using a securement device or by taping the catheter to the patient's leg ➡ **PFP8** Ensure the catheter drainage bag is positioned below the patient's bladder ➡ **PFP9**.

26. Ensure residual anaesthetic gel is removed and that the glans penis is clean. Where applicable, gently push the foreskin back over the glans penis.

27. Remove the sterile towel by tearing it on one side.

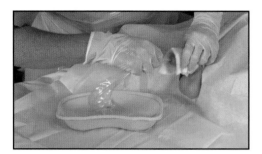

Figure 8.12 Inserting the catheter

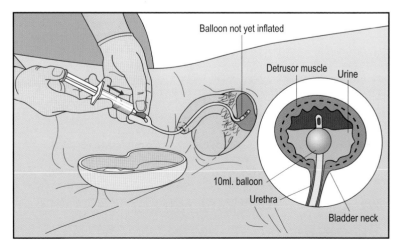

Balloon not yet inflated

Detrusor muscle

Urine

10ml. balloon

Urethra

Bladder neck

Figure 8.13 Inflating the balloon

28. Replace the patient's bedclothes and ensure he is dry and comfortable

29. Place a small amount of urine (10–20 ml) into the specimen pot and send it and the request form to the laboratory as soon as possible, for culture and sensitivity testing ➡ **PFP10**.

30. Dispose of equipment and clinical waste appropriately. Remove gloves and apron and wash hands.

31. If the patient's condition allows, encourage oral fluids ➡ **PFP11**.

32. Measure and document the amount of urine contained in the receiver.

33. Document catheterisation in the patient's records ➡ **PFP12**.

➡Points for practice

PFP1 A catheterisation pack usually contains the following sterile items: kidney dish/receiver, dressing towels, gloves, gallipot and gauze swabs. If a catheterisation pack is not available, a sterile dressing pack containing gloves can be used and the other items added as required.

PFP2 When choosing the size of catheter to be inserted, choose the smallest size possible. For most men a 12 ch/Fg or 14 ch/Fg will be adequate, although a larger size may be necessary if there is blood or sediment in the urine. Trauma from catheter insertion is commonly associated with urethral stricture formation. Trauma arises when too large a catheter is used, when the catheter is forced on insertion or when the balloon is inflated in the urethra. It can also be caused by penile erection and pain, particularly during sleep, is a common complication of having an indwelling catheter. Additional serious complications include: bleeding, swelling, urinary retention and renal problems (Nazarko 2010). Necrosis in the bladder neck may also result from an overly large catheter or balloon. Catheters come in different lengths that refer to the length of the urethra (RCN 2008). The standard length urinary catheter is better known as the male length catheter and ranges from 40 to 44 cm (Nazarko 2010). A female catheter is not long enough to reach the bladder in an male and their use in males has led to an alert by the NPSA (2009) restricting the availability of female catheters outside of specialist settings. A second catheter is useful in case catheterisation is unsuccessful with the first.

PFP3 In most hospitals, only registered nurses who have received additional training may perform male catheterisation (Doherty 2006).

PFP4 The volume of water required will be indicated on the catheter. A balloon size of 10 ml is recommended for the routine drainage of clear urine, as this is usually sufficient to retain the catheter. Larger balloon sizes may irritate the bladder and cause bladder spasm and bypassing of urine (Nazarko 2010). 30–80 ml balloons are used in specialised catheters in urology units and should not be used for routine catheterisation. It is important to use the exact amount of water as indicated on the catheter.

PFP5 Concerns about contamination of the hands during urethral cleansing and instillation of gel can be overcome by using two pairs of sterile gloves (one on top of the other) at the start of the procedure. The outer pair can then be removed after cleansing, prior to catheter insertion.

PFP6 If difficulties are encountered force or pressure must not be used. Asking a male patient to cough may allow the catheter to pass the prostate more easily (Head 2006).

PFP7 In some instances a patient may have a catheter valve fitted instead of a drainage bag. This allows the bladder the fill up and are emptied intermittently (e.g. 4 hourly). They are most suitable for patients requiring long-term catheterisation who have good bladder capacity, good cognitive function and the dexterity to manage the valve. They should not be used for patients who have poor bladder sensation, urgency or who are cognitively impaired.

PFP8 Securing a urinary catheter was identified by the RCN (2008) as being a key competency in its catheter care guidelines. There are a number of devices on the market that can be classified broadly as adhesive and non-adhesive. There are advantages and limitations to both types but what is important is that the catheter is secured sufficiently to enable the patient to move without discomfort, reduce the risk of urethral traction or catheter dislodgement and encourage good urine flow (Fisher 2010).

PFP9 Positioning the catheter drainage bag below the level of the patient's bladder aids gravity flow and prevents reflux or urine. Ensure the bag is not touching the floor as this is an infection risk (Head 2006).

PFP10 Urine from the sterile receiver or contained within the plastic wrapper can be tipped into the specimen pot.

PFP11 Traditionally people with an in-dwelling urinary catheter were encouraged to have a high fluid intake, which was thought to reduce the incidence of catheter-associated urinary-tract infections (CAUTI). This has now been discredited, but good fluid intake will result in more dilute urine, which in turn enables smaller diameter catheters to be used and so reduce the risk of urethritis (Pomfret 2006). Most acute patients will have a fluid balance chart (see p. 236).

PFP12 Ideal records of catherisation should include; the reason for catheterisation, patient consent, the date and time of catheterisation, the type of catheter (size, length, gauge), the batch number and manufacturer of the catheter (an adhesive label showing the batch number may be available), the size of balloon and the amount of water used to inflate it. A plan of care including review/assessment date should be documented.

8.17 Urethral catheter care

Preparation

Patient
- Explain the procedure, to gain consent and cooperation ➡ **PFP1**
- Ensure the patient's privacy and dignity are maintained
- Place the patient in a supine position with knees and hips flexed and slightly apart

Equipment/Environment
- Soap, water and disposable washcloth
- Clean towel

Nurse
- Wash and dry hands thoroughly
- Put on apron and gloves

Procedure

Female patients
1. Clean the vulval area from above downward using warm soapy water ➡ **PFP2**.
2. Clean the catheter by gently wiping in one direction away from the catheter–meatal junction. Rinse well.
3. Dry the area by patting with a towel.

Male patients
1. Retract the foreskin before cleaning ➡ **PFP2**.
2. Clean the shaft of the catheter away from the catheter–meatal junction and rinse well.
3. Dry the area by patting with a towel.
4. Reposition the foreskin on completion of cleaning.
5. Ensure the patient is dry and comfortable
6. Dispose of all waste appropriately
7. Remove gloves and apron and wash hands
8. Record catheter care and report any abnormalities

➡**Points for practice**

PFP1 Where possible, patients should be taught to attend to their own meatal and perineal hygiene, thus reducing the risk of cross-infection. Powders or lotions should not be used after cleansing as these trap organisms in the area.

PFP2 The main aim of cleansing is to remove secretions and encrustation. Cleansing with soap and water has been shown to be as effective as any other method. Cleaning in addition to normal hygiene practice is not necessary and daily bathing or showering is sufficient to maintain meatal hygiene unless there is excessive exudate or encrustation (RCN 2008).

8.18 Care of suprapubic catheter

Patient	Equipment	Nurse
• Explain the procedure to gain co-operation and consent ➡ **PFP1**	• If a dressing is required an aseptic dressing technique must be used	• Wash hands and dry thoroughly
• Ensure privacy and dignity are maintained	• Clean dressing trolley or other suitable surface.	• An apron should be worn
• The patient should be reclining in bed or in a chair/wheelchair	• Dressing pack, cleansing solution and new dressing according to the care plan/local policy ➡ **PFP3**	• Additional protective clothing may be necessary if indicated by the patient's condition (see Ch. 1).
• Empty the leg bag, particularly if the adhesive plaster is to be removed ➡ **PFP2**	• Sterile scissors if required to cut the dressing	

Procedure

1. Clean the trolley or other appropriate surface according to local policy and prepare a new length of adhesive strapping.

2. Take the trolley to the bed/chair area. Adjust the bed to a safe working height or sit down to avoid stooping.

3. Remove the dressing pack from its outer packaging; place it on the clean trolley/surface.

4. Using your fingertips and touching the edges of the paper only, open the pack and lay it flat to create a sterile field (see p. 285).

5. Remove the yellow waste bag and place it to one side. Touching only the edge of the glove pack (or wrist part of the gloves if loose) move them to the edge of the sterile field.

6. Taking care not to contaminate the sterile field, carefully pour the cleansing solution into the tray (Figure 9.1 on page 286). Open the dressing and sterile scissors (if required), onto the sterile field.

7. Adjust any remaining bedclothes to expose the catheter and then loosen the adhesive strapping. If a dressing is in place, loosen it but do not remove it.

8. Wash your hands or use alcohol hand-rub. Ensure your hands are completely dry before proceeding.

9. Open the yellow waste bag and put your hand inside so that the bag acts as a glove. Use this to remove the adhesive strapping and/or soiled dressing (Figure 9.2 on page 286).

10. Inspect the dressing to note the type and amount of exudate. Observe the skin around the catheter for signs of infection or cellulitis.

11. Turn the bag inside out so that the dressing is contained within it, and using the self-adhesive strip, attach the bag to the side of the trolley or other convenient place close to the wound.

12. Taking care not to touch the outside of the gloves, put on the sterile gloves (Figure 9.3 on page 287).

13. Use your non-dominant hand to hold up the catheter. In your dominant hand, use gauze swabs soaked in cleansing solution (but not dripping) to clean around the catheter to remove any encrustations. Use each swab once only.

14. Use fresh gauze swabs to dry around the catheter and apply the new dressing ➡ **PFP4**

15. Place all waste in the clinical waste bag.

16. Remove gloves and discard into waste bag.

17. Replace clothing and ensure the patient is comfortable. Use adhesive strapping to fix the catheter to the skin to prevent pulling.

18. Discard clinical waste. Remove apron and wash hands.

19. Document the dressing and conditon of suprapubic catheter and surrounding skin according to local policy.

➡ Points for practice

PFP1 A suprapubic catheter is inserted through the abdominal wall into the bladder, where a water-filled balloon holds it in place. The insertion site must be treated as a surgical wound. Patients should be encouraged to care for their own catheters where possible, to encourage independence.

PFP2 The weight of a full urine bag may pull on the catheter. Observe the urine; if soon after insertion, haematuria is common. Encourage increased oral intake if condition allows.

PFP3 A 'keyhole' type dressing the catheter will be used until discharge around the catheter ceases. If a keyhole dressing is not available, use sterile scissors to cut a 'Y' shape in the centre of a self-adhesive dressing, to fit around the catheter.

8.19 Emptying a catheter bag

Preparation

Patient

- Explain the procedure to the patient, although it should not cause any discomfort
- The patient may prefer the bed to be screened
- Patients with a leg bag who are mobile can empty the bag into the toilet

Equipment/Environment

- Measuring jug ➡ PFP1 and paper towel to cover
- Two alcohol-impregnated swabs

Nurse

- Wash and dry hands thoroughly
- Gloves and an apron should be worn
- Additional protective clothing may be necessary if indicated by the patient's condition (see Ch. 1)

Procedure

1. Take the covered jug and other equipment to the bedside.
2. If the drainage bag is on a floor stand, it does not need to be removed from the stand for emptying. If the bag is hanging on the side of the bed, it may need to be removed from its holder. Hold the bag over the jug, making sure that the drainage port does not touch the jug (Figure 8.14).
3. Clean the drainage port with an alcohol impregnated swab.

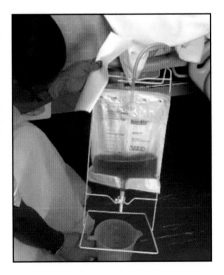

Figure 8.14 Emptying a catheter bag

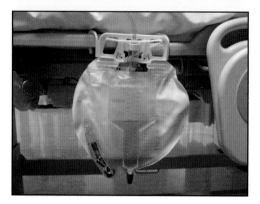

Figure 8.15 Hourly measurement catheter bag

4. Open the drainage port and allow the urine to flow into the jug. Close the drainage port and wipe the outlet tap with the second alcohol-impregnated swab.

5. Reposition the catheter bag as necessary ensuring that the drainage port is not touching the floor and the tubing is not kinked, to allow free drainage into the bag.

6. Cover the jug and take it to the sluice/dirty utility room. Measure the amount of urine and discard ➡ **PFP2**. Clean or discard the urine jug according to local policy ➡ **PFP3**.

7. Remove gloves and apron and wash hands.

8. Record the amount on fluid balance chart if appropriate.

9. If the patient's condition allows, encourage oral fluids.

➡Points for practice

PFP1 The container used to collect the drained urine will vary according to local policy; it may be disposable or one that is disinfected after each use. If using a disinfected jug it should be one that is only used for urine. This should differ in colour and design from those used for drinking water.

PFP2 If hourly urine measurement is required, a special drainage bag is used. This incorporates a small reservoir that can be emptied into the drainage bag without opening the 'closed' system (Figure 8.15).

PFP3 The cleaning of the jug will vary according to local policy. If disposable, it will be discarded. If not disposable, it may be disinfected, or placed in a bedpan washer or returned to the sterile supplies department for decontamination.

8.20 Continuous bladder irrigation

Preparation

Patient

- Explain the procedure, to gain consent and cooperation
- Ensure privacy and dignity are maintained
- The patient will be catheterised with a three-way urethral catheter

Equipment/Environment

- Clean trolley or other appropriate surface
- Sterile dressing towel
- Antiseptic skin-cleansing solution according to local policy
- Non-toothed clamp
- Sterile jug
- Sterile 'Y' shaped irrigation set and fluid as prescribed (usually 0.9% sodium chloride) at room temperature ➡ **PFP1**
- Infusion stand ➡ **PFP2**
- Large catheter drainage bag
- Sterile dressing pack containing gloves
- Alcohol hand-rub

Nurse

- Wash and dry hands thoroughly
- An apron should be worn
- Additional protective clothing may be necessary if indicated by the patient's condition (see Ch.1).

Procedure

1. Take the trolley and equipment to the bedside.

2. Open the irrigation fluid bags and hang on the infusion stand.

3. Maintaining asepsis, attach and prime the irrigation set to expel all air. Close the flow control clamp of the irrigation set ➡ **PFP3**.

4. Ask/assist the patient to adopt a supine position, and expose the catheter and catheter drainage tube.

5. Clamp the catheter using a non-toothed clamp or the clamp on the catheter-bag tubing (Figure 8.16) ➡ **PFP4**.

6. Wash and dry your hands.

7. Maintaining asepsis, open the dressing pack and other equipment, attach the disposal bag to the side of the trolley and pour antiseptic solution into the gallipot.

8. Cleanse your hands with alcohol hand-rub, allow to dry and then put on the sterile gloves.

9. Place the sterile towel underneath the irrigation inlet of the catheter.

10. Cover both the catheter and spigot with sterile gauze, and touching only the gauze, remove the spigot from the irrigation port of the catheter and discard.

11. Thoroughly clean around the irrigation port with antiseptic solution, using each swab only once and wiping in the same direction.

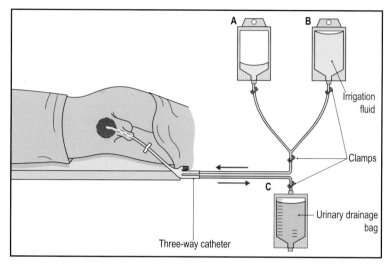

Figure 8.16 Continuous bladder irrigation

12. Maintaining asepsis, attach the irrigation set to the irrigation port, but do not open the flow control clamp.

13. Release the clamp on the catheter and allow accumulated urine to drain. Empty the contents of the catheter bag into the sterile jug (see p. 263).

14. Discard gloves.

15. Open the flow control clamp and set irrigation at the prescribed rate, ensuring that fluid/urine is draining freely into the catheter bag ➡ **PFP5** (Figure 8.16).

16. Assist the patient into a comfortable position and advise him to report any bladder distension, pain or discomfort ➡ **PFP6**.

17. Dispose of equipment and waste appropriately.

18. Measure the volume of urine and discard.

19. Remove apron and wash hands.

20. Document the time of commencement and the volume of irrigation fluid being infused on the fluid balance chart.

21. Check the volume in the catheter drainage bag at least every hour for the first 24 hours, empty as necessary and document on fluid balance chart ➡ **PFP7**.

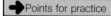 Points for practice

PFP1 3 litre bags of irrigation solution are preferable, as they require less frequent changing and interruption of the closed system. This reduces the risk of infection.

Time	Input (irrigation fluid) A	B	Total output (irrigation fluid plus urine)	Total output (running total)	Urine (total output minus input)	Urine (running total)
0600	3000		600	600		
0630			750	1350		
0700			700	2050		
0730	↓		750	2800		
0800		3000	500	3300	300	300
0830			750			
0900			750			
0930		↓	800			
1000	3000		850	3150	150	450
1030			800			
1100			750			
1130	↓		800			
1200			850	3200	200	650

Table 8.1 Example of irrigation fluid and urine output charting

PFP2 Irrigation fluid should be suspended from a separate infusion stand from that used for intravenous infusions.

PFP3 When priming the irrigation set, make sure that only one clamp (i.e. A or B, Figure 8.16) is open. This will prevent irrigation fluid running from one bottle to the other

PFP4 It is important to use a non-toothed clamp to prevent damage to the tubing.

PFP5 The rate of infusion will vary according to the degree of haematuria (blood in the urine). The aim is to obtain drainage fluid that is rosé in colour. Haematuria will be greatest in the first 12 hours following surgery and 6–9 litres of irrigation fluid is likely to be required. This should fall to 3–6 litres in the second 12 hours. Irrigation is usually discontinued on the morning following surgery. Only one bag of irrigation fluid is used at a time. When the first bag is empty the second bag can be commenced immediately ensuring continuous flow. In the meantime, the empty bag can be replaced (Steggall 2011).

PFP6 If clot retention is suspected (the output stops, there is evidence of abdominal distension and the patient complains of pain and discomfort) irrigation should be stopped immediately and the problem reported. Deflation and reinflation of the catheter balloon or a bladder washout may be required (see p. 268).

PFP7 The volume of irrigation fluid being infused and the amount of drainage in the catheter bag should be recorded on a fluid balance chart. The difference between the two figures is the urine output (Table 8.1).

8.21 Bladder washout/lavage

Preparation

Patient

- Explain the procedure, to gain consent and cooperation ➡ **PFP1**
- Ensuring dignity and privacy, position the patient to allow access to the catheter
- An absorbent, waterproof pad should be placed under the patient's buttocks

Equipment/Environment

- Sterile dressing pack containing gloves
- Sterile dressing towel
- A 50 ml bladder tip syringe ➡ **PFP2**
- Sterile jug
- Sterile washout solution (0.9% sodium chloride) at room temperature ➡ **PFP3**
- Two sterile bowls or receivers
- Antiseptic cleansing solution according to local policy
- Alcohol hand-rub or hand washing facilities
- Non-toothed clamp
- Sterile spigot if washout solution is to be retained
- New catheter drainage bag

Nurse

- Clean trolley or other appropriate surface
- Wash and dry hands thoroughly
- An apron should be worn
- Additional protective clothing may be necessary if indicated by the patient's condition (see Ch. 1)

Procedure

1. Take the prepared trolley to the patient's bedside and position it on the right or left depending on the nurse's dominant hand.

2. Maintaining asepsis, open the sterile dressing pack and additional equipment including the sterile jug, bladder syringe and sterile bowls/receivers. Pour antiseptic solution into the gallipot. Pour washout solution into the jug.

3. Open the catheter drainage bag and place it in an accessible position, leaving the cover on the catheter connector to maintain sterility.

4. Arrange the bedclothes to expose the genital area and check the absorbent pad is under the buttocks.

5. Wash and dry your hands or clean them using alcohol hand-rub, and put on the sterile gloves.

6. Draw up 30–40 ml of washout fluid into the syringe (note the amount) and expel the air.

7. Place the sterile towel between the patient's legs, creating a sterile field.

8. Place one receiver on the sterile towel.

9. Clamp the catheter.

10. Cover both the catheter and drainage tube with sterile gauze, and touching only the gauze, disconnect the catheter from the tubing. Place the end of the catheter in the sterile receiver.

11. Clean the end of the catheter with antiseptic solution and attach the bladder syringe. Unclamp the catheter and gently instil the solution into the bladder (Figure 8.17).

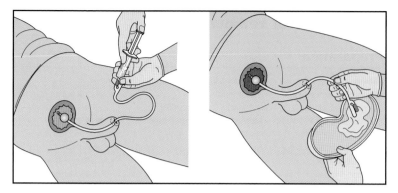

Figure 8.17 Instilling washout solution

12. Remove the syringe and allow the solution to drain out naturally into the second sterile receiver. If the solution does not drain, aspirate gently using the bladder syringe ➜ **PFP4**. Repeat the process, using 30–40 ml of solution each time, until the urine is clear and flowing freely.
13. Connect the new drainage bag.
14. Ensure the patient is comfortable and is not experiencing bladder discomfort.
15. Dispose of equipment and waste appropriately
16. Remove gloves and apron and wash hands.
17. Encourage fluids and mobilisation if condition allows.
18. Measure the input (amount of washout solution inserted) and output (drainage or aspirate) to calculate any urine output.
19. Document bladder washout and report any abnormalities.

➜Points for practice

PFP1 Bladder washout or lavage using a syringe is only undertaken to remove blood clots following urological surgery. It must not be used to unblock long-term urethral catheters as the use of bladder syringes have been shown to cause damage; even the gentlest of force in instilling and withdrawing solution has been found to cause tissue trauma (Rew 2005).

PFP2 A bladder-tip syringe differs from other syringes; the tip is large and designed to fit the opening of a urinary catheter.

PFP3 Although not used routinely, commercially prepared catheter maintenance solutions (CMS), are sometimes used in the management of long-term urethral catheters to dissolve encrustations. These solutions must not, under any circumstances be inserted into the bladder using a syringe (Mitchell 2008).

PFP4 If no fluid is returned after instillation of the first 30 ml, instil a further 30 ml. If there is still no return, seek advice.

8.22 Catheter removal

Preparation

Patient

- Explain the procedure, to gain consent and cooperation ➡ **PFP1**
- Ensure the patient's privacy and dignity are maintained throughout
- Position the patient in a supine position with knees and hips flexed and slightly apart

Equipment/Environment

- Clean trolley or tray
- A 20 ml syringe ➡ **PFP2**
- Measuring jug and paper towel to cover
- Large disposable absorbent pad
- Disposable receiver
- Clinical waste bag for disposal of catheter and catheter bag
- Specimen pot and 20 ml syringe (for catheter specimen)

Nurse

- Choose appropriate time for catheter removal ➡ **PFP3**
- Wash and dry hands thoroughly
- An apron and gloves should be worn

Procedure

1. Take the equipment to the bedside and position the clinical waste bag for easy access.
2. Take a catheter specimen of urine (see p. 246).
3. Empty the catheter bag (see p. 263)
4. Clean the urinary meatus if necessary (see p. 260)
5. Place the absorbent pad under the buttocks.
6. Check the volume of water in the balloon (usually written on the catheter or obtain from patient records), attach the syringe to the balloon port on the catheter and withdraw the water to deflate the balloon. Make sure you withdraw the full amount from the balloon ➡ **PFP4**.
7. Place the receiver between the patient's thighs.
8. Ask the patient to breathe in and out and on exhalation gently but firmly withdraw the catheter into the receiver ➡ **PFP4**.
9. Detach the catheter bag from the catheter stand (if applicable) and place it in the clinical waste bag with the receiver containing the catheter and the absorbent pad.
10. Assist the patient into a comfortable position and ensure a toilet/urinal/commode is nearby. Ask the patient to inform the nurse when urine has been passed.
11. Advise the patient regarding the possibility of frequency, urgency, haematuria and dysuria ➡ **PFP5**.
12. Advise the patient to increase oral fluid intake (2–2.5 litres in 24 hours).
13. Dispose of equipment and clinical waste appropriately.
14. Remove gloves and apron and wash hands.

15. Record the amount of urine obtained from the catheter drainage bag on the fluid balance chart.
16. Document the time of catheter removal and when the patient subsequently passes urine ➡ **PFP6**.
17. Label the catheter specimen and send it to the laboratory with the request form or refrigerate it as soon as possible.

➡ Points for practice

PFP1 The patient may be frightened of catheter removal and imagine it to be extremely painful.

PFP2 The size of syringe required will depend on the amount of water in the catheter balloon; this is written on the catheter itself or can be obtained from the patient's records.

PFP3 Catheters are usually removed first thing in the morning so that any problems that may arise can be dealt with during the day. It also means the patient will be able to more easily increase their fluid intake.

PFP4 If problems are encountered when deflating the balloon or withdrawing the catheter, medical advice should be sought. Avoid pulling back on the syringe when removing the water as this may create a vacuum and cause the balloon to 'cuff' making removal difficult (RCN 2008). It is essential that the catheter is withdrawn slowly and gently in order to reduce the trauma to the urethra caused by the creases and ridges in the balloon. Rotating the catheter as it is slowly withdrawn may also make removal easier.

PFP5 The patient may well experience feelings of wanting to pass urine following removal of the catheter. Male patients should be discouraged from placing a urinal in position 'just in case', as this may encourage frequent small volumes to be passed or 'dribbling'. A frequency chart may be requested for the first 24 hours. Haematuria (blood in the urine) may be the result of trauma following catheter removal and dysuria (pain when passing urine) may be due to inflammation of the urethra.

PFP6 The RCN catheter care guidelines recommend that detailed documentation should accompany catheter removal and include: the length of time the catheter was in situ; if the balloon deflated properly and the catheter tip and balloon were intact on removal; if encrustation was evident; if the part of the catheter that was in the bladder was clean/dirty or if there evidence of debris; if removal was painful and if there was any blood present. Any inflammation or discharge at the meatus should be reported and urine should be observed for signs of infection (e.g. cloudy, debris, colour, odour) (RCN 2008).

8.23 Stoma care

Principles

- Stoma is a greek word meaning 'opening' or 'mouth' (Rust 2007) and in the context of healthcare, refers to an artifically created opening between a body cavity e.g. intestine and the body surface (Fulham 2008).

- Stomas are generally divided into three types: input or feeding stomas, output stomas and diverting or defunctioning stomas. Input or feeding stomas e.g. gastrostomy/jejunostomy facilitate the provision of nutrition (see p. 172). Output and diverting or defunctioning stomas are surgically formed following intervention for gastrointestinal/urinary disease. The major types of surgically created stomas are: colostomy (opening into colon), ileostomy (opening into the ileum) or urostomy (e.g. ileal conduit – a stoma that drains urine). The most common type of stoma is a colostomy.

- As part of the pre-operative preparation of the patient, it is of critical importance that the optimal site for the stoma is identified. Positioning the stoma in normally done by the stoma care nurse specialist. Choosing a site is fundamental for the success of the device, patient comfort and ability to manage the stoma. If a patient is unable to manage their stoma it can negatively impact on their quality of life. Factors to be considered include:
  - using the rectus muscle to prevent prolapse of the stoma
  - finding a flat area and avoiding skin folds, bulges and rolls
  - avoiding scars, bony prominences, the umbilicus, the patient's belt or waistline
  - consideration of the patient's usual style of dress.

- In the immediate postoperative period, a baseline assessment of the stoma must be undertaken, which includes recording of the type of stoma, location, colour, size and length. In addition, while undertaking other postoperative observations, the nurse should observe the stoma (at a minimum of 4-hour intervals). It should be pink or red in colour and any discolouration, necrosis or excessive bleeding must be reported.

- The temperature of the stoma should be the same as the rest of the abdomen. This can be assessed by touching it through the transparent drainable appliance/bag that is used in the immediate postoperative period (Vujnovich 2008).

- For patients who have a colostomy or ileostomy, the stoma bags have a charcoal filter that allows flatus to escape. However, in the initial period following surgery, the filter should be covered or a filterless bag should be used so that it can be observed that peristalsis is returning by the presence of flatus in the bag.

- Day-to-day assessment should include: examination of the mucocutaneous junction (where the mucosa of the bowel joins the skin), assessment of the peristomal skin condition and the surface anatomy of the peristomal area. The stoma is secured to the peristomal skin by means of soluble or non-soluble sutures. These are not removed and will fall or out or dissolve in a number of weeks (Fulham 2008). Any separation at the mucocutaneous junction should be documented by using the numbers of a clock face to describe the location, with 12 o'clock being in line with the patient's head

- The stoma will be oedematous in the immediate postoperative period but this should gradually reduce over a number of weeks.

- Assessment of the condition of the peristomal skin includes observing for redness, inflammation or broken areas. The most common cause of excoriation or sore skin is contact with stoma output, which is more corrosive from an ileostomy or urostomy than from a colostomy (Vujnovich 2008).

- There may not be any output from an ileostomy or colostomy for the first 24–48 hours. However, a urostomy should start functioning immediately although the urine may be slightly blood stained. The usual output from an ileostomy is of a porridge-like consistency whereas that from a colostomy is semi-formed to formed faeces. Output from the stoma should be documented and any concerns about the type or volume should be reported. It is important to clearly document observations and assessment.

- Regular care and inspection of a stoma is vital so that any deterioration in the stoma, such as mucocutaneous separation (stoma detaches from the edges of the surrounding skin and can leave a cavity), necrosis, prolapse, retraction, herniation or skin excoriation is reported promptly. Delay exacerbates the problem and may cause pain and distress for the patient.

- Gloves and an apron should be worn when caring for a stoma. Additional protective clothing may be necessary if indicated by the patient's condition (see Ch. 1).

Stoma appliances

- There is an extensive range of stoma products available that are largely grouped into one-piece or two-piece, which are either closed or drainable (Vujnovich 2008). Drainable bags are used in the initial postoperative period. Subsequently, patients with an ileostomy may continue to use a drainable appliance as the output is semi-formed to liquid and may need to be emptied several times a day (Vujnovich 2008). Patients with a colostomy may be more suited to a closed appliance (Williams 2006).

- One-piece appliances have the flange and pouch as one unit whilst they are separate in two-piece appliances (Williams 2006). Hospitals tend to use transparent/clear bags that facilitate observation of the stoma. Once they are comfortable with managing their appliances, some patients prefer opaque appliances as they do not have to see the output (Fulham 2008).

- Stoma appliances should be leak proof, odour proof, unobtrusive, noiseless and disposable. As a flatus filter is not used in the first few days following surgery it is important to reassure the patient as the odour can cause distress.

- Some appliances such as the transparent bags/appliances used in hospitals come with a starter hole that allows the nurse to cut the flange to fit the size of the stoma. This is particularly useful when the stoma is irregular in shape (Williams 2006).

- When cutting the flange ensure it is cut according to the template so that it fits snugly around the stoma (Figure 8.18). If the aperture is too small it will cause friction on the delicate blood vessels of the stoma, causing bruising or bleeding. If, on the other hand, the aperture is too big, the contents of the bowel will spill out of the stoma onto the surrounding skin, causing excoriation and soreness (Fulham 2008).
- When the bag is removed, it is important to do this gently so that the skin is not pulled. Use counter-pressure with your other hand (Rust 2007).
- The skin and stoma should be cleaned whenever the bag is changed, to prevent skin soreness. A special stoma cream may be advocated if there are skin problems at the stoma site. Make sure the surrounding skin is dry before attaching a new bag.
- Ensure the bag is securely attached to the skin, thus preventing leakage and distress for the patient. Some stoma bags have a clip at the bottom to enable them to be emptied without removing the bag (drainable). Take care that the clip is securely fitted to prevent leakage.
- Many hospitals have Stoma Nurse Specialists for advice regarding care of the stoma.

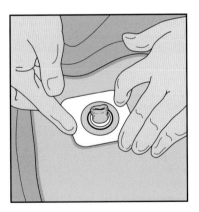

Figure 8.18 Fitting the flange around the stoma

8.24 Changing a stoma bag

Preparation

Patient

- Ask/assist the patient to sit or lie in a comfortable position ➡ **PFP1**
- Ensure privacy and dignity are maintained throughout
- Place a protective pad next to the stoma site to protect clothing

Equipment/Environment

- Clean stoma appliance/bag and flange ➡ **PFP2**
- Scissors to cut the flange or aperture of the bag to size
- Stoma template
- Disposable wipes
- Jug to dispose of the contents of the used bag (if applicable)
- Disposable protective pad
- Clinical waste bag
- Soap and water for cleansing the skin
- Barrier cream if advised

Nurse

- Wash and dry hands thoroughly
- Put on apron and gloves
- Additional protective clothing may be necessary if indicated by the patient's condition (see Ch. 1)

Procedure

1. Place the disposable protective pad next to the stoma to protect the patient's clothing. Place the clinical waste bag in a easily accessible position.

2. If the stoma bag is the type that can be emptied before removal (drainable), empty the contents into the jug.

3. Gently peel the adhesive off the skin, using the other hand to apply counter-pressure to prevent damage to the skin.

4. Remove the bag and place into the clinical waste bag.

5. Wipe the skin free of faeces and secretions using disposible wipes.

6. Clean the skin and stoma using soap and water and gently pat the skin until thoroughly dry.

7. Check the condition of the stoma and the surrounding skin (peristomal skin) for any soreness, redness, ulceration or other abnormalities.

8. Apply barrier cream if appropriate.

9. Remove gloves.

10. Cut a hole to the correct size in the bag or flange having measured the stoma or using the stoma template as a guide. Ensure there is a 3 mm clearance.

11. Place the flange and/or the bag over the stoma so that the aperture fits snugly and is well attached ➡ **PFP3** (Figures 8.18 & 8.19).

12. If drainable type is used, attach the clip to the base of the bag ➡ **PFP4**.

13. Remove the protective pad (use gloves if this is soiled) and discard into clinical waste bag.

14. Ensure the patient is comfortable and offer a hand wash if they have participated in the process.

15. Dispose of any excreta, the soiled bag and other clinical waste appropriately.

16. Leave the scissors with the patient's stoma equipment, which is often kept in the bedside locker.

17. Remove apron and wash hands.

18. Document the stoma bag change and the condition of the peristomal skin. Report any abnormalities.

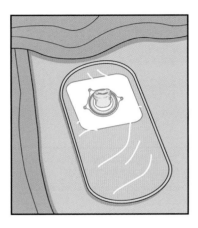

Figure 8.19 Stoma bag in position

➡Points for practice

PFP1 Patients are usually taught to care for their own stomas and so should be encouraged to participate.

PFP2 Many patients have a bag containing all the necessary equipment. Some stoma bags have a separate flange and bag; others are one-piece appliances (see p. 273).

PFP3 If a one-piece appliance is being used it should be applied from the bottom up. For a two-piece appliance, the flange should be placed directly over the stoma and then the pouch attached.

PFP4 If the bag is the type that can be emptied without removing it, there will be a special 'roll-up' clip at the bottom. Take care not to discard this when emptying the bag.

Bibliography/Suggested reading

Black, P., 2009. Managing physical postoperative stoma complications. British Journal of Nursing (Stoma Care Supplement) 18 (17), S4–S10.

This article addresses the physical complications such as parastomal hernia, prolapse, retraction, obstruction and stenosis that may occur after stoma surgery and discusses how healthcare professionals can help

Booth, F., Lee, L., 2005. A guide to selecting and using urinary sheaths. Nursing Times Plus 101 (47), 43–46.

This article provides a good overview of the issues to be considered when selecting and using urinary sheaths

Borwell, B., 2009. Rehabilitation and stoma care: addressing the psychological needs. British Journal of Nursing (Stoma Care Supplement) 18 (4), S20–S25.

This article focuses on the psychological impact of debilitating surgery on individuals. The paper proposes that addressing individual psychological needs is a challenge for healthcare professionals in a diverse, multicultural society. Strategies are presented for helping the patient achieve successful rehabilitation and psychological adaptation

Department of Health, 2001. The essence of care: continence and bladder and bowel care. Department of Health, London.

Government guidelines based on patient-focused bench-marking to ensure high quality care

Doherty, W., 2006. Male urinary catheterisation. Nursing Standard 20 (35), 57–63.

This article is part of the continuing professional development series. It examines the procedure of male catheterisation and its development as a role performed by trained nurses, regardless of gender. The reasons for urinary catheterisation, issues in relation to male sexuality and patient assessment and education are also discussed

Fisher, J., 2010. The importance of effective catheter securement. British Journal of Nursing (Continence Care Supplement) 19 (18), S14–S18.

This article examines the importance of securing/fixing indwelling urinary catheters. It explores the various types of securement devices and the advantages and disadvantages of each. The importance of individual assessment when selecting an appropriate device is emphasised

Fulham, J., 2008. A guide to caring for patients with a newly formed stoma in the acute hospital setting. Gastrointestinal Nursing 6 (8), 14–23.

This article examines the fundamental aspects of stoma care required by individuals facing surgery for stoma formation. The article provides an overview postoperative stoma care, emotional support for the patient and ongoing support following discharge. Selecting the correct appliance, common complications and the role of the stoma care nurse specialist are also addressed

Harrison, S.C.W., Lawrence, W.T., Morley, R., Pearce, I., Taylor, J., 2010. British Association of Urological Surgeons' suprapubic catheter practice guidelines. British Journal of Urology International 107, 77–85.

Although aimed at doctors, this article provides useful information about the indications for suprapubic catheterisation and care of the catheter. Very useful advice about the use of antibiotics and when this is indicated

Head, C., 2006. Insertion of a urinary catheter. Nursing Older People 18 (10), 33–36.

This article focuses on the urinary catheter insertion in older people and explores the incidence of catheter use and associated complications

Mitchell, N., 2008. Long term urinary catheter problems: a flow chart to aid management. British Journal of Community Nursing. 13 (1), 6–12.

This articles presents a flow chart to assist nurses in making a proper assessment of the causes and management of urinary bypassing, blockage and non-drainage of long term urinary catheters

Moppett, S., 2000. Which way is up for a suppository? Nursing Times 96 (19), NT Plus:12–1.

This article discusses the rationale relating to the most effective way to insert a suppository (blunt end first) in order to aid retention

National Patient Safety Agency, 2009. Female urinary catheters causing trauma to adult males.[online]. Available from: http://www.nrls.npsa.nhs.uk/resources/type/alerts (accessed 20.01.12.).

A female catheter is not long enough to reach the bladder in a male and their use in males has led to this alert by the NPSA recommending restricting the availability of female catheters except in specialist settings

Nazarko, L., 2010. Effective evidence-based catheter management: an update. British Journal of Nursing 19 (15), 948–953.

This article examines the clinical indications for catheterisation, the importance of appropriate product selection and actions needed to reduce the risk of infection

Pomfret, I., 2006. Urinary catheter care. Nursing and Residential Care 8 (10), 446–448.

This article explores the use of indwelling urinary catheters to manage urinary incontinence when all else has failed. The advantages and disadvantages are explored as well as the methods, types of drainage systems and issues in respect of maintenance of the catheter

Rew, M., 2005. Caring for catheterized patients: urinary catheter maintenance. British Journal of Nursing 14 (2), 87–92.

This article explores the evidence and opinions surrounding the ongoing problem of catheter blockage and how catheter life can be maintained. The article examines the role of pH testing, the role of the patient's general health, the use of catheter-maintenance solutions and techniques associated with instillations

Rigby, D., Gray, K., 2006. Understanding urine testing. Nursing Times 101 (12), 60–62.

This article looks at collection of urine specimens and urinalysis using reagent sticks. It also explains what abnormal findings might mean and the implications for practice

Robinson, J., 2006. Selecting a urinary catheter and drainage system. British Journal of Nursing 15 (19), 1045–1050.

Selecting a catheter and drainage system can be confusing due to the vast array of catheters, materials used and drainage systems available from various companies. This article is written to help in the selection of a urinary catheter and the drainage system which is best suited to the patient

Roodhouse, A., Wellsted, A., 2006. Safety in urine sampling: maintaining an infection-free environment. British Journal of Nursing 15 (16), 870–872.

This article reports on the needle-free port designed specifically to reduce the occupational health risk of needlestick injuries associated with urine sampling in patients with an indwelling urinary catheter

Royal College of Nursing, 2008. Catheter Care: RCN Guidance for Nurses Royal College of Nursing, London [online]. Available from: http://tinyurl.com/c23aww (accessed 20.01.12.).

This comprehensive publication contains National Occupational Standards (NOS) to guide practice in catheter care. It also includes care of suprapubic catheters

Rust, J., 2007. Care of patients with stomas: the pouch change procedure. Nursing Standard 22 (6), 43–47.

This article discusses the pouch change procedure in a ward setting immediately following surgery for stoma formation. Psychological preparation of the patient and practical preparation including the procedure for pouch change are outlined

Scales, K., Pilsworth, J., 2008. The importance of fluid balance in clinical practice. Nursing Standard 22 (47), 50–57.

This article discusses the importance of fluid balance for nurses and provides an overview of the physiology of how water is gained and lost by the body. It explains fluid balance in illness and how to assess hydration. There is also discussion about fluid balance charts, when they should be used, and nurses' professional responsibilities

Skinner, S., 2005. Understanding clinical investigations: a quick reference manual, second ed. Baillière Tindall, Edinburgh.

This excellent book provides information about a wide range of investigations such as urinalysis, why they are done, what the findings might indicate and the implications for nurses. It also provides a quick overview of the relevant physiology

Steggall, M., 2011. Nursing patients with urinary disorders. In: Brooker, C., Nicol, M. (Eds.), Alexander's nursing practice, fourth ed. Churchill Livingstone Elsevier, Edinburgh.

This chapter provides a good overview of the anatomy and physiology of the urinary system and the male reproductive system. It addresses common disorders of the renal and the rest of the urinary tract system including their treatment and nursing care

Vujnovich, A., 2008. Pre- and post-operative assessment of patients with a stoma. Nursing Standard 22 (19), 50–56.

This article outlines the pre and postoperative nursing care for patients undergoing surgery leading to stoma formation

Williams, J., 2006. Stoma care part 1: choosing the right appliance. Gastrointestinal Nursing 4 (6), 16–19.

This is the first of two articles that examine issues surrounding the choice of appliance following stoma forming surgery. This article addresses choosing the right appliance while the second article (see below) deals with choosing the right accessories for management of the stoma

Williams, J., 2006. Stoma care part 2: choosing appliance accessories. Gastrointestinal Nursing 4 (7), 16–19.

Wilson, J., 2006. Infection control in clinical practice, third ed. Baillière Tindall Elsevier, Edinburgh.

A comprehensive text that explains basic microbiology, types of organisms and how they are spread. It then provides guidance on all aspects of infection control. Ch. 13 provides advice on cleaning, disinfection and sterilisation and Ch. 10 addresses prevention of infection associated with urethral catheters.

Peri-operative care

©2012 Elsevier Ltd.

9.1 Wound assessment

Principles

The purpose of a wound assessment is to gather information about the wound and surrounding skin, to determine whether the wound is healing, unchanged or deteriorating. The assessment also enables nurses to select the most appropriate wound dressing. However, each time nurses assess a wound it is essential to also assess the patient's physical and psychological condition, and the social environment (Dealey 2005). A number of wound assessment tools exist (Benbow 2009, Vuolo 2006). These are designed to encourage a systematic approach and provide prompts, which guide the nurse to collect information around key parameters to determine the condition of the wound. An assessment tool should also identify factors that may adversely affect the person's ability to heal effectively, such as poor nutrition and poor circulation. Once the wound assessment is completed an appropriate plan of care is written, with specific objectives to guide the management of the wound.

Wound assessment tools

Most wound assessment tools will incorporate consideration of the following factors, which are known to influence wound healing:

1. **Cause and type of wound** – it is important to note the cause of the wound, and when and how the wound occurred. Any factors that may affect wound healing (e.g. grit in the wound) can be identified and addressed. Acute wounds may be described as traumatic (caused by an injury, including burns) or surgical (caused by an operation). Acute wounds usually heal quicker and without complication provided that infection does not occur. Chronic (or older) wounds may be caused by ischaemia (poor blood supply) or pressure (such as a pressure ulcer). Patients with chronic wounds often have a number of conditions that will affect the body's ability to heal a wound (see 10 below). Pressure ulcers may be graded to determine their severity (see p. 382). Leg ulcers require specialised assessment by experienced practitioners. For more information see Anderson (2007).

2. **Wound location** – the location of the wound may have considerations for the patient and influence the choice of dressing. For example, a sacral pressure ulcer may become contaminated with urine or faeces, the wound may be difficult to dress and the patient may feel uncomfortable if the dressing is too big. A deep laceration on a patient's hand may restrict their ability to work; a longer lasting water-resistant dressing may be more appropriate.

3. **Wound measurement** – measurements of the size of the wound are recorded at the initial assessment and then usually weekly using the same tool. The simplest method is to use a disposable tape measure to record the length and width of the wound. The most accurate method is to trace around the wound margins using a clear acetate sheet with a grid matrix; the surface area can then be calculated by counting the number of grid squares within the

outline. Photography can be used to produce a picture of the wound with a transparent grid overlay, or with a ruler placed alongside the wound to show the size. The patient's confidentiality, privacy and dignity must be considered at all times, and photography must be used in accordance with local policy.

4. **Wound margins** – when assessing a wound it is helpful to start looking at the wound edges (margins). In the initial stages of a wound forming the edges will usually be red and slightly raised due to the inflammatory response of the healing process. After 48–72 hours this should have settled and the wound margins will start to appear paler as healing progresses. Finally, tissue will migrate from the edges across the wound in the process of epithelialisation (see below). If wound edges look red and raised in the later stages of wound healing (>72 hours from the wound forming) this may indicate a wound infection.

5. **Appearance of the tissue type in the wound bed** – there are five different tissue types found in the wound bed, which give an indication of the stage of healing. These can be described by colour or descriptors.

   - Red – granulation tissue. This indicates a healing wound.
   - Pink/pale purple – epithelisation: this indicates the latter stages of wound healing as new protein cells help to complete the wound repair.
   - Green – infected: Indicates the presence of an infection.
   - Yellow – sloughy: this is devitalised tissue that may need a special dressing designed to lift it from the wound bed.
   - Black – necrotic: this is dead, ischemic tissue that usually requires surgical removal.

   Many wounds will present with more than one tissue type. When a wound presents with a combination of tissue types, each must be documented with an estimated percentage. For example, 70% granulation, 10% slough and 20% epithelialisation

6. **Presence of exudate** – this refers to the type of exudate (colour, appearance and viscosity) and volume of exudate. Colour, appearance and viscosity can be assessed by inspecting the dressing when it is removed. However, assessing the volume of exudate is more subjective and is usually documented using descriptors such as minimal, moderate, or large. A more accurate measurement can be obtained by recording the number of dressing changes to determine if these have become more or less frequent. This is important as infection may be present if the exudate in the wound increases and the patient experiences an increase in wound pain.

7. **Odour** – the presence of a newly detected odour may indicate infection. Heavily infected wounds can cause an offensive odour that can be detected when standing near to the patient, as well as when the dressing is removed, and continues once the wound is cleaned. Patients who experience a distinct odour from their wound are likely to feel embarrassed and uncomfortable in front of nurses, visitors' and other patients. Activated charcoal dressings can be helpful in absorbing odour.

8. **Condition of the surrounding skin** – it is important to note the condition of the surrounding skin as this will provide additional information about the patent's general health status, and changes will alert the nurse to any new problems. For example: dry, flaky and itchy skin may indicate eczema; dry and scaly skin may indicate dehydration; redness may be a sign of inflammation or injury (often present in the first 48 hours following an acute wound), or skin may appear white and spongy due to maceration (where the skin has become soggy). It is also good practice to determine the skin temperature by feeling the skin with the back of the hand.

9. **Pain** – the presence of pain will affect the comfort and wellbeing of the patient, and is also likely to indicate a potential infection. As pain is unique to the individual, it is important to incorporate a pain assessment to determine the severity of the pain and any related issues (p. 66).

10. **Factors affecting healing** – many things will affect the wounds ability to heal. These include: intrinsic factors such as age, malnutrition, dehydration, smoking, poor circulation, and the patient's medical condition. Also, extrinsic factors such as sustained pressure, medication, infection, poor surgical technique, poor wound management and the patient's environment. Psychological factors relating to body image, anxiety and grief may also affect the person's ability to look after their wound.

9.2 Aseptic dressing technique

Preparation

Patient

- Explain the procedure, to gain consent and cooperation
- Assess the wound dressing ➡ **PFP1**
- Check patient comfort, e.g. convenience, position, need for toilet, etc.
- Administer analgesics as appropriate and allow time to take effect
- Adjust bedclothes to permit easy access to the wound but maintain warmth and dignity ➡ **PFP3**

Equipment

- Dressing trolley or other suitable surface
- Dressing pack, syringe (for irrigating the wound), cleansing solution and new dressing according to the care plan/local policy ➡ **PFP2**
- Other equipment (e.g. scissors) as required
- Alcohol hand-rub or hand washing facilities
- Draw screens around the bed for privacy and ensure adequate light. Clear the bed area, close windows, turn off fans, etc.
- Draw screens around the bed for privacy and ensure adequate light. Clear the bed area, close windows, turn off fans, etc.

Nurse

- Consult care plan to determine the type of dressing required, frequency of change, etc.
- Make sure hair is tied back securely
- Wash and dry hands thoroughly
- An apron should be worn. Additional protective clothing may be necessary if indicated by the patient's condition (see Ch. 1).

Procedure

1. Clean the trolley or other appropriate surface according to local policy ➡ **PFP4**.

2. Gather the equipment, check the sterility and expiry date of all equipment and solutions. Place these on the bottom of the trolley or somewhere convenient.

3. If scissors are needed to cut non-sterile tape, wash your own scissors, dry thoroughly, clean with an alcohol-impregnated swab and place on the bottom of the trolley. If sterile scissors are needed (e.g. to cut a sterile dressing), these are usually packed separately.

4. Take the trolley to the bed area ➡ **PFP5**. Adjust the bed to a safe working height to avoid stooping.

5. Remove the dressing pack from its outer packaging; place it on the clean trolley/surface.

6. Using your fingertips and touching the edges of the paper only, open the pack and lay it flat to create a sterile field (Figure 9.1).

7. Carefully pick up the edge of the waste bag and place it at one corner of the sterile field

8. Touching only the corner of the pack (or wrist part if not packed) carefully move the gloves to the edge of the sterile field ➡ **PFP6**.

9. Taking care not to contaminate the sterile field, carefully pour the cleansing solution into the tray (Figure 9.1). Open the dressing, syringe, etc., onto the sterile field. If non-sterile tape is required, cut/tear it now and attach it to the trolley in a convenient place for use later.

10. Adjust any remaining bedclothes to expose the wound then loosen the existing dressing, but do not remove it ➡ **PFP7**.

11. Wash your hands or use alcohol hand-rub. Ensure your hands are completely dry before proceeding.

12. Open the yellow waste bag and put your hand inside so that the bag acts as a glove. Use this to remove the soiled dressing (Figure 9.2).

13. Inspect the dressing to determine the type and amount of exudate.

14. Turn the bag inside out so that the dressing is contained within it, and using the self-adhesive strip, attach the bag to the side of the trolley or other convenient place close to the wound ➡ **PFP8**.

15. Taking care not to touch the outside of the gloves, put on the sterile gloves (Figure 9.3).

16. Fold the dressing towel over your fingertips to avoid contamination with the bedclothes or skin, and place close to the wound, if required.

17. Use a gauze swab dipped in cleansing solution to clean *around* the wound to remove blood, etc. ➡ **PFP9**.

18. If the wound itself needs cleaning, use a syringe primed with solution in one hand and a gauze swab on the skin below the wound in the other (Figure 9.4). Making sure that neither the syringe nor gauze come into contact with the wound, allow the solution to flow into the wound, collecting the solution in the gauze swab held below the wound ➡ **PFP10**.

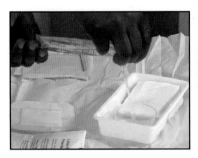

Figure 9.1 Pouring cleansing solution.

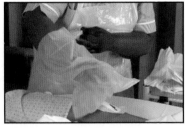

Figure 9.2 Using clinical waste bag as glove to remove dressing.

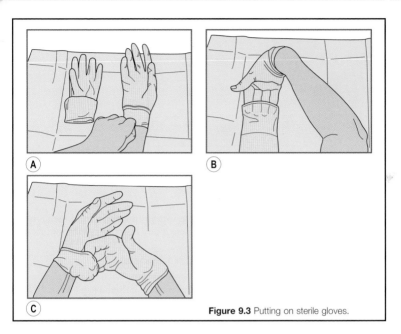

Figure 9.3 Putting on sterile gloves.

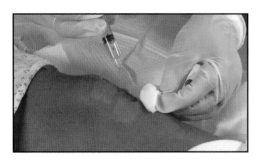

Figure 9.4 Irrigating the wound.

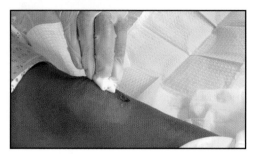

Figure 9.5 Drying around the wound.

19. Use fresh gauze swabs to dry *around* the wound (not the wound itself), using each swab once only (Figure 9.5). If there is any infection, swab from clean towards infected areas.

20. Gently apply the new dressing making sure it is secure.

21. Place any sharps, e.g. stitch cutters, in a sharps bin. Wrap all used disposable items in the sterile field and place in the waste bag. Remove gloves and discard in waste bag. This should then be sealed/tied and placed in the clinical waste.

22. Replace the bedclothes and assist the patient as necessary into a comfortable position. Readjust the bed to a safe height.

23. Remove apron, discard in the clinical waste and wash hands.

24. Return any unused items to the stock cupboard. Clean the trolley according to local policy.

25. Document the dressing change and condition of the wound. Report any abnormalities.

▶Points for practice

PFP1 Examine the care plan and the current dressing to determine what type is being used and whether it has been adequate, e.g. whether more padding to absorb exudate is needed. If necessary, assess the wound before the dressing (see p. 282)

PFP2 The type of dressing pack will vary according to availability, individual preference and the type of wound. If necessary, warm the solution according to local policy to prevent wound cooling.

PFP3 Do not leave the patient unattended on a raised bed. Leave the screens only partly drawn until you return if there are concerns about patient safety.

PFP4 The trolley or surface used must be cleaned thoroughly before use. Local policies may vary, but hot soapy (detergent) water is recommended and the surface must then be dried thoroughly to discourage the growth of microorganisms (Wilson 2006). If alcohol wipes are indicated in the policy, those designed for hard surfaces (not skin wipes) must be used and allowed to dry thoroughly.

PFP5 In some hospitals, dressings are performed in a clean treatment room rather than at the bedside, to reduce the risk of cross-infection.

PFP6 Some practitioners put their hand inside the clinical waste bag and use it as a 'glove' to arrange the sterile equipment on the trolley. Unsterile gloves are then used in step 12 to remove the soiled dressing.

PFP7 Leave the existing dressing in place to minimise wound exposure to airborne organisms and minimise wound cooling as this affects wound healing (Wilson 2006). If the dressing is heavily bloodstained unsterile gloves should be used to loosen it.

PFP8 The waste bag should be positioned so that used swabs can be discarded without passing over the sterile field.

PFP9 Gauze should not be used to clean inside the wound as this has been shown to damage the delicate granulating tissue of a healing wound. In some hospitals the solution is warmed to prevent cooling and vasoconstriction at the wound site.

PFP10 A syringe (usually 10 ml unless the wound is very large) should be used to gently irrigate any wound that needs cleaning. There is a lack of agreement regarding the recommended pressure to use when irrigating the wound (Spear 2011).

9.3 Removal of skin closures: sutures/staples

Preparation

Patient
- Explain the procedure, to gain consent and cooperation
- Check patient comfort, e.g. position, convenience, need for toilet, etc.
- Administer analgesics if appropriate and allow time to take effect ➡ **PFP1**
- Adjust the bedclothes to permit easy access to the wound but maintain warmth and dignity ➡ **PFP2**

Equipment
- Dressing pack containing sterile gloves
- Sterile scissors/stitch cutter and forceps or staple remover as appropriate
- Alcohol hand-rub or hand washing facilities
- Draw screens around the bed and ensure adequate light. Clear bed area, close windows, turn off fan, etc.

Nurse
- Consult the care plan to determine when the sutures/staples are due for removal, the dressing type, etc.
- Make sure hair is tied back securely
- Wash and dry hands thoroughly. An apron should be worn
- Additional protective clothing may be necessary if indicated by the patient's condition (see Ch. 1)

Procedure

1. Follow the procedure for the aseptic dressing technique to step 9 (see p. 285).
2. Taking care to maintain sterility, open the stitch cutter and forceps or staple remover onto the sterile field (Figure 9.6).
3. Adjust any remaining bedclothes to expose the wound then loosen the existing dressing but do not remove it.
4. Wash your hands or use alcohol hand-rub. Make sure that your hands are completely dry before proceeding.
5. Open the sterile waste bag and put your hand inside so that the bag acts as a glove (see Figure 9.2). Use this to remove and inspect the old dressing.

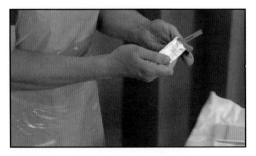

Figure 9.6 Opening stich cutter onto sterile field.

6. Turn the bag inside out so that the dressing is contained within it, and using the adhesive strip, attach the bag to the side of the trolley or other convenient place close to the wound ➡ **PFP3**.

7. Taking care not to touch the outside of the gloves, put on the sterile gloves (see Figure 9.3).

8. Inspect the wound for signs of healing. If the wound looks inflamed or there is any exudate (pus) present, advice should be sought from an experienced nurse. It may be necessary to remove just one or two sutures/staples to allow the pus to drain ➡ **PFP4**.

9. Do not clean the wound before removing the sutures/staples, as cleansing solution may seep into the holes made by the sutures/staples when removed.

10. If the wound is longer than 15 cm, remove alternate sutures/staples and check that the wound is fully healed before removing the rest ➡ **PFP5**:

    • **Individual sutures** – use the forceps to lift up the knot of the suture. In your other hand, hold the scissors or stitch cutter flat against the skin and slide it under the suture to cut it (Figure 9.7A). The place where you cut it is important; in order to prevent infection the part of the suture that has been lying on the skin must not be drawn underneath the skin.

    • **Staples** – a special instrument is used to remove staples (Figure 9.7B). This should be placed under the centre of the staple and squeezed hard. This bends the staple so that it comes out of the skin easily and does not have to be 'hooked' out. The staple can be steadied, if necessary, by holding it with forceps.

    • **Continuous suture** – this means the incision is held together with one thread, which passes under and over the incision about every centimetre. There is a knot at each end. Use the forceps to lift the knot at one end and cut the first 'suture' at the end furthest from the knot (Figure 9.8A). Lift the knot to remove the loose end from under the skin and cut close to the skin (Figure 9.8B). Slide the forceps under the next stitch (Figure 9.8C), raise it to remove the underlying thread and cut it close to the skin. Repeat this process with all the others, making sure that the part that has been on the skin is not pulled underneath the skin. Never cut both ends of a suture or you will be unable to remove the hidden part underneath the skin.

    • **Subcutaneous suture** – this is a continuous suture but it is not visible above the skin. There is usually a bead at each end. Cut the thread holding one bead and gently pull the other until the whole thread is removed from under the skin.

11. Use a gauze swab dipped in cleansing solution to clean and then dry <u>around</u> the wound if necessary (not the wound itself).

12. If there are any small areas where the skin edges are not completely healed together, skin-closure strips may be applied ➡ **PFP6**.

13. If appropriate, apply the new dressing.

14. Place any sharps, e.g. stitch cutters, in a sharps bin. Forceps, if not disposable, should be returned to the sterile supplies department for decotamination.

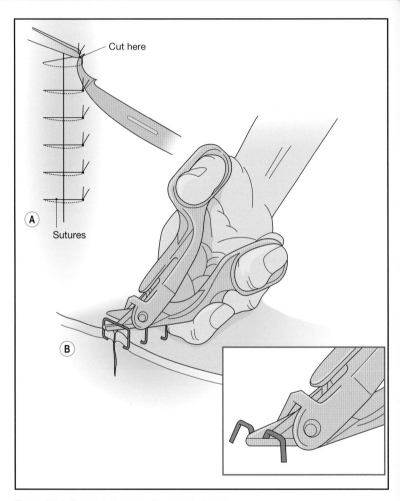

Figure 9.7 A: Removal of sutures; B: removal of staples.

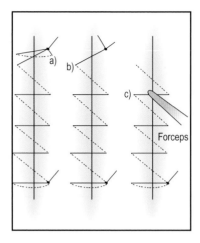

Figure 9.8 Removal of continuous suture.

15. Wrap all non-sharp disposable items in the sterile field and place in the waste bag. Remove gloves, discard into the clinical waste bag and tie securely.

16. Replace the bedclothes and assist the patient as necessary into a comfortable position, and readjust the bed to a safe height.

17. Remove apron, discard in the clinical waste bag and wash hands.

18. Return any unused items to the stock cupboard. Clean the trolley according to local policy.

19. Document the care given and the condition of the wound. Report any difficulties with the procedure, changes or abnormalities.

▶ Points for practice

PFP1 The removal of sutures or staples should not be painful, although the patient may anticipate pain or discomfort. Explanation and careful positioning may alleviate this.

PFP2 Do not leave the patient unattended on a raised bed. Leave the screens only partly drawn until you return if there are concerns about patient safety.

PFP3 The waste bag should be positioned so that used swabs can be disposed of without passing over the sterile field.

PFP4 If the wound is longer than 15 cm or if the incision is in a place where there may be a strain on the skin and underlying tissues, it is better to remove

---

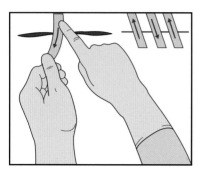

Figure 9.9 Applying skin-closure strips.

alternate sutures/staples, starting with the second one along. This allows you to check that the wound does not begin to gape at any point before the rest are removed. If the wound begins to gape, the remaining sutures/staples may be left until the following day and reassessed. In some instances the number of sutures/staples removed needs to be documented. With continuous sutures (see step 10), if the wound begins to gape do not remove any more. Make sure it is clear where the free end is and the rest can be left in place.

PFP5 When removing sutures only make one cut until you can determine where the loose end is and it is visible. Cut the suture as close to the skin as possible. The part of the suture that has been lying on the skin must not be pulled under the skin during removal as this will introduce microorganisms into the skin.

PFP6 Skin-closure strips are used to pull the edges of the wound together to promote healing. Starting at the centre of the wound, attach the strip to the skin on one side of the wound and making sure that the skin edges are aligned without creating excessive tension, lay it over the wound and attach it to the skin on the other side. The next and any subsequent strips should be attached first to alternate sides of the wound (Figure 9.9). This will apply even pressure to the wound edges (Lynch and Cole 2006).

9.4 Wound drainage

Principles

Open system

* This refers to a hollow tube or corrugated piece of rubber or plastic that is situated in the wound to promote drainage into the dressing (Figure 9.10). If there is a large amount of drainage, the end of the drain may be inserted into a stoma bag (see p. 273). This is designed to keep the wound area free from drainage and thus reduce the risk of infection and to prevent damage to the skin.

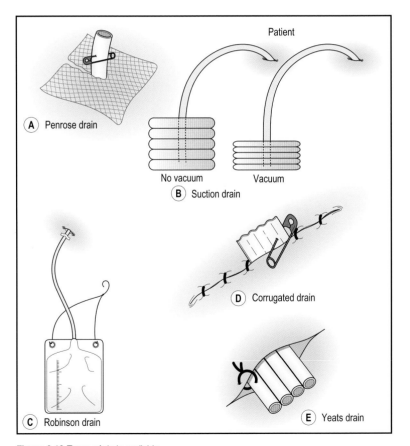

Figure 9.10 Types of drain available.

Closed system

- This refers to a system whereby the drain is attached to tubing and a bag for the collection of drainage. This means that the system is 'closed' and thus the risk of infection is greatly reduced. Many closed systems incorporate a vacuum to encourage active drainage (Figure 9.11).

- The bag or bottle should be supported by attachment to the bed or patient's clothing to prevent pulling, kinking, blockage and accidental dislodgement of the drain.

- Asepsis must be maintained when changing the bag or bottle (see p. 3).

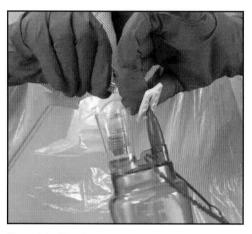

Figure 9.11 Changing a vacuum drainage bottle.

9.5 Changing a vacuum drainage bottle

Preparation

Patient
- Explain the procedure, to gain consent and cooperation
- Adjust the bed to a safe working height. Take care not to dislodge the drain

Equipment
- New sterile vacuum drainage bottle (check that a vacuum is present)
  ➡ **PFP1**
- Orange/Yellow clinical waste bag

Nurse
- Wash and dry hands thoroughly
- Put on apron and clean gloves
- If there is a danger of splashing, goggles should be worn
  ➡ **PFP2**

Procedure

1. Detach the drainage bottle from the bed, taking care not to let the bottle slip or the drainage tube may be pulled out.
2. With the clamps that are provided as part of the system, clamp off both the drainage tube (above the connection to the bottle) and the bottle.

Bottle system

1. Carefully remove the drainage tube from the 'old' bottle, taking care not to touch the last 2–3 cm to keep it sterile.
2. Note the volume of drainage, then discard the bottle with its contents into the clinical waste bag ➡ **PFP3**.
3. Using an aspetic non-touch technique (p. 3) connect the tubing firmly into the new bottle and release the vacuum clamp (Figure 9.11). Release the clamp on the drainage tubing.

Small concertina system

1. If it is necessary to empty the drainage and replace the vacuum container, detach the container, empty into a jug taking care to avoid splashing.
2. Squeeze the container flat, push the tubing firmly back into container and release the clamp on the drainage tubing.
3. If drainage is no longer required, remove the drainage tubing and insert the stopper. Discard into the clinical waste system
4. Secure the container to the bed or patient's clothing to prevent pulling. Check the vacuum is present (Figure 9.12).
5. Remove gloves, discard into clinical waste bag and close securely.
6. Ensure the patient is comfortable and the drain is not pulling. Adjust the bed to a safe height.
7. Dispose of equipment and clinical waste appropriately.
8. Remove apron, discard in the clinical waste and wash hands.
9. Document the amount and type of drainage according to local policy.

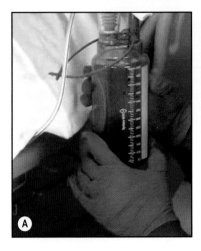

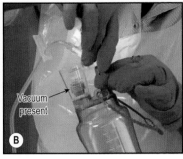

Figure 9.12 Vacuum drainage system. A: Vacuum lost; B: vacuum present.

➡Points for practice

PFP1 The presence of a vacuum is usually indicated by the small concertina of plastic folds at the top of the bottle; when the vacuum is no longer present, the concertina effect is lost (Figure 9.12). If only a small amount of drainage is expected, a small concertina container may be used. This is squeezed flat to create a vacuum and then the stopper is replaced to maintain the vacuum.

PFP2 If there is a risk of splashing during the bottle change, goggles should be worn. However, nurses who wear spectacles do not need to wear goggles (see Ch. 1).

PFP3 The used bottle, once clamped, should be discarded into the clinical waste bag. It should not be emptied because of the risk of splashing and contact with blood.

9.6 Removal of wound drain

Preparation

Patient
- Explain the procedure, to gain consent and cooperation.
- Prepare the patient as described on page 285.

Equipment/Environment
- As for the aseptic dressing technique (see p. 285) plus:
  - Sterile stitch cutter or sterile scissors.
  - Sterile disposable forceps.
  - Sterile dressing towel

Nurse
- Wash and dry hands thoroughly
- Put on apron
- Ensure hair is tied back securely
- Additional protective clothing may be necessary if indicated by the patient's condition (see Ch. 1)

Procedure

1. Prepare the patient, bed area and equipment as described for the aseptic dressing technique (see p. 285).

2. Note the amount of drainage. If the drain has a vacuum bottle attached, clamp the tubing with the clamp provided to prevent suction during removal of the drain ➡ **PFP1**.

3. Put on sterile gloves and clean the site, if necessary, so that the knot of the suture holding the drain in place is visible and accessible ➡ **PFP2**. Place the sterile towel under the tubing.

4. Lift up the knot of the suture with the sterile forceps, and using the stitch cutter, cut the suture close to the skin, and remove the suture (see p. 290).

5. Fold a gauze swab several times to create an absorbent pad and hold this over the site.

6. Warning the patient of a pulling sensation, gently remove the drain onto the sterile towel. Use counter-pressure on the skin with the other hand if resistance is felt ➡ **PFP3**.

7. Maintain pressure over the site until bleeding/drainage is minimal. Cover the site with a sterile dressing.

8. Detach the bottle from the bed/clothing. Wrap the bottle and the tubing in the sterile towel and discard into the clinical waste bag.

9. Place any sharps e.g. stitch cutter, in the sharps bin. Scissors, if not disposable, should be returned to the sterile supplies department for decontamination. Remove gloves and discard with dressing pack into the clinical waste bag and close securely.

10. Ensure the patient is comfortable and readjust the bed height.

11. Remove apron and wash hands.

12. Document the time and date of removal, the amount and type of drainage, and the condition of the wound

> **Points for practice**
>
> **PFP1** Clamping the tubing prevents suction during removal, which may be painful for the patient.
>
> **PFP2** If the drain site appears inflamed or purulent, a swab for culture and sensitivity should be taken (see p. 17).
>
> **PFP3** Check that the entire drain has been removed. If the drain cannot easily be removed, leave it in position and report it to the nurse in charge.

9.7 Topical negative pressure wound therapy

Principles

- Topical negative pressure (TNP) wound therapy (also known as vacuum assisted closure therapy®) is increasingly being used to promote and accelerate the closure of wounds.

- TNP wound therapy provides a uniform negative pressure to the wound bed to stimulate blood flow and generate the formation of granulation tissue. TNP therapy also draws off excess exudate to promote an optimum moist wound bed environment, reduces the number of bacteria (bacterial load) from the wound bed, removes odour, and reduces oedema from the surrounding tissues (Dealey 2005). At the same time, the negative pressure draws the wound edges together to encourage wound contraction.

- A range of different devices is available from a number of manufacturers and detailed information on each device, its application, and relevant materials will be found in the manufacturer's instruction manua. Inapporpriate or wrongly applied TNP wound therapy can harm the patient and it is the nurse's responsibility to ensure they are familiar with the device to ensure safe and accurate practice. Help and support is avaiable in many hospitals from the Tissue Viability Specialist. Nurses can also contact the manufacturer's representative for advice, training and education.

- TNP wound therapy can be applied to wounds that are slow to heal, have excessive wound fluid (exudate), or wound cavities. TNP wound therapy has been found to be effective for patients with acute, or traumatic wounds (e.g. dehisced surgical wounds, flaps, skin grafts, and partial thickness burns), and chronic wounds (e.g. pressure ulcers, diabetic ulcers and venous leg ulcers). Not all wounds will benefit from TNP wound therapy; it may have a detrimental effect on patients with fistulae, malignancy, presence of necrotic tissue, and osteomyelitis, (Benbow 2005, Ousey 2005)

- The equipment used to apply TNP wound therapy generally consists of a wound contact dressing (e.g gauze material or foam), drainage tubes, and a wound drainage collection canister, which is attached to the powered vacuum pump. A transparent film dressing is used to cover the contact dressing to ensure a tight seal around the edges of the wound. It is important to refer to the manufacturer's instructions for the device being used.

- As with all wound management, an initial wound assessment must be undertaken before TNP wound therapy is applied. It is also important to assess its effectiveness each time the dressing is changed.

- Dressings are usually changed every 48–72 hours using an aseptic technique. If the wound is infected the dressing may need to be changed every 12–24 hours.

- When the vacuum pump is switched on with the prescribed pressure the TNP wound therapy dressing contracts and becomes hard as the air pressure beneath the dressing is removed. When setting the prescribed negative pressure always take advice from the manufacturer's recommendations to ensure the correct pressure is used. If the pressure is incorrect, the patient may experience pain and bruising at the wound bed, which will adversely affect the healing process. The negative pressure may need to be increased slowly to reach the required level according to the patient's tolerance and comfort. The device can be programmed to apply continuous or intermittent negative pressure (Preston 2008).

- Document the assessment of the wound according to local policy. This should include: any concerns about the condition of the wound or treatment, the amount of drainage in the canister, when the TNP wound therapy dressing was changed and the pressure setting.

- The nurse must regularly inspect the device to ensure it is working correctly to avoid complications. Always check the manufacturer's instructions about the alarms, which may be visual or audible. For example, alarms may be triggered when the canister is full, the drainage tubes are blocked or kinked, the transparent film dressing is leaking or the battery life is low. Portable devices need the batteries recharging as requird; static devices must be connected to the wall socket but usually have a backup battery for short-term use.

9.8 Peri-operative care

Principles

There are three phases to the patient's surgical journey: pre-operative, intra-operative and postoperative. Together, these phases are known as the peri-operative period. Surgery can be classified as elective (planned) or emergency (unplanned). When patients are admitted for planned surgery (e.g. cholecystectomy, hysterectomy) a full assessment is undertaken in the pre-admission clinic, and any potential complications are addressed to ensure the patient's optimum health before surgery. However, this is not the case for emergency procedures, where the time available to prepare the patient is usually short. Emergency surgery may be due to trauma and accidents (e.g. head injury or ruptured spleen), obstruction of the gastrointestinal tract (strangulated hernia, bowel cancer) or perforated viscera (e.g ulcer, appendix) (Gilmore 2010).

There have been significant advances in the types of techniques used for surgery and many procedures are now undertaken using key hole, robotic or laparoscopic surgery. The nurse has an important part to play in the physical and psychological preparation of the patient before surgery and their continuing care during the post-operative phase. This is because it is recognised that patients who well prepared for surgery will experience fewer postoperative complications and an enhanced recovery (Garretson 2004).

The following principles focus on the care of a patient undergoing elective surgery although many are equally relevant to emergency procedures.

Pre-operative care

Pre-operative care involves the physical and psychological care of a patient before surgery, and preparation of the environment and bed area. When preparing the patient for surgery the nurse must address a number of considerations.

Consent

The surgeon is ultimately responsible for obtaining the patient's consent before any surgical procedure. For consent to be valid, patients must have the capacity to understand and retain information about the procedure long enough to decide whether they wish to proceed with the surgery. Patients must also be able to weigh up the consequences of the surgical procedure and communicate their decision to the medical staff (Department of Health 2009). Patients must give their consent willingly, without influence or pressure from family, friends or medical staff. Under no circumstances should any pre-operative medication be given before the consent is confirmed (Department of Health 2009). It is the nurse's responsibility to check that the patient's consent is completed correctly before they go to theatre.

Anxiety

It is generally accepted that undergoing surgery is an anxiety provoking time that can make patients feel vulnerable, nervous or even distressed. Determining the factors that triggers these feelings helps the nurse to address the patient's fears and concerns. These often include: fear of the unknown (what to expect, diagnosis), fear of the anaesthetic, fear of pain, feeling ill, dying, change in body image, separation from children and family, loss of security (Sterling 2006). Giving pre-operative patient education and support is vital to help the patients understand their surgery and what is expected of them, but it also helps to reduce anxiety, stress, and pain, which may promote the patient's well-being (Boore 1978). It is important to describe the recovery phase including any equipment to expect (e.g. catheter, IV fluids, naso-gastric tube), the method of pain control (e.g. PCA, p. 71), and information about mobility, when they can eat and drink, postoperative nausea and vomiting and breathing exercises (Garretson 2004).

Pre-operative hygiene

Effective hygiene prior to surgery will reduce the number of microorganisms on the skin and minimise the risk of a postoperative surgical site infection (Pratt et al. 2007). Most patients will be asked to shower surgery using an anti-bacterial solution the night before and the morning of surgery. The patient will then need to change into a theatre gown as this allows access to the operation site. Some patients may be able to wear cotton or disposable underwear to maintain dignity according to the local Trust policy.

Pre-operative checklist

A pre-operative check list is completed by the nurse according to local policy before the patient is taken to the operating theatre department. This usually includes the following:

- **Identification namebands** must contain the patient's full name, date of birth and NHS number (NPSA 2007). This information must correspond with the patient's medical notes to ensure that the correct patient is identified. Many Trusts require two namebands (one on the wrist and the other on the ankle) so that the patient can still be identified if one is removed e.g. when a cannula is inserted.

- **Allergies** It is important to ask whether the patient has any allergies (e.g skin preparation solution (iodine), dressings and plasters, medications, antibiotics, and latex) to reduce any potential harm to the patient during surgery. If an allergy is known the patient must wear an allergy alert nameband and any known allergies must be documented in the patient's notes (NPSA 2007). It is also important to indicate any adverse reactions to previous blood transfusions or blood products.

- **Baseline observations** The patient's respiratory rate, pulse rate, blood pressure and temperature must be recorded (see Ch. 2) to establish a baseline for intra and postoperative comparison. The patient's weight will be required by the anaesthetist in order to calculate the correct dose of anaesthetic medication.

- **Pregnancy test** With the women's consent, a pregnancy test should be performed on all women of childbearing age. An unknown pregnancy during the first trimester may pose an adverse risk to the woman and the fetus (NPSA 2010).

- **Marking the operation site** It is the surgeon's responsibility to mark the operation site. The operation site must be marked with an indelible pen and correspond with the patient's medical notes (NPSA 2009).

- **Pre-operative fasting** The nurse must document when the patient last ate and drank. It is important that the patient has no food for at least 6 hours and no fluids for 2 hours before going to theatre (RCN 2005). Sweets and chewing gum must not be eaten on the day of surgery as these stimulate gastric juices. This safeguards the patient from the risk of regurgitation and aspiration of gastric contents whilst undergoing a general anaesthetic. If the patient is prescribed regular oral medication this can be given with a small amount of fluid 2–3 hours before surgery. However, if the nurse is unsure, it is their responsibility to check with the medical team or anaesthetist.

- **Dental** The presence of dental crowns, caps, bridgework or loose teeth must be documented as these may obstruct the airway if they accidentally become dislodged and inhaled during the induction of anaesthesia. Dentures are normally removed and stored in a labelled denture pot.

- **Jewellery and piercings** Body piercings and jewellery must be removed or securely taped accoring to local policy. These may become dislodged and lost when the patient is moved and the use of diathermy may harm the patient (diathermy burns) if wearing metal jewellery. Wedding/partnership rings and other items of jewellery that cannot be removed must be secured to avoid loss. Some local Trust policies may allow certain items of jewellery for cultural reasons if they do not compromise the patient's safety. These must be documented in the patient's notes.

- **Nail varnish, false nails and make-up** Nail varnish and false nails must be removed as they will affect the accuracy of the oxygen saturation result (p. 350). Make-up must also be removed as this will make it difficult to assess the patient's skin colour.

- **Spectacles, hearing aids, contact lenses and prostheses** The presence of any prosthesis must be noted and, if appropriate, removed. Contact lenses can become dry and cause corneal abrasions if left in place for prolonged periods. A hearing aid should remain in place to allow the patient to communicate and understand what is happening before they are anesthetised. Spectacles should be removed when the patient is in the anaesthetic room. Prostheses such as false limbs should be removed before leaving the ward and if unable to be removed (e.g. cardiac pacemaker) this must be documented on the pre-operative checklist.

- **Urinalysis and empty bladder** A routine urinalysis should be performed to detect any abnormalities as further treatment may be required (see p. 242). Check that the patient has passed urine before surgery to avoid urinary incontinence and contamination of the sterile field whilst anesthetised. This also prevents the bladder being accidentally damaged during surgery.

- **Venous thromboembolism risk assessment** must be done to identify the patient's risk factors and determine the most appropriate treatment to reduce the risk of a deep vein thrombosis (p. 384) (NICE 2010). When anti-embolic stockings are used these must be correctly measured and applied (p. 386).

- **Hair removal** may be necessary when the surgeon's view of the operation site is restricted or where it is difficult to apply the ECG adhesive pads or dressings/plaster. The nurse should consult their local policy for the method of hair removal e.g. shaving, electric clippers or depilatory creams. If shaving of the operation site is required this is done as close as possible to the time of the operation.

- **Medical notes, X-rays, blood tests etc.** The nurse must ensure that the medical notes, X-rays, scans, blood results, consent form, prescription chart, observation chart, and any other relevant documents accompany the patient to the operating theatre department. This will facilitate a safe and accurate handover to the theatre staff and provide the surgeon with all the information necessary before the surgery begins.

- **Pre-medication** Once the pre-operative checklist has been completed, if prescribed, the nurse will administer the pre-medication to help the patient relax and reduce their anxiety. As this is a sedative the patient needs to remain in bed and use the call bell if they require any assistance.

Intra-operative care

This refers to the physical and psychological care given to the patient whilst in the anaesthetic room, operating theatre and the recovery area. Before the patient returns to the ward it is important that the nurse assesses the patient and receives a comprehensive handover from the theatre staff. This should include: the type of surgery, any concerns or complications, any blood transfusions, any medications administered in recovery, any special instructions (when they can eat and drink), vital signs, level of consciousness, pain management, wound and wound drainage, intravenous fluids, and the urine output. The patient must not be transferred to the ward until they are conscious, able to maintin their own airway and their clinical observations are stable.

Postoperative care

This includes the physical and psychological care given to the patient to ensure they are safely discharged from the recovery area and transferred back to the ward. Once back in the ward it is vital that the nurse performs a full nursing assessment. Using the ABCDE approach enables the nurse to systematically assess the patient's condition, determine the priorities of care and recognise the early deterioration of the patient (see p. 76). These observations provide a baseline for the patient's postoperative care and should be compared with the pre and intra-operative recordings. Frequency of the observations will be determined by the patient's condition. Many organisations have local polices which stipulate the frequency of postoperative observations but it is important that nurses use professional judgement to interpret the observations to closely minotor the patient's condition. Use of an early warning score (p. 76) will alert the nurse should the patient's condition start to deteriorate.

ABCDE assessment of A postoperative patient

Some specific aspects of this assessment will depend on the type of surgery. For example, following orthopaedic or vascular surgery assessment might include neurovascular assessment (p. 60). The systematic ABCDE assessment on page 76 should be used for postoperative assessment. In addition the following are important for most postoperative patients.

- **Level of consciousness** should be assessed using AVPU (p. 53). When a more comprehensive neurological assessment is needed (e.g following neurological surgery) the Glasgow coma scale (p. 48) should be used. Unconscious patients need careful monitoring. Snoring or noisy breathing indicates a partially obstructed airway and must be reported.

- **Psychological suppport** Although most patients will be prepared for surgery they are likely to feel anxious, and will continue to need reassurance. Information relating to the outcome of the surgery, any attachments, equipment, the use of PCA, or any other concerns or worries will need to be addressed (e.g. altered body image). The involvement of the family is equally important during the postoperative phase.

- **Oxygen** Many patients will be prescribed oxygen by mask or nasal cannula (p. 338) postoperatively, and some will require oxygen for a longer period. The number of litres of oxygen may be prescribed as a range (e.g. 4–6 litres) and this adjusted in response to the patient's oxygen saturation (p. 350). The target oxygen saturation for the patient will be documented on the prescription chart.

- **Intravenous fluids** It is important to ensure that IV fluids run at the prescribed rate and the cannula is inspected regularly using the visual infusion phlebitis (VIP) score (p. 122). All input and output will be documented on a fluid balance chart.

- **Antibiotics** Check the prescription chart for any additional medications e.g prophylactic antibiotics; often a single dose is prescribed after the operation. As with all medicines, it is important to check for allergies.

- **Wounds and drains** Observe the wound site and any wound drainage and note the amount and type of drainage (p. 295) If the operation is per vagina, record the blood loss by noting the number of sanitary pads. If the operation in transurethral, there will be continuous bladder irrigation (p. 265).

- **Nasogastric tube** This may be on free drainage or require manual aspiration. The amount and type of aspirate must be documented.

- **Nil by mouth** All patients will be unable to eat and drink for a period of time. Instructions regarding when they can commence oral fluids will be part of the operation notes. If the surgery has involved the bowel it will be necessary to wait for bowel sounds to return before the patient can start drinking. Inspect the mouth (p. 318) and provide regular mouth care/mouth washes while the patient is unable to take oral fluids.

- **Pain** Assess the patient's pain using a pain score (p. 66) and the effectiveness of the pain management system used, e.g patient controlled analgesia (p. 71). Ensure patients know how to use the PCA or request analgesics before the pain becomes severe.

- **Postoperative nausea and vomiting (PONV)** Many patients experience PONV and this should be assessed when assessing pain. Many patients report that PONV is one of the most distressing aspects of their hospital stay. Ensure the patient has anti-emetics prescribed. Prophylaxis is often prescribed for patients at moderate to high risk for PONV (Gibson and Magowan 2011).

- **Urine output** If the patient is catheterised, it is important to closely monitor the urine output. Output of less than 0.5 ml per kg per hour should be reported. If the patient is not catheterised it is important to document when the patient first passes urine.

- **Temperature** Many patients will have a low temperature following surgery and so need to be slowly warmed see page 34. It is important to continue to monitor the patient's temperature as a raised temperature may be the first indication of an infection.

- **Blood glucose level** If the patient has diabetes he/she may be prescribed an insulin infusion that is titrated according to their blood gluscose level. A variable dose regimen (sliding scale) will be prescribed.

- **Complications of reduced mobility** Most patients will be able to mobilise very soon after the operation but those with reduced mobility require re-assessment for pressure ulcer risk using a recognised assessment tool e.g. Waterlow (p. 377) and the risk of venous-thromboembolism risk (p. 384). Inspect the patent's anti-embolism stockings to ensure that they are applied correctly (p. 386).

Bibliography/Suggested reading

Anderson, I., 2007. Use of Doppler ultrasound in assessing leg ulcers. Nursing Standard 21 (47), 50–56.

This article provides a comprehensive overview of the use of Doppler ultrasound in assessing patients with leg ulcers, and includes the use of equipment, the procedure, calculating ABPI and the implications of the results

Baxter, H., 2003. Management of surgical wounds. Nursing Times 99 (13), 66, 68.

A useful article that examines the intrinsic and extrinsic factors that affect wound healing, such as skin preparation and shaving, and complications such as dehiscence

Benbow, M., 2005. Evidence-based wound management. Whurr, London.

This is a useful book that includes the origins of wound care, wound assessment, classification and types of wounds and wound management treatment and therapies. Each chapter provides a concise source of resources and research to underpin the principles addressed within this book

Benbow, M., 2009. Woundcare: the basics. Practice Nurse 37 (6), 20–25.

This article provides an overview of the basic principles relating to wound care and includes an overview of wound assessment, a description of wound bed preparation using the TIME framework, which identifies barriers to wound healing, and documentation.

Boore, J., 1978. Prescription for recovery. RCN, London.

This seminal piece of research still has relevancy today to demonstrate that pre-operative patient education can have a positive outcome to the patient during the postoperativephase of their recovery. It shows that effective pre-operative preparation reduces anxiety, pain, and infection to enhance the patient's recovery

Bowers, K., Barrett, S., 2009. Wound-related pain: features, assessment and treatment. Nursing Standard 24 (10), 47–56.

A useful article that forms part of the Continuing Professional Development series and provides an overview of the different types of pain, and pain assessment and management for a patient with a wound

Collier, M., 2003. The elements of wound assessment. Nursing Times 99 (13),48–49.

This article provides a good overview of the holistic assessment of wounds and includes classification, assessment of the surrounding skin, using photographic records and documentation

Dealey, C., 2005. The care of wounds, a guide for nurses, 3rd edn. Blackwell, Oxford.

A comprehensive book that covers the history of wound care, physiology of wound healing, types of dressings, wound management interventions and all types of wounds and even skin care for patients undergoing radiation

Department of Health, 2009. Reference guide to consent, examination and treatment, 2nd edn. HMSO, London. [online]. Available from: www.dh.gov.uk (accessed 06.08.11.).

This document updates the previous 2001 edition and provides specific guidance for consent for individuals having physical interventions. There document sets out clear standards for seeking consent and covers issues relating to the mental capacity of adult, consent with children and young adults and withdrawing consent

Fletcher, J., Anderson, I., 2011. Tissue viability and managing chronic wounds. In: Brooker, C., Nicol, M. (Eds.), Alexandra's nursing practice, 4th edn. Churchill Livingstone Elsevier, Edinburgh.

Although Chapter 23 addresses some issues relating to chronic wounds, it provides a comprehensive guide to wound healing, wound assessment and the management of different types of wounds

Garettson, S., 2004. Benefits of pre-operative information programmes. Nursing Standard 18 (47), 33–37.

This article discusses the benefits of pre-operative information and how nurses can develop resources and programmes to improve patient outcomes before surgery

Gibson, C., Magowan, R., 2011. Nursing the patient undergoing surgery. In: Brooker, C., Nicol, M. (Eds.), Alexander's nursing practice, 4th edn. Churchill Livingstone Elsevier, Edinburgh, Ch 26.

This comprehensive chapter explores all aspects of peri-operative care including pre-operative assessment, safety in the operating theatre, anaesthesia, recovery from anaesthesia and postoperativecare. The risk factors for PONV are explained. The accompanying website contains case studies and a postoperativecare plan

Gilmore, D., 2010. Peri-operative care. In: Pudner, R. (Ed.), Nursing the surgical patient, 3rd edn. Bailière Tindall, Edinburgh.

This is a useful text that covers the main principles of surgical care for adults to include an overview of the principles of perioperative care with a depth overview of some related issues, nutrition and wound healing. The book also covers different surgical procedures and identifies the principles of care for each area

Hart, S., 2007. Using an aseptic technique to reduce the risk of infection. Nursing Standard 21 (47), 43–47.

This article stresses the importance of hand washing in reducing HCAI and discusses the difference between, and indications for, surgical aseptic technique and aseptic non touch technique (ANTT)

Hoban, V., 2005. Wound care; what every nurse should know. Nursing Times 101 (12), 20–22.

An interesting article that argues that wound care is every nurse's responsibility, not just the responsibility of the specialist tissue-viability nurses. It discusses evidence-based practice, type of dressing and their uses and the early warning signs that something is going wrong

Lynch, T., Cole, E., 2006. Techniques for acute wound closure. Nursing Standard 20 (21), 55–64.

Although the focus is on acute wounds most of the article is equally applicable to other wounds. It covers wound assessment, wound cleansing and different types of wound closure

Myers, B., 2011. Wound management principles and practice, 3rd edn. Pearson, New Jersey.

This is a comprehensive text that includes wound healing, wound assessment, types of wounds and wound therapies and interventions. At the end of each chapter there is a summary of key points with questions to answer. A website can be accessed to compliment the book and provides images, video clips and references

National Institute for Health and Clinical Excellence, 2010. Venous thromboembolism: reducing the risk of venous thromboembolism (deep vein thrombosis and pulmonary embolism) in patients admitted to hospital. NICE, London [online]. Available from: http://guidance.nice.org.uk/CG92/Guidance (accessed 04.08.11.).

This guidance sets out the care and treatment of all patients who are at risk from a deep vein thrombosis while in hospital. The guidance covers those who are at risk and the care and treatment that may be necessary whilst in hospital and on discharge

National Patient Safety Agency Alert, 2007. Standardising wristbands improves patient safety. [online]. Available from: www.nrls.npsa.nhs.uk/resources/?entryid45=59842 (accessed 07.08.11.).

This alert gives guidance of the use of and information required for wristbands for patients in hospitals. It is stipulated that wristbands should now be electronically generated

National Patient Safety Agency, 2009. WHO Surgical checklist. [online]. Available from: www.nrls.npsa.nhs.uk/resources/?entryid45=59860 (accessed 07.08.11.).

Although this resource provides an overview of best practice recommendations for safety in the operating department, it outlines the recommendation for marking the operation site

National Patient Safety Agency Alert, 2010. Checking pregnancy before surgery. [online]. Available from: www.nrls.npsa.nhs.uk/alerts/?entryid45=73838 (accessed 05.08.11.).

This NPSA alert provides a background for checking all females of childbearing age before surgery

Ousey, K., 2005. Pressure area care. Blackwell, Oxford.

Although this book primarily focuses on pressure area care and pressure ulcers, some of the key principles within this text can be related to different types of wound. There are some easy to understand explanations around wound therapies and types of dressing

Pratt, R.J., Pellowe, C.M., Wilson, J.A., et al., 2007. Epic2: national evidence-based guidelines for preventing healthcare-associated infections in NHS hospitals in England. Journal of Hospital Infection 65 (1), suppl 1, S1–S64.

These national evidenced-based guidelines set out the broad principles of best practice for preventing HCAI in NHS hospitals in England. The document describes key principles for preventing infections and the required interventions

Preston, G., 2008. An overview of topical negative pressure therapy in wound care. Nursing Standard 23 (7), 62–68.

This article provides an overview of topical negative pressure wound therapy, and discusses some of the current issues that need to be considered with the increasing range of commercial devices now available from different manufacturers. The article also sets the scene for the future and acknowledges that further evidence is needed in this particular area of wound care

Royal College of Nursing, 2005. Peri-operative fasting in adults and children: Practice guideline. RCN, London [online]. Available from: www.rcn.org.uk_data/assets/pdf_file/009/78678/002800.pdf (accessed 05.08.11.).

These practice guidelines provide a comprehensive overview of pre-operative fasting with recommendations for best practice

Spear, M., 2011. Wound cleansing: solutions and techniques. Plastic Surgical Nursing 31 (1), 29, 31.

Reviews the literature on the use of tap water versus normal saline in wounds and the different techniques. Concludes that there is insufficient robust evidence to either support or refute the use of tap water. Likewise there are some different opinions on the amount of pressure and volume required for wound irrigation

Sterling, L., 2006. Reduction and management of pre-operative anxiety. British Journal of Nursing 15 (7), 359–361.

This article discusses the importance of addressing pre-operative anxiety for patients undergoing surgery. It considers the impact of anxiety on the patient and the undesirable consequences on their recovery and includes a description of the possible techniques that can be used to reduce the level of anxiety

Vuolo, J., 2006. Assessment and management of surgical wounds in clinical practice. Nursing Standard 20 (52), 46–56.

An interesting article that provides an overview of surgical wound classification, wound assessment and methods of wound closure for patients with a surgical wound

Wilson, J., 2006. Infection control in clinical practice, 3rd edn. Baillière Tindall, London.

A comprehensive text that explains basic microbiology, types of organisms and how they are spead. It then provides guidance on all aspects of infection control. Chapter 23 provides advice on cleaning, disinfection and sterilisation

Zois, J., 2005. Postoperativenausea and vomiting. [online]. Available from: http://www.slideshare.net/drpritesh/ponv (accessed 15.8.11.).

A well presented powerpoint presentation that exlpains the physiology of PONV and preventative strategies. It also includes the pharmacology of a number of anti-emetics

Chapter 10

Patient hygiene

©2012 Elsevier Ltd.

10.1 Assisting with a bath or shower

Preparation

Patient
- Discuss the patient's preference for a bath or a shower ➡ **PFP1**
- Discuss/assess how much the patient is able to do for themselves and how much assistance may be required
- Ascertain whether the patient wishes to use the toilet before taking them to the bathroom
- Explain the procedure, to gain consent and cooperation

Equipment
- Shower gel or antiseptic cleansing agent, according to local policy ➡ **PFP2**
- Flannel/sponge and towels
- Brush and/or comb
- Toothbrush, toothpaste and denture pot if appropriate
- Shampoo (if required).
- Clean clothing
- Toiletries, make-up, etc., according to individual preference
- Shower stool or plastic chair.
- Hoist and/or other aids to mobility as required

Nurse
- Put on plastic apron
- Additional protective clothing may be necessary if indicated by the patient's condition (see Ch. 1)

Procedure

1. Check that the bathroom is available and that the bath/shower is clean.
2. Run the bath water / check shower is working.
3. Help the patient to collect together clothes and toiletries.
4. Assist the patient to the bathroom and make sure that access by others is restricted, to ensure privacy.
5. For bathing: use your elbow to check that the bath water is the appropriate temperature (40° C) for the patient or a bath thermometer may be used ➡ **PFP3**.
6. Assist the patient with undressing, maintaining dignity by covering them with a towel.
7. Observe the condition of the patient's skin, especially at the pressure points such as heels and sacrum (see p. 377). Note any signs of inflammation, bruising, discoloration or rash. Note the integrity of the skin and its hydration, whether dry, clammy or sweaty, etc.
8. *For bathing:* assist the patient to get into the bath. A mechanical hoist is likely to be required for immobile patients.

   For showering: assist the patient to sit on the shower stool or chair and adjust the water flow to the correct temperature.
9. Assist the patient to wash. Encourage patients to do as much as they can themselves ➡ **PFP4**.
10. If required, assist the patient to wash their hair, using the flannel as an eye-guard to avoid getting shampoo in the eyes.

11. Assist the patient out of the bath or shower, using a hoist if required. Cover the patient with a towel as soon as possible, to provide warmth and maintain dignity.

12. Help the patient to: dry themselves; apply toiletries as requested; dress in chosen clothing; brush or comb their hair; clean their teeth or dentures as appropriate.

13. Assist the patient to return to bed, chair or day room, using a mechanical hoist if required. Check the patient is comfortable.

14. Return/replace towels and toiletries as appropriate.

15. Clean the bath or shower and then wash hands.

16. Document the care noting how much assistance the patient required, the state of their skin and pressure areas and the patient's general condition. Report any significant changes.

➡Points for practice

PFP1 If a shower is not available some patients may prefer to use running water while sitting in an empty bath. This is may be a culturally determined practice related to the requirement to perform ablutions prior to prayer.

PFP2 Some Trusts require patients to use antiseptic cleansing solution rather than soap, as prophylaxis against methicillin-resistant *Staphylococcus aureus* (MRSA).

PFP3 The hands can usually tolerate higher temperatures than the rest of the body. The elbow is more sensitive and will minimise the risk of the water being too hot. The safest option is to use a bath thermometer.

PFP4 If leaving patients to wash themselves make sure they have access to a call bell for assistance.

10.2 Bed bath

Preparation

Patient

- Discuss the procedure, to gain cooperation and consent
- Ascertain if the patient wishes to use a bedpan/urinal or commode prior to their bed bath
- The patient requiring a bed bath will be quite dependent and may possibly be confused or unconscious
- Ensure privacy, warmth and dignity

Equipment

- Close windows and switch off fans
- Cleansing wipes or antiseptic cleansing agent ➡ **PFP1**
- Flannel and disposable cloths
- Two towels
- Toiletries, make-up, etc., according to individual preference
- Brush and/or comb
- Toothbrush and toothpaste, tumbler of water and bowl/receiver
- Bowl of water (hand hot)
- Clean night clothes
- Trolley or suitable work surface
- Linen bag and bags for fouled or infected linen if required.
- Clean bed linen
- Clinical waste bag

Nurse

- An understanding of the patient's individual needs and preferences
- A plastic apron should be worn
- Clean hands
- Gloves are not necessary to wash the body unless required by the patient's condition, e.g. MRSA or *Clostridium difficile* or if the patient has been incontinent ➡ **PFP2**
- Two nurses may be required for this procedure ➡ **PFP3**

Procedure

1. Assist the patient into a comfortable position. Clear space at bedside for bowl of water and toiletries. Adjust bed to a suitable working height.

2. Assist the patient to remove any night clothes, ensuring the patient is covered with a sheet or blanket to maintain warmth and dignity.

3. Assist the patient to wash the face, ears and neck. If soap is used, rinse well and dry thoroughly.

4. Wash, rinse and dry the body in a logical order, exposing only the part of the body to be washed. The suggested order is arms, chest, abdomen, genital area, legs, feet and then back ➡ **PFP4**; however, this should be discussed with the patient to ascertain any preferences. Change the water as it cools or becomes dirty. If two nurses are present, one should wash and rinse while the other dries the body and applies toiletries as requested, e.g. talc, deodorant or body cream. This reduces the amount of time the body is exposed.

5. As the patient is washed, observe the condition of the skin. Note any signs of inflammation, bruising, discoloration or rash. Note the integrity of the skin and its hydration, e.g. whether dry, clammy or sweaty, etc.

6. Put on gloves and assist the patient to wash, rinse and dry the genital area using a disposable cloth. Remember to wash from the front of the perineal area to the back. In males, ensure that the foreskin is repositioned after washing and dry underneath it. If a urinary catheter is in place, wash carefully around the urethral meatus and catheter tubing, moving away from

the meatus, and dry carefully (see p. 260). Change the water after washing the genital area.

7. Once the back and genital areas are washed the bottom sheet can be changed. This will require two nurses.To change the bottom sheet, loosen the sheet and roll it into the centre of the bed, as far as possible under the patient. Open out the clean sheet lengthwise and leaving sufficient to tuck in, roll the rest into the centre of the bed. Secure the corners and tuck in the middle to anchor the sheet. Holding the top sheet to ensure the patient is covered ask the patient to roll over to the opposite edge of the bed. The old sheet may now be removed and put in the laundry bag the clean sheet pulled through and tucked in.

7. Assist the patient to put on night clothes.

8. Remake the bed.

9. Assist the patient to clean teeth or dentures (see p. 320). If the patient is going to sit out of bed after the bed bath, it is often easier to clean the teeth when sitting in a chair.

10. Assist the patient to brush or comb hair and to clean and file nails if necessary (see p. 328).

11. Lower bed.

12. Ensure the patient is left comfortable and has belongings within easy reach.

13. Wash and dry the bowl. Rinse out the flannel if this has been used and leave to dry. Discard any disposable wipes used into the clinical waste. Return the linen bag to its collection point.

14. Remove apron and wash hands.

15. Record the procedure in the nursing documentation, noting how much the patient could do without assistance and the condition of the skin, eyes, mouth, etc.

➡ Points for practice

PFP1 Some Trusts require patients to use an antiseptic cleansing solution instead of soap as part of their infection control policy. Patients may prefer not to use soap on their face and, if they have any skin condition, may use an emulsifying ointment in the water instead of soap. Increasingly, disposable wipes impregnated with a cleansing solution are used.

PFP2 Gloves should be worn when washing the genital area as there is a risk of being contaminated with body fluids. Discard gloves prior to continuing to wash other parts of the body.

PFP3 A bed bath can be carried out by one nurse, but for severely weak or unconscious patients two nurses are required.

PFP4 The back is left until last so that it can be washed and the clean sheet inserted at the same time, to prevent unnecessary movement for the patient. One nurse can often manage until this point, but will need assistance to roll the patient and make the bed with clean linen.

10.3 Oral assessment

Preparation

Patient
- Explain the procedure, to gain consent and cooperation
- Ask the patient to sit upright if their condition allows

Equipment
- Pen torch or other suitable light source
- Tongue depressor

Nurse
- Wash and dry hands thoroughly
- Gloves and an apron should be worn
- Additional protective clothing may be necessary if indicated by the patient's condition (see Ch. 1).

Procedure

1. Raise bed to safe working height.

2. Observe the patient's lips, noting whether they are normal or dry and whether there is any evidence of ulcers, sores, cracks or bleeding.

3. Ascertain whether the patient has any dentures. Note their fit and then ask/assist the patient to remove them. Note the condition of the dentures: whether they are clean, stained, warped or cracked.

4. Place the dentures in water, as they will become warped if left dry for long periods.

5. Put on gloves and using the torch, inspect the patient's teeth, noting any decay, white patches (oral thrush), plaque or debris (food) that may be trapped between the cheek and the gum ➜ **PFP1**. Identify any worn or loose teeth.

6. Using the tongue depressor and torch, inspect the inside of the mouth, paying attention to the gums, tongue and mucous membranes ➜ **PFP2**. Observe whether they are moist, pink and healthy looking or whether there are any blistered, ulcerated or cracked areas. Note any inflammation, swelling or bleeding of the gums and mucous membranes. Note the presence of any halitosis.

7. While inspecting the mouth, note the consistency and amount of any saliva that is present ➜ **PFP3**.

8. Ascertain whether the patient has any difficulty with speech, chewing or swallowing.

9. Discuss the patient's usual oral hygiene measures and assess whether assistance will be required with oral hygiene.

10. Offer the patient water to rinse the mouth.

11. Explain any further interventions that might be required.

12. Ensure the patient is left feeling comfortable and lower bed to a safe height.

13. Clear away any equipment. Remove apron and gloves and discard in the clinical waste.

14. Wash and dry hands.
15. Document the assessment in the nursing records ➡ **PFP4**.
16. Liaise with appropriate staff if any medication or referrals are required.

➡ Points for practice

PFP1 Following a stroke patients often need assistance to check that food is not trapped as they may be unable to detect it.

PFP2 If the patient is unconscious, two nurses may be required – one to carry out the assessment and one to support the patient's jaw during inspection.

PFP3 In older patients xerostomia (reduced salivary flow) is particularly common.

PFP4 Several oral assessment tools are available for use, check local policy.

10.4 Mouth care for a dependent patient

Preparation

Patient

- Explain the procedure, to gain consent and cooperation
- Ensure privacy
- Help the patient into a comfortable sitting position. If the patient is unconscious, position them on their side and cover the bed/pillow with a waterproof cover and a towel

Equipment

- Towel and tissues
- Small, soft toothbrush
- Toothpaste/denture cleaning paste
- Container for dentures if required
- Beaker of water and bowl or receiver
- Mouth care pack
- Chlorhexidine mouthwash if prescribed ➡ **PFP1**
- Cleansing agent (e.g. weak sodium bicarbonate) if required ➡ **PFP2**
- Additional foam sticks if required ➡ **PFP3**
- Lip lubricant if required
- Suction equipment if required
- Clinical waste bag

Nurse

- Wash and dry hands thoroughly
- Put on gloves and apron
- Additional protective clothing may be necessary if indicated by the patient's condition (see Ch. 1)

Procedure

1. Raise bed to a suitable working height.

2. Cover the patient's chest with a towel and place clinical waste bag in a convenient place that allows easy access.

3. If applicable, remove the patient's dentures and place them in clean water, open mouth care tray and pour water into the gallipot/beaker.

4. Using a toothbrush and small amount of toothpaste, clean the teeth, gums and tongue, taking care not to cause any trauma to the mouth. Small up and down or circular strokes are the most effective ➡ **PFP4**. Remember to clean the inner and outer aspects and biting surfaces of the teeth.

5. If the mouth is encrusted with tenacious mucus or trapped food, a weak solution of sodium bicarbonate may be used ➡ **PFP2** – dip foam sticks into a freshly made solution and gently wipe these around the mouth ➡ **PFP3**. Discard foam sticks into clinical waste.

6. Following cleaning, the mouth should be rinsed with water to remove any debris or remaining toothpaste, which can have a drying effect on the oral mucosa. The patient should be encouraged to rinse vigorously and then spit the fluid into a bowl. If the patient is unconscious, the mouth should be rinsed by using foam sticks dipped in water. Gentle suction may be used to remove fluid or excess secretions (see p. 354).

7. If the patient has dentures, these should be cleaned with a toothbrush and denture-cleaning paste and rinsed thoroughly before giving them back to the

patient ➡ **PFP5**. Ordinary toothpaste should not be used as this is too abrasive. Do not dry the dentures as this makes them difficult to insert ➡ **PFP6**.

8. Use the towel to dry around the patient's mouth.

9. If the lips are dry, a thin layer of petroleum jelly or lip balm may be applied.

10. Lower bed and ensure patient is comfortable.

11. Clean the toothbrush and replace in locker with toothpaste.

12. If frequently used, cover the mouthcare tray/ cleansing solution and place on locker.

13. Remove gloves and apron and discard in clinical waste. Wash and dry hands.

14. Write date and time on mouthcare pack cover so that it is discarded within 24 hours.

15. Document any improvement or abnormal findings.

➡ Points for practice

PFP1 Some patients may prefer to rinse their mouth with a mouthwash solution after their teeth and mouth have been cleaned. Chlorhexidine gluconate may be incompatible with some ingredients in toothpaste; leave an interval of at least 30 minutes between using mouthwash and toothpaste (British National Formulary 2011)

PFP2 If sodium bicarbonate solution is required, a weak solution should be prepared by mixing a very small amount (equivalent to 1 teaspoon in 500 ml) in a tumbler of water. If the solution is too strong it may damage the oral mucosa.

PFP3 Foam sticks are not effective at removing plaque from the surface of the teeth, but they are useful for rinsing or refreshing the mouth.

PFP4 If using a battery powered toothbrush, set to minimum setting to avoid trauma to the oral mucosa.

PFP5 If patients have oral thrush (*Candida albicans*), their dentures should be soaked in a chlorhexidine solution for at least 10 minutes to minimise the risk of re-infection.

PFP6 Unconscious patients should not wear their dentures, as these may obstruct the airway. The dentures should be cleaned and stored in water in a labelled denture pot.

10.5 Facial shave

Preparation

Patient

- Ascertain the patient's preferences for shaving and incorporate this into the hygiene routine accordingly
- If possible, the patient should be sitting up

Equipment

- Bowl of hot water
- Flannel/disposable cloth and towel
- Shaving cream or soap
- Razor ➡ **PFP1**
- Aftershave/cologne according to individual preference

Nurse

- Wash and dry hands thoroughly
- Put on apron
- Additional protective clothing may be necessary if indicated by the patient's condition (see Ch. 1)

Procedure

1. Raise bed to a suitable working height. Drape a towel across the patient's chest.
2. Ask/assist the patient to wash their face. Inspect the face for any raised areas, such as moles or sores.
3. Apply the shaving cream or soap to the face, creating a good lather.
4. Using short strokes of the razor in the direction of the hair growth, shave the face starting with the cheeks and moving down towards the neck ➡ **PFP2**. Avoid any raised area such as moles or blemishes.
5. The nurse's free hand should be used to pull the skin taut (Figure 10.1).
6. Rinse the razor after each stroke.
7. When the entire face and neck have been shaved, rinse the face in clean water and pat dry with a towel.

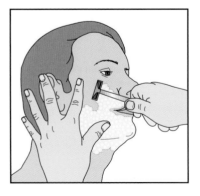

Figure 10.1 Holding the skin taught when shaving.

8. Apply aftershave or cologne if desired.
9. Lower bed and ensure the patient is comfortable.
10. Wash and dry the bowl and replace it in the appropriate storage area. Rinse facecloth thoroughly or discard disposable wipes in the clinical waste.
11. Replace patient's personal equipment in their locker.
12. Remove apron and wash hands/use alcohol hand rub.
13. Document the procedure, noting how much the patient could do for themselves.

➡️Points for practice

PFP1 Many patients will have their own electric razor and so will not require a wet shave. Communal electric razors should not be used, because of the risk of cross-infection. Some depilatory creams are available for the face, but these must be patch tested 24 hours prior to use in case of allergic reaction.

PFP2 Patients can often help by making facial movements that tighten the skin being shaved, e.g. filling out cheeks with the tongue.

10.6 Washing hair in bed

Preparation

Patient

- Explain the procedure, to gain consent and cooperation
- Ascertain the patient's preferences regarding hair care
- Ensure warmth and privacy

Equipment

- Plastic sheeting and absorbent pad or towel to protect the bed
- Shampoo and conditioner if used
- Comb and/or brush
- Flannel/disposable cloth and towels
- Two large plastic bowls (one full of hand-hot water, the other empty) or one shaped bowl for hairwashing ➡ **PFP1**
- Clean jug
- Hairdryer if available

Nurse

- A second nurse may be needed, to support the patient's head and neck
- An apron should be worn
- Additional protective clothing may be necessary if indicated by the patient's condition (see Ch. 1)

Procedure

1. Remove the head of the bed and raise the bed to a suitable working height.

2. Place the plastic sheeting and the absorbent pad or towel over the pillows, and place the empty bowl on a chair at the top of the bed.

3. Ask/assist the patient to lie on their back at the very top of the bed, with pillows supporting the shoulders and the head positioned over the bowl. Cover the shoulders with a towel.

4. Observe the condition of the hair and scalp ➡ **PFP2**. Wet the patient's hair by taking warm water from the bowl into the jug and pouring it over the hair, allowing the water to run into the bowl on the chair.

5. Gently massage shampoo into the hair.

6. Rinse the hair with clean water, ensuring that the patient protects their eyes with the flannel or disposable cloth to avoid shampoo getting in. Repeat the process if the patient would like two applications of shampoo and/or conditioner.

7. If conditioner is used, comb it through the hair and leave for 2–3 minutes before rinsing.

8. After the final rinse, wrap the patient's hair in a towel and remove the bowl of water.

9. Assist the patient into a sitting position (if their condition allows) and towel dry the hair.

10. Lower the bed to a safe height and replace the bed head.

11. Brush or comb the hair into the desired style, using a hairdryer if one is available ➡ **PFP3**.

12. Leave the patient comfortable, and if no hairdryer is available, in a warm environment until the hair is dry.

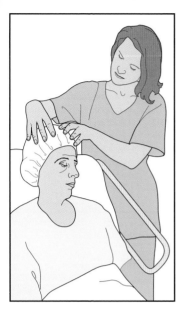

Figure 10.2 Washing the hair using no-rinse shampoo cap.

13. Clean, dry and replace the used equipment as per local policy.
14. Remove apron and discard in clinical waste. Wash hands/use alcohol hand gel.
15. Document the procedure.

Points for practice

PFP1 Some hospitals have large bowls specifically designed for hairwashing which have a gap for the neck so wáter is less likely to spill. Some provide disposable caps that contain a 'no rinse' shampoo (Figure 10.2). These do not require the use of bowls or wáter as the hair is massaged through the cap. The cap can be warmed in a microwave before use if desired. Once the cap is removed the hair can be dried and styled as required.

PFP2 Before washing the hair, the nurse should assess the condition of the scalp, noting any inflammation, dryness or redness. The condition of the hair should also be noted.

PFP3 Some patients may like products applied to their hair after washing to prevent dryness and help with styling.

10.7 Eye care

Preparation

Patient

- Explain the procedure, to gain consent and cooperation ➡ **PFP1**
- Assist the patient into a comfortable position, with the head tilted backwards

Equipment

- Sterile eye-care pack containing gallipot, gauze swabs and gloves ➡ **PFP2**
- Extra gauze swabs if required
- Sterile 0.9% sodium chloride (normal saline) solution
- Clinical waste bag

Nurse

- Cleanse hands
- An apron should be worn.
- Additional protective clothing may be necessary if indicated by the patient's condition (see Ch. 1)

Procedure

1. Raise bed to a suitable working height. Open the eye-care pack and arrange all equipment on a suitable work surface. Place clinical waste bag in a convenient position close to the patient.

2. Pour the saline solution into the gallipot. Put on the setrile gloves.

4. Fold four swabs into quarters and dip into saline solution.

3. Ask the patient to close their eyes, and explain which eye is to be cleaned first. Always clean an infected eye last ➡ **PFP3**.

4. Using the point of the folded swab gently clean the lower lid from the nose outwards, ensuring that it does not touch the cornea.Use another swab to clean the upper lid.

5. Using a new swab each time, repeat stage 4 until any discharge or encrustation has been removed. Discard used swabs in the clinical waste bag.

6. Dry the lid by gently wiping with a dry swab.

7. Repeat steps 4–6 with the other eye ➡ **PFP3**.

8. Remove gloves and put all used equipment in the waste bag ➡ **PFP4**.

9. Ensure the patient is left comfortable and lower the bed.

10. Discard the used pack in clinical waste. Remove apron and wash hands.

11. Document eye care, noting the condition of the eyes.

➡ Points for practice

PFP1 Eye care may be required prior to the administration of eye drops or ointment (see p. 208).

PFP2 If an eye care pack is not available individually packed sterile equipment can be assembled.

PFP3 If both eyes are infected, two separate eye-care packs should be used and the hands washed before cleaning the second eye.

PFP4 Because of the risk of infection, eye-care packs should not be kept for repeated use. A new pack should be used each time.

10.8 Caring for fingernails and toenails

Preparation

Patient

- Explain the procedure, to gain consent and cooperation ➡ **PFP1**
- Ascertain usual nail-care habits
- Carry out this procedure following a bath if possible, as soaking may soften the nails

Equipment

- Bowl of warm water
- Nail clippers, nail file or emery board
- Orange stick
- Hand cream or lotion according to patient preference
- Towel

Nurse

- Wash and dry hands thoroughly
- Put on plastic apron. Additional protective clothing may be necessary if indicated by the patient's condition (see Ch. 1)
- Knowledge of local policy regarding nail care ➡ **PFP1**

Procedure

Fingernails

1. Inspect the hands, fingers and nails, noting any signs of dryness and the condition of the nails and cuticles.

2. If patient has not recently had a bath, wash the hands in a bowl of warm soapy water ➡ **PFP2**

3. Clean under the fingernails with an orange stick or nail file while washing the hands. Dry the hands.

4. If nail clippers are available, clip the nails. Clip small sections of the nail ➡ **PFP3**. After clipping, file the fingernails until they are level with the top of the finger. The nails can then be smoothed to the shape of the finger. If nail clippers are not available, file the nails; do not use scissors.

5. Push the cuticles back gently with an orange stick and apply hand cream or lotion as appropriate.

Toenails

1. Sit in a comfprtable position so that the patient's feet can rest on a towel on your lap.

2. Inspect the feet and toenails, noting any dryness, inflammation or cracking. Also note any calluses or ulcerated areas and the colour and temperature of the feet to assess adequacy of circulation.

3. If the patient has not recently had a bath, wash the feet in a bowl of warm soapy water.

4. If clippers are available clip the toenails ➡ **PFP1**, ➡ **PFP3**. Clean and file the toenails as for fingernails, but do not file the corners as this may encourage ingrowing nails.

5. Apply moisturising lotion as required.

Finger and toenails

1. After cleaning, clipping and filing the nails leave the patient comfortable.

2. Clean any reusable equipment as per local policy and discard waste in clinical waste.

3. Remove apron and wash and dry hands.

4. Document care, noting the condition of the nails, and report any abnormal findings. Refer to chiropodist if required ➡ **PFP1**.

➡ Points for practice

PFP1 Some Trust policies state that patients must be referred to chiropody or podiatry services for toenail care. This is especially important in patients with diabetes and peripheral arterial disease who may have peripheral neuropathy and, therefore, be unaware of any trauma to the toes. However, if the nails are not deformed or thickened then the nurse should be able to clean and trim them.

PFP2 Do not soak the nails as this increases the likelihood of trauma when clipping or filing the nails.

PFP3 Cut the nails straight across or follow the curve of the finger or toe, but do not cut down into the sides of the nails as this may cause trauma.

10.9 Last offices

Preparation

Patient

- Death will have been confirmed
  ➔ PFP1
- Relatives will have been informed and given the opportunity to see the deceased and may wish to participate in the last offices
- Attention must be paid to the beliefs and wishes of deceased patients and their relatives. Religious requirements should be observed. Advice from religious personnel may be required
  ➔ PFP2
- Screen the bed securely as soon as death occurs to ensure privacy and dignity

Equipment

- Prepare the bed area to ensure sufficient space is available
- Equipment for bed bath (see p. 316)
- Cotton wool, gauze or padding if there are any leaking wounds
- Clean sheet and shroud
- Tape for securing the sheet
- Two name bands
- Two labels from the 'deceased patients book' **➔ PFP3**
- Property book
- Linen bag and clinical waste bag
- Cadaver bag (if required)
  ➔ PFP4

Nurse

- Last offices require two nurses working together quietly
- Be familiar with hospital policy regarding last offices
- An apron should be worn and gloves should be available. Additional protective clothing may be necessary if indicated by the patient's condition (see Ch. 1)

Procedure

1. Take the equipment to the bedside and secure the screens, to prevent accidental opening. Raise the bed to a suitable working height.

2. Wash the front of the patient. If the patient is male, the second nurse could shave the patient whilst the first nurse washes **➔ PFP5**. Leave/replace dentures if they fit.

3. Spigot any tubes, catheters and infusions unless otherwise indicated, e.g. post mortem (autopsy) requirements **➔ PFP6**.

4. If leakage is apparent from wounds or orifices, use packing or padding, according to local policy **➔ PFP6**. It may be necessary to express urine from the bladder into a receiver.

5. With the second nurse as a witness, remove all jewellery from the body unless advised otherwise, e.g. Sikhs – leave bracelet (kara). If jewellery is left, this should be covered with adhesive tape or tied in position to prevent loss. Document removal and add to property list.

6. Place the shroud on the patient, with the fastening at the back. Roll the patient onto their side to wash back and fasten shroud.

7. If local policy requires, pack the mouth with gauze.

8. Place a clean sheet diagonally under the patient, leaving enough sheet to fold over the head and feet **➔ PFP7**

9. Place one label on the chest, attached to the shroud with adhesive tape.

10. Check there is one nameband on the wrist and place the other on one ankle or according to local policy.
11. Before wrapping the patient in the sheet, check whether the relatives wish to view the body ➡ **PFP8**.
12. Wrap the body in the sheet and secure with tape.
13. Place the other label on the chest.
14. If there is a risk of infection, the body may be placed in a cadaver bag.
15. Complete the property form. Both nurses must document and sign for any valuables. Any valuables left on the body should also be noted on the death form. Store property according to local policy, e.g. in the bereavement office.
16. Clear away equipment and dispose of clinical waste safely. Remove protective clothing and wash hands.
17. Contact porters or mortuary technicians to remove the body. Ensure that the other patients are screened when the body is removed, and a calm and quiet approach is adopted.
18. Ensure all documentation has been completed according to local policy.

➡ Points for practice

PFP1 After death, the body is usually left for an hour before last offices are commenced, during which time a doctor or senior nurse will have certified the death. A pillow may be used to support the jaw, to prevent the mouth falling open, and the eyes closed with wet gauze swabs if necessary. The limbs should be straightened if necessary.

PFP2 Religious/cultural preferences must be ascertained prior to last offices, e.g. who can touch the body, non-removal of religious objects or jewellery, etc.

PFP3 The labels used to identify the body are found in the 'deceased patients' or 'death notice' book and must be completed before being torn out, to ensure that all copies are completed at the same time. In some Trusts, the labels are provided with other items (e.g. shroud) in a 'last offices' pack.

PFP4 A cadaver bag is required for infected patients. The bag is labelled 'danger of infection' in addition to the name of the infection.

PFP5 Care should be taken when shaving a dead person, as doing so when they are still warm can cause bruising or marking which does not appear until a few days later.

PFP6 It is important to prevent leakage from the body, as this is unpleasant and potentially dangerous for porters and mortuary technicians. Refer to local policy regarding removal of drains/catheters/tubing and packing the body to prevent leakage. This should not be performed if a post mortem examination (autopsy) is required. The medical team will advise on the need for a post mortem examiniation.

PFP7 When rolling the patient to put in the clean sheet, a deep sigh may be heard. This is due to air being forced out of the lungs.

PFP8 If the patient is to be seen by the family after last offices leave the face uncovered. A coloured counterpane makes the bed look less clinical.

Bibliography/Suggested reading

Berridge, M., 2009. Guidance on maintaining personal hygiene in nail care. Nursing Standard 23 (41), 35–38.

Guidance on how to perform routine nail care and a review of factors that have impacted on nurses' reluctance to perform nail care

British National Formulary (BNF). BMJ Publishing Group Ltd., Royal Pharmaceutical Society of Great Britain and RCPCH Publications, London.

This is published twice a year and so the most recent edition should be used. This publication lists all medications and their classification. It identifies indications, cautions, contraindications and dose for each medication. (Available at www.bnf.org - in order to access the latest edition, registration is necessary at this website, but there is no charge for this).

Department of Health, 2010. Essence of care 2010 Benchmarks for the fundamental aspects of care. Benchmarks for personal hygiene. The Stationary Office, London.

These guidelines identify best practice benchmarks for all asepects of caring for a patient's hygiene needs

Hills, M., Albarran, J., 2009. Evaluating last offices care and improving services offered to newly bereaved relatives. Nursing Times 105 (23), 14–16.

This article discusses the results of an audit into last offices and makes recommendations for improving practice

Hills, M., Albarran, J., 2010. After death 2: exploring the procedures for laying out and preparing the body for viewing. Nursing Times 106 (28), 22–24.

This article examines the procedures for laying out and preparing the body for viewing

Huskinson, W., Lloyd, H., 2009. Oral health in hospitalised patients: assessment and hygiene. Nursing Standard 23 (36), 43–47.

This article provides an overview of good oral care and identifies an oral assessment tool.

Massa, J., 2010. Improving efficiency, reducing infection and enhancing experience. British Journal of Nursing 19 (22), 1408: 1410–1414.

This article highlights the benefits of a 'wipe-based' bed bath method compared with the use of soap and water

NHS National End of Life Care Programme, 2011. Guidance for staff responsible for care after death (last offices). [online]. Available from: http://www.endoflifecareforadults.nhs.uk/publications/guidance-for-staff-responsible-for-care-after-death (accessed 25.6.11.).

This guide aims to provide a consistent view that accommodates the UK's diverse religious and multicultural beliefs

Robinson, J., 2009. Information on practical procedures following death. Nursing Standard 23 (19), 43–47.

This article discusses the procedures required after death and examines funeral arrangements. This information may be helpful to both nurses and relatives

Royal College of Nursing. 2011. Promoting older people's oral health. RCN, London.

This guide is intended to improve nurses' knowledge of oral care for oder people. It has a useful glossary of terms and covers problems often experienced by older patients. It includes standards, assessment tools and examples of good practice

Chapter 11

Respiratory care

©2012 Elsevier Ltd.

11.1 Assessment of breathing and counting respirations

Preparation

Patient
- The patient should be relaxed and resting, or recent activity should be noted. Get the patient into as upright a posture as is possible and comfortable (see p. 336)
- Do not inform the patient when you will be assessing breathing ➡ **PFP1**

Equipment
- Watch with a second hand

Nurse
- The hands should be clean
- Additional protective clothing may be necessary if indicated by the patient's condition (see Ch. 1)

Procedure

1. Observe the movement of the chest wall for symmetry of chest movement – this is best observed in front of the patient rather than at the side ➡ **PFP2**.
2. Observe whether accessory muscles are being used ➡ **PFP3**.
3. Observe the rhythm and depth of respirations ➡ **PFP4**.
4. Count the respirations for 60 seconds.
5. Observe for the following:
   - difficulty in, or struggling with, breathing
   - pain on breathing and its location
   - noisy respiration – whether there is any wheeze or stridor (high pitched sounds).
   - cough – whether dry or productive.
   - sputum – amount, colour and consistency (see p. 352).
6. Observe the patient's colour for signs of cyanosis ➡ **PFP5**.
7. Document the respiratory observations according to local policy and report any abnormalities (see p. 52 for an example of charting).
8. Adjust the frequency of observations as necessary.
9. Ensure the patient is comfortable. Breathless patients may be most comfortable sitting in a chair.

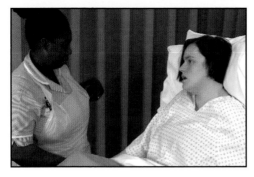

Figure 11.1 Monitoring the respiration rate while apparently counting the pulse.

➡️Points for practice

PFP1 A more accurate observation is obtained if the patient is unaware that their respirations are being counted. Many nurses achieve this by pretending to be feeling the radial pulse when in fact observing the movement of the chest wall (Fig. 11.1).

PFP2 The chest should rise and fall equally or symmetrically. If one side does not move as well as the other, this could indicate a pneumothorax (collapsed lung), bronchial obstruction or injury.

PFP3 Accessory muscles are the sternocleidomastoid and trapezius muscles in the neck and shoulders. If these are being used (noticed by movement of these muscles), it indicates that the patient is unable to use the diaphragm and external intercostal muscles adequately (Esmond 2011).

PFP4 If breathing is very shallow and difficult to observe, lightly rest your hand on the patient's chest or abdomen to feel movement. The normal rate for an adult is 12–20 breaths per minute.

PFP5 Cyanosis is a blue discoloration of the skin and mucous membranes and is most noticeable around the lips, earlobes, mouth and fingertips. In dark-skinned patients, signs of poor perfusion or cyanosis may be detected if the area around the lips or nail beds is dusky in colour.

11.2 Positioning the breathless patient

Preparation

Patient
- Explain the procedure, to gain consent and cooperation
- The patient may be anxious because of the difficulty in breathing

Equipment
- Bed with adjustable backrest or electric raising mechanism
- Four or five pillows
- Bed table with brakes
- Firm, supporting armchair
- A hoist or sliding aid may be needed if the patient is unable to move up the bed unaided

Nurse
- Two nurses may be needed
- An apron should be worn if assisting the patient to move
- Additional protective clothing may be necessary if indicated by the patient's condition (see Ch. 1)

Procedure

1. Explain to the patient exactly what is planned so that movement is reduced to a minimum.

2. Ask/assist the patient to sit forward. A second nurse may be needed to support the patient while the backrest is adjusted and the pillows are arranged ➡ **PFP1**.

3. Adjust the backrest or raise the head of the bed.

4. Arrange the pillows so that the patient feels supported (Fig. 11.2). This will vary according to patient preference, but you should ensure that the lumbar region is supported ➡ **PFP1**.

5. If the foot of the bed can be raised slightly, this may help to prevent the patient slipping down.

6. For a short period, the patient may get relief by leaning forward with the forearms resting on a pillow on a bed table.

7. If able to get out of bed, the breathless patient is often most comfortable sitting in an armchair, and many prefer to sleep in this position.

8. As you help the patient to re-position observe for changes in respiratory pattern, cough, colour, etc. (see p. 334).

9. Ensure drink, call bell, etc., are close to hand.

10. If sitting for long periods, a pressure-relieving mattress or cushion may be needed to prevent pressure ulcers ➡ **PFP2**.

11. Document the care given and report any change in condition.

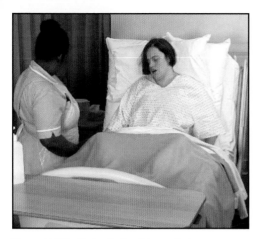

Figure 11.2 Positioning the breathless patient.

➡️ Points for practice

PFP1 When positioning the breathless patient, the aim is to maximise respiratory functioning while reducing physical effort; therefore, the patient must be comfortable and well-supported. Ensure the pillows are supporting the small of the back so that the patient does not sink into them and thus restrict chest movement (Fig. 11.2).

PFP2 In the patient with poor or restricted mobility, regular re-positioning is necessary to prevent pressure ulcers (see Ch. 12).

11.3 Face masks and nasal cannulae

Preparation

Patient

- Explain the procedure, to gain cooperation and consent
- Prepare the patient pre-operatively if oxygen therapy is planned postoperatively
- Patients, visitors, family or carers must be made aware of the dangers of smoking when oxygen is being administered ➡ **PFP1**

Equipment

- Piped oxygen or oxygen cylinder ➡ **PFP2**
- Oxygen tubing ➡ **PFP3**.
- Prescription chart ➡ **PFP4**
- Mask or nasal cannulae as prescribed ➡ **PFP5**

Nurse

- The hands should be clean when handling oxygen equipment
- Additional protective clothing may be necessary if indicated by the patient's condition (see Ch. 1)

Procedure

1. Except in an emergency situation, oxygen therapy must be prescribed by a doctor.

2. Turn on the oxygen flow meter and set the flow rate (Figs 11.3 & 11.5) ➡ **PFP6**.

3. Place the mask over the patient's nose and mouth with the elastic strap over the ears to the back of the head. Adjust the length of the strap to ensure the mask fits securely (Fig. 11.4A).

4. If using nasal cannulae (sometimes called nasal specs/nasal speculae), place 2 cm of tubing into the nostrils; the other tubes go over the ears and either under the chin or behind the head (Fig. 11.4C).

5. Observe the patient's respiratory pattern and oxygen saturations to ensure that the therapy is working ➡ **PFP7**.

6. Document oxygen therapy according to local policy.

7. Offer drinks or if more appropriate mouth care ➡ **PFP8**.

8. Tubing and masks may be reused several times for the same patient. It should be disposed of in the clinical waste when no longer required.

9. If using an oxygen cylinder, ensure that a replacement cylinder is available when the volume when the volume indicator gauge shows a quarter full.

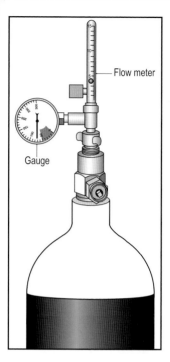

Flow meter

Gauge

Figure 11.3 Oxygen cylinder.

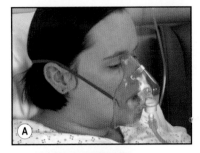
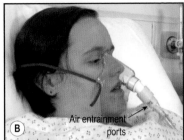

Air entrainment
ports

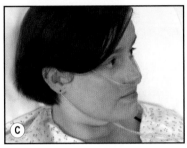

Figure 11.4 A Hudson mask; B Mask with venturi system; C Nasal cannula.

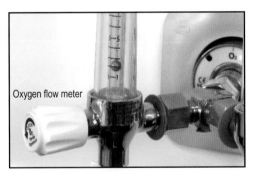

Oxygen flow meter

Figure 11.5 Oxygen flow meter set at 2 L per minute.

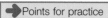

Points for practice

PFP1 Oxygen is highly inflammable.

PFP2 An oxygen cylinder has a black base with white shoulders and has 'oxygen' written on it (Figure 11.3).

PFP3 Oxygen tubing may come in prepacked lengths as a continuous roll with a 'bubble' (widened portion) at regular intervals. Cut through the centre of the bubble and then further trim as necessary to ensure a secure fit onto the flow meter and mask. The length should allow freedom of movement for the patient, but not be so long that it may become kinked or touch the floor.

PFP4 The National Patient Safety Agency (NPSA 2010) emphasise that oxygen therapy is a medication and therefore must be prescribed, except in emergency situations.

PFP5 If a percentage of oxygen has been prescribed, a special mask that incorporates a Venturi system is used (Fig. 11.4B). These are colour-coded and specify the flow of oxygen required to deliver 24%, 28%, 35%, 40% and 60% oxygen.

    Other devices are known as variable performance devices where oxygen is prescribed and delivered using litres per minute (l/min) rather than fixed percentages (Esmond 2011). Examples include the Hudson mask, which is used to deliver a high concentration of oxygen and 8–10 l/min is usually prescribed, and the non rebreathe mask with reservoir bag, which is used to deliver very high concentrations of oxygen and 10–15 l/min is usually prescribed. If nasal cannulae are used, the flow rate of the oxygen must not exceed 2 l/minute or it will damage the nasal mucosa.

PFP6 The centre of the ball in the flow meter must sit at the level of the flow rate prescribed (Fig. 11.5).

PFP7 The British Thoracic Society (2008) states that oxygen should be prescribed to achieve a target range of saturations, e.g. 88–92% or 94–98% dependent on the patients condition. The effectiveness of therapy can therefore be monitored by using the prescribed saturation range.

PFP8 Oxygen therapy dries the mucous membranes of the mouth. Frequent drinks should be taken or frequent mouth care provided if the oxygen is not being humidified. Humidification should always be considered if oxygen therapy is required for prolonged periods and for patients with respiratory infections who have difficulty expectorating sputum (Esmond 2011) (see p. 342).

11.4 Humidified oxygen

Preparation

Patient
- Explain the procedure, to gain consent and cooperation

Equipment
- Piped oxygen or oxygen cylinder
- Large-bore 'elephant' tubing
- Humidifier and water reservoir

Nurse
- The hands should be clean and the principles of asepsis maintained when handling the water reservoir of the humidifier

Procedure

1. Check the prescription regarding the percentage of oxygen to be administered ➜ **PFP1**.

2. Connect the humidifier to the oxygen flow meter according to the manufacturer's instructions ➜ **PFP2**.

3. Connect the wide-bore tubing to the mask and set the flow meter to the flow required to achieve the prescribed percentage of oxygen ➜ **PFP3**.

4. A fine mist should appear in the mask. Ask/assist the patient to put on the mask and adjust the retaining strap to prevent pressure on the ears. The nose part of the mask may need to be adjusted to prevent mist going into the eyes (Figure 11.6).

5. Ensure the patient is comfortable. The humidified oxygen may encourage the patient to cough so a sputum pot and tissues should be provided.

6. Document humidified oxygen therapy according to local policy.

7. If using an oxygen cylinder, monitor the amount remaining and order a replacement when it is down to quarter full.

8. Check regularly to see if water is collecting in the tubing ➜ **PFP4**. The water reservoir should be replaced when empty. The tubing and mask should be changed every 24 hours.

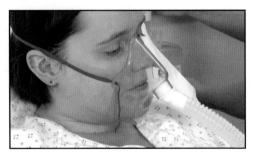

Figure 11.6 Humidified oxygen.

> **Points for practice**

PFP1 Except in an emergency situation, all oxygen therapy must be prescribed.

PFP2 Connection will vary according to the type of humidifier. Usually it is achieved by removing the connector at the base of the flow meter, attaching the humidifier by screwing it into position.

PFP3 It is important that the flow is set at the rate indicated to achieve the prescribed percentage of oxygen. This is usually indicated on the top of the humidifier where it attaches to the flow meter. There may also be a valve adjustment, which should be turned to the correct setting.

PFP4 Water that collects in the wide-bore tubing should be emptied or the tubing changed according to local policy.

11.5 Use of nebuliser

Preparation

Patient
- Explain the procedure, to gain consent and cooperation
- The patient should be in a comfortable position, sitting upright

Equipment
- Air, air compressor or oxygen (piped or cylinder) according to prescription ➡ **PFP1**
- Nebuliser and face mask or mouthpiece ➡ **PFP2**
- Nebuliser solution and prescription chart ➡ **PFP3**

Nurse
- The hands should be clean and the principles of asepsis maintained when handling the nebuliser and solution
- Additional protective clothing may be necessary if indicated by the patient's condition (see Ch. 1)

Procedure

1. Check the expiry date and check the nebuliser solution and the patient's identity with the prescription (p. 183-185).

2. Unscrew the base of the nebuliser and add the solution (this is usually in a plastic ampoule that is squeezed to expel the liquid), then screw together again (Figure 11.7A).

3. Make sure the mouthpiece or face mask is securely attached to the nebuliser.

4. Set the flow meter on the air cylinder to 6 l/minute. A fine mist should appear in the mask and a hissing sound will be heard. If the mist does not appear, turn the flow meter to 8 l/minute ➡ **PFP4**.

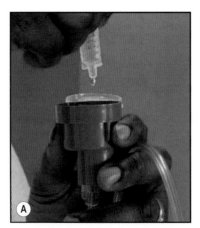

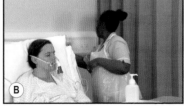

Figure 11.7 A: adding nebuliser solution; B: nebuliser therapy.

5. Ask/assist the patient to use the mouthpiece or put on the mask by placing the retaining strap over the ears and back of the head (Figure 11.7B).

6. The patient should remain sitting upright until all the solution has been vaporised. This may take up to 15 minutes.

7. The nebuliser is likely to encourage the patient to cough, so a sputum pot and tissues should be provided.

8. Document nebuliser therapy according to local policy.

9. A peak expiratory flow rate may be requested before and after the nebuliser (see p. 346).

10. If the nebuliser is to be used again, it should be left clean and dry and stored in a plastic bag on the patient's locker.

➡Points for practice

PFP1 The use of air or oxygen will depend on the underlying disease process. Most patients with asthma will be prescribed oxygen, whereas those with chronic obstructive pulmonary disease (COPD) are usually prescribed nebulisers with air. If using a cylinder, check that it is at least a quarter full. Air cylinders are grey-green in colour with black and while shoulders. Oxygen cylinders have a black base with white shoulders (see Figure 11.3). Some patients have compressed air boxes to 'drive' the nebuliser, operated with a simple on/off switch.

PFP2 Wherever possible, a mouthpiece is the preferred option as it provides better deposition of the drug into the lungs and reduces side-effects (Esmond 2011). If the patient is having nebuliser therapy regularly, the mask or mouthpiece will be kept at the bedside between uses. Nebuliser therapy is usually administered 2–4 times per day.

PFP3 Drugs to be nebulised (e.g. a bronchodilator) must be prescribed and this must be checked according to local policy (see p. 183-185).

PFP4 A nebuliser converts the liquid medication into an aerosol for the patient to inhale. This is dependent on the flow of gas through the liquid and although manufacturer's guidance should be followed generally the flow needs to be above 6 l/min to produce the small aerosol particles (BTS/SIGN 2009, Kelly and Lynes 2011). Flow rates above 8 l/min are generally too forceful and may cause the oxygen tubing to disconnect from the nebuliser pot.

11.6 Peak expiratory flow rate

Preparation

Patient

- Explain the procedure, to gain consent and cooperation
- Ideally, the patient should be standing. If the patient's condition does not allow this, they should sit as upright as possible ➡ **PFP1**
- The patient should be rested, as recent exertion may affect the accuracy of the measurement

Equipment

- Peak flow meter
- Disposable mouthpiece
- Chart to record measurement

Nurse

- The hands should be clean
- An apron should be worn if assisting the patient to move
- Additional protective clothing may be necessary if indicated by the patient's condition (see Ch. 1)

Procedure

1. Peak expiratory flow rate measurement may be required before and after a nebuliser to montior the patient's condition, or during patient assessment.

2. Attach disposable mouthpiece to the peak flow meter and set the pointer to zero.

3. Instruct the patient to inhale deeply, place their lips around the mouthpiece to form a tight seal, and holding the meter horizontally, exhale forcibly (Figure 11.8). Make sure that the patient's fingers do not occlude the pointer ➡ **PFP2**.

4. Note the measurement.

5. Repeat steps 2–4 twice more ➡ **PFP3**.

6. Following the procedure, ensure the patient is comfortable.

7. Document the highest of the three measurements (Figure 11.9). Pre- and post-nebuliser recordings may be recorded in different colours or different symbols to differentiate between them (Figure 11.9) ➡ **PFP4**.

8. Report any abnormality or significant variation from previous recordings ➡ **PFP5**.

9. The disposable mouthpiece may be reused for the same patient. Keep dry and protected from dust.

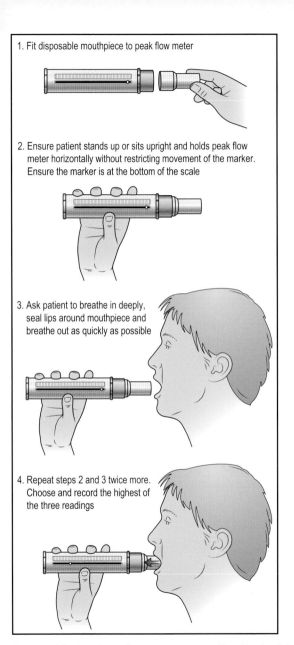

1. Fit disposable mouthpiece to peak flow meter

2. Ensure patient stands up or sits upright and holds peak flow meter horizontally without restricting movement of the marker. Ensure the marker is at the bottom of the scale

3. Ask patient to breathe in deeply, seal lips around mouthpiece and breathe out as quickly as possible

4. Repeat steps 2 and 3 twice more. Choose and record the highest of the three readings

Figure 11.8 Peak expiratory flow rate measurement. From Brooker C & Nicol M: Nursing Adults (Mosby, 2003) with permission.

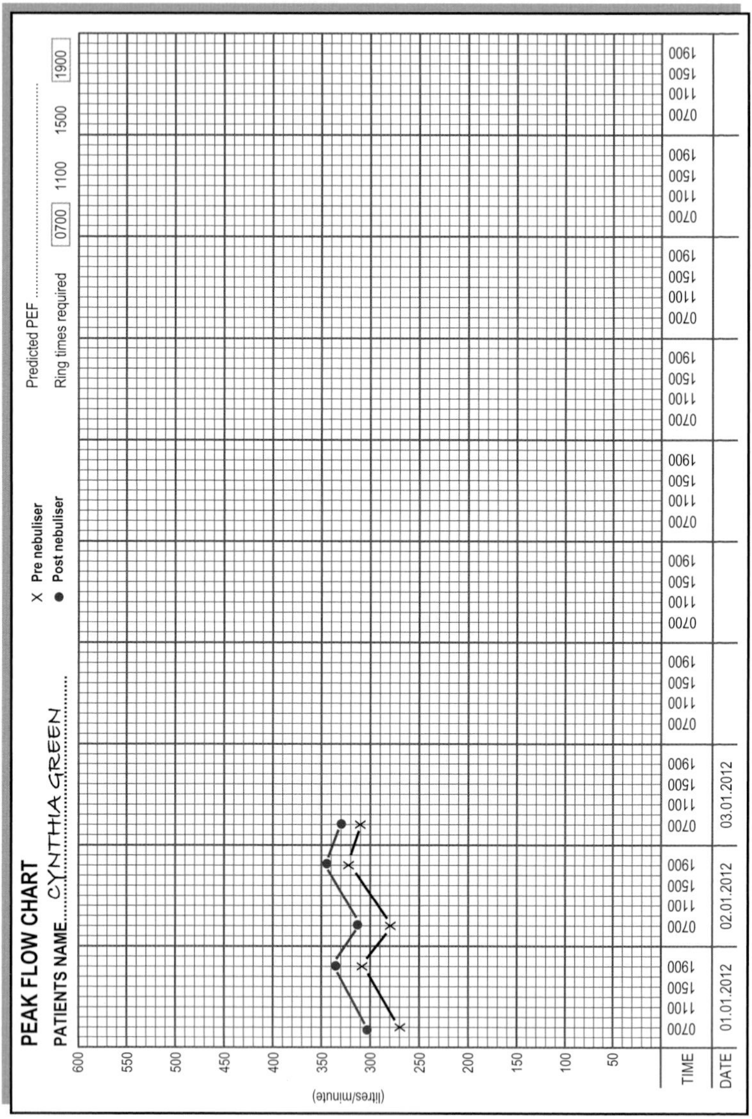

Figure 11.9 Peak flow chart.

➡️Points for practice

PFP1 The patient should adopt the position they usually adopt when recording peak expiratory flow rate, but sitting upright or standing is best (Higgins 2005).

PFP2 Peak expiry flow rate (PEFR) measures the best expiratory flow rate. Remind the patient to exhale as hard as they can. It may be useful to demonstrate this to a patient who has not performed a PEFR before.

PFP3 If the patient is extremely breathless or the procedure causes the patient distress (e.g. excessive coughing or wheezing), do one recording only. Document this on the chart.

PFP4 If the peak expiratory flow rate is to be measured after a nebuliser, this should be done 30 minutes afterwards (Higgins 2005).

PFP5 The peak expiratory flow rate is measured in litres per minute and varies according to age, sex and stature. In order to find out what is normal for an individual a chart is used to estimate what the patient's PEFR should be. There is a useful website that explains how to do this: http://www.peakflow. com/top_nav/normal_values/PEFNorms.html

11.7 Pulse oximetry (oxygen saturation)

Preparation

Patient
- Explain the procedure, to gain co-operation and consent
- Patient's hands should be clean

Equipment
- Pulse oximeter to measure oxygen saturations (SpO₂)
  ➡ **PFP1**
- Sensor appropriate to patient's size and condition

Nurse
- The hands should be clean and an apron should be worn
- Additional protective clothing may be necessary if indicated by the patient's condition (see Ch, 1)

Procedure

1. Assess the patient's peripheral circulation in order to choose an appropriate sensor. The most usual are those that clip onto the patient's finger, although sensors that clip onto the ears or adhesive nasal sensors are available.

2. Before applying the sensor, check that the patient's skin is clean and dry.

3. If using a finger sensor, remove nail polish or false nails, as this could give a false reading ➡ **PFP2**. Avoid placing the finger probe on the same arm as a blood pressure cuff as the reading will be inaccurate during inflation of the cuff.

4. Turn on the machine and ensure the cable is plugged into the machine. Apply the sensor by clipping it on to the end of the finger (Figure 11.10)

5. Observe waveform fluctuations to ensure that the pulse waveform and oxygen saturation levels are registering and note the reading (Figure 11.10) ➡ **PFP3**.

6. Set alarm limits on pulse oximeter if not pre-set by manufacturer.

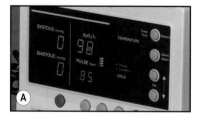

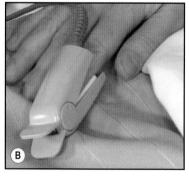

Figure 11.10 Pulse oximeter and finger sensor.

7. If continuous oxygen saturation measurements are required, change the sensor site every 4 hours to prevent pressure damage or irritation from adhesive sensors.

8. If intermittent oxygen saturations are being measured, remove the sensor between readings and switch off the machine. Ensure the patient is comfortable.

9. Clean the machine and sensor according to local policy. Store the machine and cable as per manufacturer's instructions after use.

10. Remove apron and wash hands/use alcohol hand gel.

11. Document oxygen saturations, noting whether the patient is receiving oxygen therapy. Report any changes or abnormalities.

➡️Points for practice

PFP1 The pulse oximeter is used to measure oxygen saturation (SpO_2) levels. The normal level is 95–99% (Clark and Giuliano 2006). The pulse oximeter will also show the pulse rate, but it is important to feel the patient's pulse rate to be able to monitor its rhythm and strength.

PFP2 Patients with jaundice may give falsely high readings due to high serum bilirubin levels. If the patient has recently had any investigations that involve the injection of radio-opaque dyes, then this may cause spurious readings.

PFP3 Some models of pulse oximeter do not show a pulse waveform, just a digital readout.

11.8 Observation of sputum

Preparation

Patient
- Explain the procedure, to gain consent and cooperation
- Ensure privacy – the patient may be distressed or embarrassed at having to expectorate

Equipment
- Disposable sputum carton with lid
- Tissues
- Clinical waste bag

Nurse
- Hands should be clean
- Gloves and apron should be worn if the patient needs assistance with expectoration, use of tissues, etc.
- Additional protective clothing may be necessary if indicated by the patient's condition (see Ch. 1).

Procedure

1. Expectoration will be easier if the patient is sitting up, supported by pillows, or is sitting in an armchair.

2. Encourage the patient to expectorate into the sputum pot rather than swallowing the sputum ➡ **PFP1**. 'Huffing' may help the patient to expectorate.

3. Observe the sputum for the following:
   - quantity
   - consistency: whether watery, frothy or tenacious (sticky)
   - colour: clear (normal mucous); white and frothy (pulmonary oedema); yellow/green (pus- infected); black flecks (smoke inhalation)
   - fresh blood (haemoptysis – trauma, tuberculosis or tumour)
   - odour: foul-smelling sputum may indicate a lung abscess.

4. A mouthwash or drink should be offered after expectoration.

5. Replace lid and remove used sputum pot after observation and discard in clinical waste bin.

6. Provide the patient with clean sputum pot and ensure they are comfortable. They may feel very tired after a bout of coughing.

7. Remove gloves and apron and wash hands.

8. Document findings and report any changes or abnormalities.

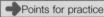 Points for practice

PFP1 The assistance of a physiotherapist may be necessary to teach the patient how to breathe deeply and expectorate without strain rather than coughing ineffectively.

11.9 Obtaining a sputum specimen

Preparation

Patient
- Explain the procedure and the number of specimens required
  ➡ **PFP1**

Equipment
- Universal specimen pot
- Plastic specimen bag and label or laboratory request form
- Drinking water and mouthwash
- Tissues

Nurse
- Gloves and apron should be worn if the patient needs assistance with expectoration, use of tissues, etc.
- Additional protective clothing may be necessary if indicated by the patient's condition (see Ch.1).

Procedure

1. Ask the patient to rinse their mouth thoroughly with water ➡ **PFP2**.
2. Ask/assist the patient to expectorate into the sterile pot ➡ **PFP3**.
3. Seal the lid and complete the label with the date, patient's full name, hospital number, ward and type of specimen.
4. Place the pot and the laboratory request form in a plastic specimen bag and dispatch to the laboratory straight away ➡ **PFP4**.
5. Ensure the patient is comfortable and offer a mouthwash and/or tissues as appropriate.
6. Dispose of any waste appropriately.
7. Remove gloves and apron. Wash hands.
8. Document that the specimen has been obtained. Note colour, smell and consistency of specimen.

➡ Points for practice

PFP1 Three consecutive early-morning specimens may be requested for acid-fast bacilli (tuberculosis) or for cytology (malignant cells).

PFP2 The mouth should be rinsed with water (not mouthwash) before expectoration, to reduce contamination of the specimen with food.

PFP3 When obtaining the specimen it is important to ensure that it is mucoid or mucopurulent, which indicates that it is sputum and not just saliva.

PFP4 If a bar-coded computer-generated label is available, a laboratory request form is not required. Sputum specimens must be sent to the laboratory immediately as respiratory pathogens will not survive for long periods. If refrigerated for more than 12 hours *Haemophilus influenzae* and *Streptococcus pneumoniae* may die and gram negative organisms over-grow in the specimen.

11.10 Oral suctioning

Preparation

Patient
- Explain the procedure, to gain consent and cooperation
- The patient requiring oral suctioning may be semiconscious or unconscious. If so, they should be positioned on their side, facing the nurse ➡ **PFP1**

Equipment
- Suction machine (if piped suction is not available).
- Suction tubing and oral sucker, e.g. Yankauer suction device (Figure 11.11).
- Sterile distilled water ➡ **PFP2**.

Nurse
- The hands must be washed and dried thoroughly.
- An apron and gloves should be worn. Additional protective clothing may be necessary if indicated by the patient's condition (see Ch. 1).
- Goggles will be required if airborne secretions are likely.

Procedure

1. Switch on the suction machine and attach the tubing and oral sucker, ensuring a good fit to prevent loss of suction pressure ➡ **PFP3**.

2. If able to cooperate, ask the patient to open their mouth.

3. The Yankauer suction device has a hole in the shaft, which when occluded by your thumb enables suction to be applied. If an alternative oral sucker is used and has no suction-control mechanism, kink the suction tubing so that suction is not applied until required.

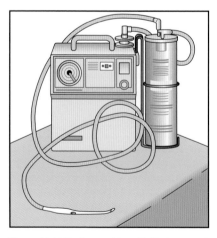

Figure 11.11 Suction machine with Yankauer sucker attached.

4. Gently insert the suction device into the mouth, taking care not to make the patient 'gag' by inserting it too far. This can be achieved by not losing sight of the tip of the suction device ➡ **PFP4**.

5. Apply suction but occluding the hole, moving the sucker around the mouth as necessary.

6. Release suction and remove the suction device from the mouth.

7. After the procedure ensure the patient is comfortable. Mouth care may be required following oral suctioning (see p. 320).

8. Clean the oral sucker and suction tubing by suctioning sterile water through it until all traces of secretions have gone.

9. The oral sucker may be used again on the same patient providing it is left clean and covered by a plastic bag between uses. The sucker and tubing should be replaced every 24 hours.

10. Remove gloves and apron and wash hands.

11. Document oral suctioning, noting the amount and appearance of the secretions.

12. If the suction machine has a reusable bottle, this should be emptied at least every 24 hours – or according to local policy. Goggles should be worn when emptying it. If it has a disposable sealed container, this does not need to be emptied but sealed and discarded when full or when the patient no longer requires suctioning.

➡ Points for practice

PFP1 Oral suctioning may be required by patients who are able to cough, but are too weak to expectorate. It may also be necessary during cardiopulmonary resuscitation and in unconscious patients if there are copious secretions.

PFP2 The sterile distilled water is used to clean the suction tubing after use and must be kept closed to discourage bacterial growth. The bottle must be changed every 24 hours. If poured into a bowl, the bowl must be kept clean and dry when not in use.

PFP3 There is little supporting evidence for correct suction pressure for oral suctioning, but it is suggested that 120 mmHg/28 kPa is the maximum pressure used (Moore 2003).

PFP4 There is a risk of stimulating the patients gag reflex if the suction device is inserted too far. This can cause the patient to vomit, which may cause aspiration into the lungs in unconscious or semi-conscious patients. It is best to 'only suck as far as you can see', i.e. keep the tip of the suction catheter in view at all times.

11.11 Care of a tracheostomy

Preparation

Patient

- Explain the procedure, to gain consent and cooperation
- Tracheostomy care is easier if the patient is recumbent or semi-recumbent in bed

Equipment

- Sterile dressing pack containing gloves
- Extra gauze swabs may be needed
- Dressing trolley or other suitable surface
- Keyhole dressing according to local policy
- Self-fastening tracheostomy tapes
- Cleansing solution according to local policy ➡ **PFP1**
- Tracheal dilators ➡ **PFP2**
- Alcohol hand-rub or hand washing facilities
- Scissors to cut tapes

Nurse

- The hands must be washed and dried thoroughly
- An apron should be worn. Additional protective clothing may be necessary if indicated by the patient's condition (see Ch. 1)
- Two nurses will be needed when changing the tapes (one to hold the tube)

Procedure

1. It is a good idea to perform tracheal suction (see p. 358) prior to the dressing change, to minimise the risk of coughing and possible dislodgement of the tube.

2. Prepare the trolley and equipment as for an aseptic dressing (see p. 285).

3. Raise the bed to a safe working height. Remove any humidification/oxygen apparatus from the tracheostomy site, but leave the tapes tied ➡ **PFP3**. If possible hold/position the oxygen mask close to the tracheostomy throughout the dressing change.

4. Wash your hands/use alcohol hand gel.

5. Open the dressing pack, keyhole dressing (➡ **PFP4**) and cleansing solution, and use the yellow waste bag as a 'glove' to remove the old dressing (see p. 286).

6. Attach the waste bag to the side of the trolley nearest the patient. Re-wash your hands or clean them using alcohol hand-rub. Put on the sterile gloves.

7. Use gauze swabs and cleansing solution to clean around the tracheostomy as necessary. Use gauze swabs to gently dry the site.

8. Apply the keyhole dressing (Figure 11.12).

9. With a second nurse holding the tube in position ➡ **PFP5**, undo one velcro fastener, and pass the tape behind the patient's neck to the other nurse. Remove the other velcro fastener and remove the tape.

10. Use the old tape to measure and cut the new tape to size. Thread the velcro fastener of the long length of padded tape through one side of the

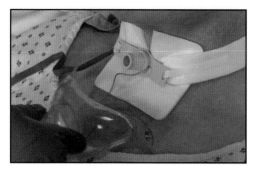

Figure 11.12 'Keyhole' tracheostomy dressing.

tracheostomy tube and secure. Pass the tape behind the patient's neck. Attach the velcro fastener of the short tape to the other side of the tracheostomy tube and then attach it securely to the long tape using the velcro provided.

11. Ensure that there it is a snug fit but not too tight. It should be just possible to slip a finger between the tape and the patient's neck.

12. Replace any humidification/oxygen equipment.

14. Ensure the patient is comfortable and there is no respiratory distress.

15. Discard all clinical waste appropriately.

16. Remove apron and wash hands.

17. Document the dressing change, noting the appearance of the tracheostomy site.

Points for practice

PFP1 The cleansing solution may vary according to local policy, but 0.9% sodium chloride is usually sufficient.

PFP2 Tracheal dilators should always be kept by the patient's bedside in case the tracheostomy is dislodged. However, once the tracheostomy is well established, the opening is unlikely to close if the tube is temporarily removed.

PFP3 If the patient is on a ventilator, this must not be disconnected during the dressing change. The second nurse will be needed to support the tubing etc., to facilitate the dressing change.

PFP4 Tracheostomy dressings can be a source of infection (Harkin 2011) so aseptic dressing technique is essential. Dressings must be changed as soon as soiled and skin can be protected by barrier cream or film.

PFP5 Two nurses are needed to safely change the tracheostomy tapes, so that one can hold the tube in position to prevent dislodgement if the patient coughs or moves unexpectedly.

11.12 Tracheal suctioning

Preparation

Patient

- Explain the procedure, to gain consent and cooperation.
- The patient will have an endotracheal (ET) tube or tracheostomy in situ ➡ **PFP1**

Equipment/Environment

- Suction machine (if piped suction is not available)
- Suction tubing
- Correctly sized sterile suction catheters with a diameter of no more than half that of the tracheostomy tube (Harkin 2011) ➡ **PFP2**
- Sterile distilled water ➡ **PFP3**
- Supply of single sterile gloves ➡ **PFP4**
- Yellow clinical waste bag/bin

Nurse

- Wash and dry hands thoroughly
- Wear non-sterile gloves on both or just your non-dominant hand and an apron ➡ **PFP4**
- Goggles ➡ **PFP5**

Procedure

1. Turn on the suction machine and test the suction pressure ➡ **PFP6**.

2. Open the suction-control end of a suction catheter, but leave it in its packet. Attach the end to the suction tubing, ensuring a good fit so that suction pressure is not lost.

3. Place the tubing and suction catheter (still in its packet) in a convenient position ready for use.

4. Open a sterile glove and put it on your dominant hand.

5. With your non-dominant hand, remove any humidifying/oxygen apparatus from the ET tube/tracheostomy ➡ **PFP7**.

6. With the same hand, pick up the suction tubing and carefully pull the suction catheter out of its packet.

7. As the suction catheter emerges, take hold of it in your sterile-gloved hand 10–15 cm from the end of the catheter. Do not allow the catheter to touch anything.

8. Insert the suction catheter into the ET tube/tracheostomy and, after warning the patient, advance it until it reaches the bifurcation of the right and left main bronchi (Figure 11.13). This will make the patient cough ➡ **PFP8**.

9. When the patient coughs, withdraw the suction catheter 1–2 cm and then apply suction by occluding the suction-control apparatus with the thumb of your non-dominant hand ➡ **PFP9**.

10. Continue to apply suction and gradually withdraw the catheter, rolling it between your fingers and thumb as you do so. The patient cannot breathe during suction therefore it should be performed for no more than 10–15 seconds each time (Harkin 2011)

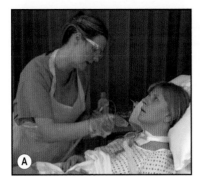
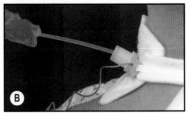

Figure 11.13 Tracheal suctioning.

11. Remove the catheter from the ET tube/tracheostomy and wrap it around the fingers of your sterile-gloved hand. Remove the glove, turning it inside out with the catheter contained within it.

12. Disconnect the catheter from the suction tubing and discard.

13. Repeat as necessary using a new catheter and sterile glove each time ➡ **PFP10**, allowing the patient time to recover before it is repeated.

14. Replace any humidification/oxygen equipment.

15. Ensure the patient is comfortable and breathing has returned to its usual rate.

16. Clean the suction tubing by suctioning sterile water through it until all traces of sputum have gone. The tubing should be replaced every 24 hours.

17. Ensure that there are more suction catheters available closeby to the patient ready for the next trachael suction.

18. Replace the cap on the bottle of sterile distilled wáter. Remove the goggles and leave ready for future use.

19. Remove gloves and apron and wash hands.

20. Document suctioning, noting the amount and appearance of the secretions.

21. Monitor the amount in the suction container. If the suction machine has a disposable sealed container, this does not need to be emptied, but sealed and discarded when full or when the patient no longer requires suctioning. If it has a reusable bottle, this should be emptied at least every 24 hours. Goggles should be worn when emptying it as there is a high risk of splashing (see Ch. 1).

Points for practice

PFP1 Tracheal suctioning should be carried out regularly to clear secretions from the tracheostomy tube (Harkin 2011). The frequency will depend on the patients condition. Nurses caring for patients with a tracheostomy should have supervision and training in this skill until deemed competent (Paul 2010).

PFP2 The suction catheter diameter should be no more than half the size of the diameter of the tube to allow for adqequate flow of oxygen around the catheter during suction (Harkin 2011).

PFP3 The sterile distilled water is used to clean the suction tubing after use and must be kept closed to discourage bacterial growth. The bottle must be changed every 24 hours. If the water is poured into a bowl, the bowl must be kept clean and dry when not in use.

PFP4 A new single sterile glove is used with each suction catheter. Non-sterile glove should be worn on your non-dominant hand to prevent contact with tracheal secretions when the suction-control apparatus is occluded with your thumb. If the catheter does not have an integral suction-control mechanism, a 'Y' connector may be inserted to serve the purpose. If non-sterile gloves are worn on both hands, a thin sterile glove can be placed over the glove on your dominant hand.

PFP5 It is recommended that goggles are worn because of the risk of airborne secretions when the patient coughs or the suction catheter is withdrawn.

PFP6 Suction pressure should be 80–120 mmHg/12–16 KPa (Moore 2003)

PFP7 If the patient is on a ventilator, the top of the ET tube/tracheostomy should be removed at the last minute and replaced immediately after each suctioning. Suction should be performed swiftly, no more than 1–15 seconds, as the patient is unable to breathe unaided. A guide is to hold your own breath as you insert the catheter and aim to complete suctioning by the time you need to breathe again.

PFP8 When the suction catheter touches the tracheal wall, the patient will cough, sometimes violently. Patients find this unpleasant and often distressing, but it is important to induce coughing to prevent stasis of secretions in the lungs.

PFP9 The suction catheter should be rolled between the fingers as it is withdrawn, to facilitate the removal of secretions and to prevent high pressure being applied to any part of the tracheal wall. The tips of most suction catheters are designed to minimise this.

PFP10 Suctioning can be repeated until the ET tube/tracheostomy is clear of secretions and the breathing sounds clear. However, this may be distressing and so it may be necessary to allow time for the patient to rest during the procedure. No more than three suction passes should be made at any one time.

11.13 Insertion and management of chest drains

Preparation

Patient

- Explain the procedure, to gain cooperation and consent
- Explain positioning of the tube and subsequent limitations to mobility
- Explain the importance of not raising the bottle higher than the patient's chest ➡ **PFP1**
- Ask/assist the patient to move into the required position – usually upright, sitting forward resting on a table for support
- Raise the bed to a safe working height
- Ensure privacy and dignity are maintained throughout

Equipment

- Dressing trolley or clean surface
- Sterile chest drain insertion pack or dressing pack
- Hypoallergenic adhesive tape and sterile dressing
- Goggles, sterile gown and gloves for doctor
- Antiseptic skin-cleansing solution according to local policy
- Local anaesthetic as prescribed
- Syringes and needles for administration of local anaesthetic
- Sterile disposable scalpel
- Suture material (usually silk) for closing and retaining suture
- Sterile chest drain and introducer/ trochar
- Sterile drainage equipment (usually disposable) and sterile water
- Two tubing clamps ➡ **PFP2**
- Sharps bin

Nurse

- The nurse's role during chest drain insertion is to observe and support the patient and assist the doctor
- Record the patient's blood pressure, pulse, respiratory rate and oxygen saturation as baseline measurements
- Wash and dry hands thoroughly
- Put on apron. Additional protective clothing may be necessary if indicated by the patient's condition (see Ch. 1).

Procedure

1. Assess the patient's pain and administer analgesic or sedation 20 minutes before the procedure.

2. Maintaining the principles of asepsis, assemble the drainage equipment and add the sterile water. Make sure that the tube to be attached to the chest drain tubing is 4–5 cm below the water level (Figure 11.14) ➡ **PFP3**.

3. Open the sterile pack and add the sterile gown, gloves, syringe, scalpel and suture material.

4. Pour the antiseptic skin-cleansing solution into a gallipot. The doctor will now wash and dry their hands and put on the goggles, sterile gown and gloves.

5. When requested by the doctor, open the sterile needle for attachment to the syringe and hold the ampoule of local anaesthetic for the doctor to check and then draw into the syringe. This will then be used to numb the proposed insertion site.

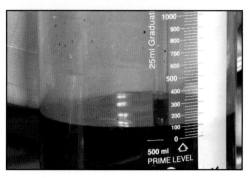

Figure 11.14 Underwater seal chest drain.

6. When requested by the doctor, open the packaging of the chest drain and introducer/trochar. The introducer will be placed inside the chest drain and then inserted into the chest wall.

7. During insertion of the chest drain explain each step of the procedure to the patient and observe the patient for signs of discomfort or respiratory distress.

8. Once the chest drain is inserted it should be attached to the drainage bottle immediately. The tubing may be clamped to prevent further lung collapse prior to attachment to the drainage bottle. Once securely attached, remove clamp.

9. The drain is then secured in place with a retaining suture and a 'closing' suture is inserted by the doctor ➡ **PFP4** and ➡ **PFP5**. The drain should be further secured to the chest wall with adhesive tape and the site covered with a dry sterile dressing ➡ **PFP6**.

10. Check that the drainage system is functioning by observing for swinging movement of water in the tubing as the patient breathes. There should be bubbling in the water with respiration in the case of a pneumothorax, and drainage of blood into the bottle in the case of a haemothorax ➡ **PFP7**.

11. If suction has been prescribed, the suction tubing is attached to the short tube in the bottle, the one that does not touch the water ➡ **PFP8**.

12. Ensure that the patient is comfortable and that the tubing of the chest drain is not pulling or kinked.

13. Discard needles, scalpel and the chest drain introducer into the sharps bin.

14. Safely dispose of all clinical waste and apron in the clinical waste bin

15. Wash and dry hands thoroughly.

16. A chest X-ray is required to confirm the position of the chest drain.

17. Document the chest drain insertion and, if applicable, the amount of suction required.

18. Record the patient's blood pressure, pulse, respiratory rate, temperature and oxygen saturation at least 4-hourly, and reassess the patient's pain. Continue to monitor the drainage, whether the fluid level is 'swinging', and if any air leak/ bubbling is seen in the chest drain bottle.

20. Encourage the patient to mobilise and sit up where possible. Deep breathing and coughing promote pleural drainage ➡ **PFP9**.

➡ Points for practice

PFP1 The drainage bottle should always be kept below the level of the patient's chest to prevent siphoning of fluid into the pleural space (Briggs 2010).

PFP2 Chest drain tubes should only be clamped if accidental disconnection occurs or when bottles are being changed. Unnecessary clamping of tubes may cause a tension pneumothorax.

PFP3 The end of the long tube in the bottle must be underwater to prevent air being drawn into the lungs during inspiration. It should be no more than 4–5 cm beneath the water level as this may make expansion of the lung more difficult.

PFP4 The retaining suture (know as the 'stay'suture) secures the chest drain in position, and the 'closing' suture seals the insertion hole when the chest drain is removed. A closing suture may not be necessary if a small chest drain tube is used (Laws et al 2003).

PFP5 If more than one drain has been inserted, make sure they are clearly labelled (e.g. basal and apical).

PFP6 The tubing can be secured to the patient's clothing by wrapping tape around the tubing and placing a safety pin through the tape. This can prevent kinks in the tubing, which will prevent drainage.

PFP7 To facilitate measurement of the rate of drainage, a piece of tape placed vertically next to the calibrated scale of the bottle can be marked at suitable intervals. If the bottle requires changing because it is nearly full, a new bottle should be prepared as in procedure point 2. The chest drain should be double clamped close to the chest and the tubing disconnected from the full bottle. The new bottle is then attached, ensuring that there is an underwater seal before unclamping the chest tube. The full bottle should be emptied (goggles should be worn) and discarded in the clinical waste. The amount of drainage should be recorded.

PFP8 A suction pressure of 5 kPa is usually used (Thorn 2006). Do not turn off the suction without disconnecting the tubing from the chest drain as this has an effect similar to the tube being clamped and may cause a tension pneumothorax.

PFP9 Take care that the drainage bottles are not damaged when raising or lowering the bed.

11.14 Chest drain removal

Preparation

Patient

- Explain the procedure, to gain consent and cooperation
- Instruct the patient to practise deep breathing and holding their breath ➡ **PFP1**
- Ask/assist the patient to adopt an upright position which is comfortable.
- Ensure privacy

Equipment/Environment

- Dressing trolley or clean work surface
- Sterile dressing pack containing gloves.
- Extra pair of non-sterile gloves for the assisting nurse
- Sterile dressing towel
- Skin-cleansing solution according to local policy ➡ **PFP2**
- Sterile dressing to cover site
- Sterile stitch cutter
- Alcohol hand-rub or hand-washing facilities
- Large clinical waste bag
- Sharps bin

Nurse

- Two nurses are required for this procedure
- The hands should be washed and dried thoroughly
- Aprons should be worn
- Additional protective clothing may be necessary if indicated by the patient's condition (see Ch. 1)
- Both nurses should wear goggles

Procedure

1. Administer any prescribed analgesic or sedative ➡ **PFP3**.

2. Take the equipment to the bedside and raise the bed to an appropriate height to avoid stooping.

3. Maintaining the principles of asepsis, open the dressing pack and pour the cleansing solution into a gallipot or fluid tray. Open the stitch cutter and dressing onto the sterile field.

4. Loosen the dressing around the drain site but do not remove.

5. Wash your hands or clean them using alcohol hand-rub.

6. Using the waste disposal bag as a 'glove', remove the dressing (see p. 286).

7. Put on sterile gloves and clean around the drain site to remove any dried blood or exudate that may impede removal of the drain.

8. Prepare the 'closing' suture so the ends are free and ready to be tied when the drain is removed. Cut and remove the suture holding the drain in place (see p. 290).

9. Ask the assisting nurse to put on gloves and hold the end of the closing suture ➡ **PFP4**.

10. Instruct the patient to take two deep breaths and hold the third breath (this should have been practised beforehand) ➡ **PFP1**.

11. While the patient is holding their breath, the nurse quickly and smoothly removes the chest drain. The assisting nurse pulls the closing suture tight and ties it with a double knot. Speed is essential.

12. On completion, instruct the patient to breathe normally.

13. Ask the assisting nurse to disconnect the chest drain tubing and discard it in the clinical waste bag ➡ **PFP5**.

14. Clean any fluid or exudate from the drain site and cover it with a dry dressing.

15. Ensure the patient is comfortable and sitting upright. Lower the bed ➡ **PFP6**.

16. Measure the final drainage and dispose of all waste and equipment appropriately. The chest drain bottle and tubing is usually disposable and can be discarded in the clinical waste.

17. Remove gloves, apron and goggles and wash hands.

18. Document chest drain removal noting, the final measurement and any difficulties during the procedure.

19. A chest X-ray may be ordered following the removal of the chest drain to ensure a pneumothorax has not recurred

20. Instruct the patient to report any breathlessness/difficulty in breathing

---

➡ Points for practice

PFP1 One of the main complications of chest drain removal is recurrent pneumothorax. The risk of this occurring increases if the patient breathes in whilst the drain is being removed (Bruce et al. 2006).

PFP2 The skin-cleansing solution used may vary according to local policy, but 0.9% sodium chloride is usually sufficient.

PFP3 The doctor may prescribe analgesia or a sedative prior to chest drain removal; this should be given at least 20 minutes before the procedure. Some units now use entonox during the procedure.

PFP4 If the drain was attached to suction, this should be disconnected before chest drain removal.

PFP5 If two chest drains are connected to one bottle, clamp each drain close to the patient's chest and disconnect the tubing from the bottle prior to removal.

PFP6 The closing suture can be removed after 5 days.

11.15 Non-invasive ventilation

Principles

Non-invasive ventilation (NIV) refers to the provision of ventilatory support through the patient's upper airway using a mask or similar device (RCP National Guidelines 2008). Other forms of ventilation delivered by an endotracheal tube, tracheostomy tube or laryngeal mask are described as invasive ventilation.

NIV is used for a range of respiratory conditions but is an essential component of the care of patients with chronic obstructive airways disease (COPD) when there has been no improvement following conventional therapy of bronchodilators, oxygen, steriods and antibiotics (Leave 2011). Nurses caring for patients recieving NIV need to be experienced in the use of the equipment according to local policy. This is a specialist area of care that requires in-depth knowledge of respiratory physiology, pulse oximetry and arterial blood gas analysis.

NIV assists breathing by giving the patient a mixture of air and oxygen through a tightly fitting facial or nasal mask. This helps the patient to take a full breath, thus providing an adequate oxygen supply to the body. NIV is usually prescribed as either CPAP or BiPAP.

Continuous Positive Airway Pressure (CPAP)

CPAP delivers a continuous flow of oxygen at a prescribed pressure which remains constant during inspiration (breathing in) and expiration (breathing out) (Figure 11.15). The constant pressure increases lung volume and keeps the alveoli at the end of each breath to allow more time for gaseous exchange (Esmond, 2011).

Bilevel Positive Airway Pressure (BiPAP)

In contrast, BiPAP provides a higher pressure when breathing in, and a lower pressure when breathing out. This works in the same way as CPAP but has been shown to decease the work of breathing more than CPAP alone (Ho and Wong, 2006). For more information on CPAP and BiPAP see Royal College of Physicians (2008).

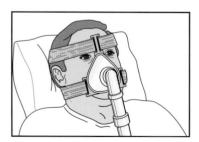

Figure 11.15 Patient with CPAP mask.

Bibliography/Suggested reading

Briggs, D., 2010. Nursing care and management of patients with intrapleural drains. Nursing Standard 24 (21), 47–55.

This article provides a good overview of the indications for chest drains and underwater seal drainage and discusses some of key issues in relation to the nursing care of a patient with a chest drain

British Thoracic Society, 2008. Working example of oxygen section for a hospital prescription chart. [online]. Available from: http://www.brit-thoracic.org.uk/Portals/0/Clinical%20Information/Emergency%20Oxygen/Emergency%20oxygen%20guideline/Chart3.pdf (accessed 24.01.12).

The British Thoracic Society have excellent easy to follow guidance on many respiratory diseases and types of oxygen therapy. This webpage illustrates how oxygen should be prescribed. The website is full of useful resources and is highly recommended

British Thoracic Society, Scottish Intercollegiate Network (BTS/SIGN), 2009. British guideline on the management of asthma: a national clinical guideline. [online]. Available from: http://www.sign.ac.uk/guidelines/fulltext/101/index.html (accessed 26.01.12).

This website provides an excellent resource for clinicians caring for asthmatic patients. It provides clinical guidance based on best available evidence

Bruce, E., Howard, R., Franck, L., 2006. Chest drain removal pain and its management: literature review. Journal of Clinical Nursing 15, 145–154.

An extensive review of the evidence in relation to pain management for chest drain removal

Clark, A., Giuliano, K., 2006. Pulse oximetry revisited: 'But his O2 sat was normal!' Clinical Nurse Specialist 20 (6), 268–272.

A very good article explaining exactly what pulse oximetry measures and its limitations. Issues learned from legal cases are highlighted and discussed

Cleave, L., 2011. Chronic obstructive pulmonary disease. In: Clarke, D., Ketchell, A., (Eds.), (2011) Nursing the acutely ill adult. Priorities in assessment and management. Palgrave Macmillan, Basingstoke.

This in-depth chapter describes the pathophysiology, assessment and treatment of a patient with COPD. A case study is used to illustrate key concepts. Oxygen therapy, non invasive ventilation and other treatments are discussed

Esmond, G., 2011. Nursing patients with respiratory disorders. In: Brooker C., Nicol, M., (Eds.), Alexander's nursing practice, fourth ed. Churchill Livingstone Elsevier, Edinburgh.

This chapter provides a comprehensive resource for all aspects of respiratory nursing from the relevant A&P and respiratory assessment to smoking cessation, respiratory medication, support techniques and oxygen therapy to nutrition, pulmonary rehabilitation and end-stage management of respiratory disease

Harkin, H., 2011. Nursing patients with disorders of the ear, nose and throat. In: Brooker, C., Nicol, M., Alexander's nursing practice, fourth ed. Churchill Livingstone Elsevier, Edinburgh.

This chapter provides a section on the nursing management of a tracheostomy – from pre-and post operative care to changing and removing tubes

Higgins, D., 2005. Measuring PEFR. Nursing Times 101 (10), 32–33.

This article discusses the measurement of and factors that influence peak expiratory flow rate (PEFR)

Ho, K.M., Wong K., 2006. A comparison of continuous and bi-level positive airway pressure non-invasive ventilation in patients with acute cardiogenis pulmonary oedema: a meta-analysis. Critical Care 10 (2), R49 [online]. Available from: http://ccforum.com/content/pdf/cc4861.pdf (accessed 11.08.11).

This paper explains the difference between the two and reports the findings of a meta-analysis to investigate the potential benefits and adverse effects of CPAP compared with BiPAP

Jevon, P., Humphrey, N., 2007. Respiratory procedures: use of spacer device. Nursing Times 103 (35), 24–25.

A good overview of the advantages and indications for use of a spacer and the principles of its use in adults and children. Includes diagrams

Kelly, C., Lynes, D., 2011. Best practice in the provision of nebuliser therapy. Nursing Standard 25 (31), 50–56.

This easy to follow paper discusses how and when nebuliser therapy should be used, it acknowledges the current evidence and limitations of the treatment and describes the patient experience

Laws, D., Neville, E., Duffy, J., 2003. Pleural Disease Group. Standards of Care Committee, British.

Thoracic Society, 2003. BTS Guidelines for the insertion of a chest drain. Thorax 58 (suppl 2), ii53–ii59.

The main purpose of these guidelines is to provide an overview of the key principles in relation to the insertion of chest drains. Good practice is identifed with supporting evidence. These are the most up to date guidelines from the British Thoracic Society, but it is worth looking at the website periodically to see if any new guidance has been recommended

Moore, T., 2003. Suction techniques for the removal of respiratory secretions. Nursing Standard 18 (9), 47–53.

This article discusses techniques for a variety of suctioning methods. It describes the procedures, rationale and potential complications

National Patient Safety Agency (NPSA), 2010. Making oxygen use safer. Nursing Times 106 (19), 10–11.

This brief paper clearly discusses the safety aspects of oxygen therapy. It provides guidance and advice on best practice

Paul, F., 2010. Tracheostomy care and management in general wards and community settings: literature review. Nurs Crit Care 15 (2), 76–85.

This paper identifies current research regarding the management of adult tracheostomy patients being cared for in general wards and the community.It emphasises patient safety and the need for skilled, trained nursing

Peakflow.com, 2004. Predicting PEFR. [online]. Available from: http://www.peakflow.com/top_nav/normal_values/PEFNorms.html (accessed 24.01.12).

This website guides you through the process of predicting a PEFR

Royal College of Physicians (RCP), 2008. Non invasive ventilation in chronic obstructive pulmonary disease: management of acute type 2 respiratory failure. Concise guidance for good practice. National guidelines, Number 11. RCP, London. [online]. Available from: http://www.brit-thoracic.org.uk/Portals/0/Clinical%20Information/NIV/Guidelines/NIVinCOPDFullguidelineFINAL.pdf (accessed 24.01.12).

These comprehensive guidelines discuss the care and management of COPD and type 2 respiratory failure, focussing on the use of NIV. Whilst written for doctors, they are of relevance for all health care professionals looking after patients receiving NIV

Thorn, M., 2006. Chest drains: a practical guide. British Journal of Cardiac Nursing 1 (4), 180–185.

A good overview of the indications for and principles of chest-drain management

Valdez-Lowe, C., Ghareeb, S., Artininan, N., 2009. Pulse oximetry in adults. American Journal of Nursing 109 (6), 52–59.

This article identifies what pulse oximetry is measuring and highlights current guidelines. whilst this is a US journal, the information is relevant to UK practice

Chapter 12

Reduced mobility

©2012 Elsevier Ltd.

12.1 Principles of moving and handling

Principles

Many patients experience a loss of mobility and independence through disease, illness or disability and it is likely that during this time, the patient will need the assistance of competent nurses to move or reposition them safely. However, every time nurses undertake any patient handling activity they are at risk from a musculoskeletal injury (Edlich et al. 2004). This risk becomes greater when poor practices and/or inappropriate techniques are used. Inconsistencies in practice may also increase the patient's vunerability and compromise patient safety and wellbeing. Nurses have an important role to play in preventing injuries associated with moving and handling. An important part of this role is to understand the principles associated with patient handling and apply these in practice. A description of all the legislation and techniques involved in moving and handling is beyond the scope of this book but the employer and employee responsibilites of key legislation and principles of risk assessment and safe posture are addressed here.

Legal requirements

Both employer and employee have defined responsibilities under Health and Safety legislation. The major legislation is summarised below.

The Manual Handling Operations Regulations (MHOR) (Health and Safety Executive 1992, amended 2004)

Implementation of this European Directive in 1992 led to important changes in health and safety requirements in relation to manual handling and moving in the workplace. This directive stipulates that employers have a duty, so far as reasonably practicable, to ensure the safety of all employees involved in moving and handling activities. Where this is not possible, employers are required to make a thorough assessment and implement measures to reduce the risk to the lowest level that is reasonably practicable. Where risk is unavoidable, they must take steps to minimise the risk.

The Health and Safety at Work Act (1974)

This stipulates that employers must ensure the health, safety and welfare of all employees, as far as it is reasonably practicable. Employers must not only provide a safe working environment but also ensure that safe working systems are implemented to prevent accidents. Employers have a responsibility to make equipment and appropriate training and supervision available to all staff. They also have a responsibility to make sure that equipment is properly maintained, and safety measures are implemented when equipment is handled, used, stored or transported.

Employees have an obligation to obey 'reasonable and lawful' instructions and to act with 'reasonable care and skill' (Health and Safety at Work Act 1974; MHOR

2004). Thus, employees have a responsibility to attend training sessions provided by employers and to use equipment and handling aids according to the manufacturers' instructions. However, it is vital that the employee never attempts to use any equipment or handling aids without the proper training and supervision. Employees also have a responsibility to inform the employers of any work situation that may require employees to work in a way that is dangerous, and may affect the health and safety of themselves or others. Although employers have a duty to perform risk assessments, employees equally have a responsibility to bring such situations to the employers' attention.

The Lifting Operations and Lifting Equipment Regulations (LOLER) (1998)

LOLER specifies that employers must ensure that any lifting equipment used in the workplace to move or lift patients (e.g.bath hoist, transfer hoist, slings) is safe and 'fit for purpose'. Employers have a responsibility to position and install equipment that safeguards the empoyee from injury. Equipment must be strong and stable, and employers must ensure that all lifting equipment is marked to indicate the safe working load. Employers have the responsibility to ensure that all the equipment used for lifting is inspected by a competent person at prescribed intervals, recorded and labelled to indicate the next inspection date. It is important that only competent staff use the equipment and all equipment must be thoroughly examined for signs of wear. The inspection label must be checked before equipment is used.

The Provision and Use of Work Equipment Regulations (PUWER) (1998)

In addition to LOLER, the PUWER regulations stipulate that any other equipment (e.g electric beds, transfer boards, sliding sheets) provided and used by an employee for work purposes must be suitable for use, and for the purpose and condition in which it is used. Equipment must be maintained in a safe condition to safeguard employees from risk of injury and inspected by a competent person to ensure that it is safe for use.

Risk assessment

Under Health and Safety Executive (HSE 1992) guidelines it is the employer's responsibility to ensure that their employees are not at risk of injury from manual handling and to implement a policy and code of practice for the workplace that are based on advice from experts in occupational health and ergonomics. They must also employ a 'competent' person, such as a back care advisor, and carry out formal handling assessments in the work place that look at: the task, the individual nurse or carer, the load and the environment.

These are important categories to remember because nurses also need to consider them in their risk assessments; the acronym TILE will help you to remember. A risk assessment addressing these four areas must be completed before every moving and handling activity. When assessing the risk you need to begin by asking the question: Is it necessary? Once you have established that it is necessary (i.e. the patient is not able to move him- or herself), you then need to complete the risk assessment.

Task (what is it that you need to do?)

- Can the patient move themselves or would the use of equipment be safer and more effective?
- Do you need help and/or equipment?
- Does it involve stooping, bending or twisting? If the answer is yes then you must find another way to do it to reduce the risk.
- Is there sufficent time so that neither you nor the patient is rushing? For example, if a patient wants to go to the toilet urgently it may be better to get them there quickly in a wheelchair and encourage them to walk back.
  - How long will it take? If the activity takes a long time it is likely that you and the patient will become fatigued
  - What is the distance? Where possible try to reduce the distance e.g. if you are helping a patient to walk down a corridor it may be better to position a chair half way so the patient can rest.

Individual (nurse or carer)

- What are your own capabilities (fitness, state of health, fatigue) ?
- Do you have appropriate knowledge, skills and training (use of equipment and techniques)?
- Do you have appropriate communication skills to explain and give instructions clearly to the patient and colleagues.
- Is your clothing appropriate? (Can you move freely? Is it clean?)
- Do you need any additional personal protective equipment (p. 2)?
- Are your shoes appropriate (low heel, non-slip sole, securely fastened and must cover the whole foot) ?
- Long hair should be tied back so that it does not fall in your face and distract you or the patient.
- Nails should be short as these may scratch the patient.
- Jewellery should not be worn as this may injury the patient.
- If you are working with another nurse or carer it is best if you are of a similar height, if at all possible.

Load (patient)

- Diagnosis/condition of the patient – is the patient 'allowed' to mobilise?
- What is the patient's height and weight?
- Physical ability of the patient – can the patient balance, weight bear on one or both legs, does the patient have any weakness in their arms or legs, are they immobilised?

- If the patient is walking, has the patient got suitable footwear and clothing? Slippers are rarely supportive; outdoor shoes are better.
- Does the patient use any aids to mobility such as a walking stick or Zimmer frame?
- Is the patient able to understand and cooperate, e.g. what is the patient's mental capacity, do they have any sensory deficits or language barriers?
- Is the patient in pain? This could lead to sudden unexpected movement and so analgesics should be administered and time allowed for this to take effect.
- Are there any intravenous infusions, drains, catheters, plaster cast etc., to consider?
- What is the condition of the patient's skin?
- How old is the patient?
- Does the patient have any cutural/religious needs (gender of nurses/handlers)?
- If the load is not a person you need to consider if it is bulky, stable/unstable, heavy, long, wide, difficult to hold onto, hot to touch, has sharp edges or is wet/slippery.

Environment

- Is there enough space to move freely without twisting or bending?
- Is the floor free of obstacles such as trailing wires, rugs, steps, furniture?
- Is the floor dry and not slippery?
- Is the equipment/furniture working properly, especially the brakes, height adjustment? Does the equipment have an inspection date and a safe work load label? Are there any signs of wear?
- Is there adequate light to see what you are doing?
- Is there excessive noise to prevent you from communicating with the patient and colleagues?
- Is the temperature ambient? Being very hot makes us feel weak and very cold makes us tense our muscles.
- Does the space provide sufficient privacy? If not, screens may be required.

Principles of safe handling and good posture

Many hospitals and other institutions have adopted safe-handling or no lifting policies.

This requires the proper training and periodic updating of all staff in the use of mechanical lifting equipment (hoists, sliding transfer aids etc.) and patient handling techniques. This means that all nurses must attend a mandatory programme before undertaking any patient handling activities. It is essential that nurses adopt the principles of good posture when moving or repositioning patients to minimise the risk of musculoskeltal injury. The key principles are:

Safe posture

- Keep your back in its natural position throughout its length as this allows the muscles to correctly move, control, support and protect the spine during any movement or activity.

- Avoid twisting or bending sideways as this will restrict the body's ability to move correctly. Keep your head in aligment with your spine (i.e.looking forward) to maintain the natural curvature of your back.

- Adopt a stable stance. Stand with your feet about hip-width apart, with one foot slightly in front of the other to form a wide base of support.

- Keep your knees 'soft' (relaxed) and slightly bent to allow flexibility and movement. Flexing the knees and using the quadriceps muscles prevents the back and shoulder msucles being used.

- Keep the load as close to your body as possible at waist height. Holding a load at a distance, away from the the body, will make the load feel heavier and will cause the shoulder and back muscles to ache.

12.2 Risk assessment of pressure ulcers

Principles

Pressure ulcers have long been seen as costly both in terms of patients' health and in cost to the health service. When assessing patients' susceptibility to developing pressure ulcers, a number of factors must be taken into consideration. These are generally grouped into two categories: external factors and internal factors.

External factors

- **Pressure** is the most important factor and occurs when the soft tissue of the body is compressed between a bony prominence and a hard surface.

- **Shear** occurs when the soft tissues and the skeleton move, but the skin does not, e.g. sliding down the bed.

- **Friction** occurs when two surfaces rub together and the top layer of the skin is scraped off, e.g when the body is rotating to sit on the side of the bed, the feet and sacrum slide on the bed sheets.

Internal factors

- **Physical factors** include the patients' general health, sensory impairment, nutrition and hydration status, level of mobility, skin condition, previous history of pressure damage and restfulness/restlessness.

- **Medical/surgical factors** consider patients' cardiovascular system, level of consciousness, level of pain, continence status, medications, surgery, acute, chronic or terminal illness, specific predisposing diseases, infections and allergies.

- **Psychological factors** incorporate an assessment of patients' mental and emotional status that may affect sleep or motivation.

- **Lifestyle factors** include smoking and weight and build.

- **Unchangeable factors** are those such as age.

In order to provide consistent information and enable nurses to plan appropriate prevention strategies, a number of assessment tools have been developed (e.g. Norton et al. 1975, Waterlow 2005). These assessment tools differ, but most consider the majority of factors outlined above. What is important is that the nurse uses clinical judgement in conjunction with the chosen assessment tool as it is often the existence of a combination of factors that increases patients' susceptibility to pressure ulcer formation.

Assessing the patient

Patients should receive an initial and ongoing risk assessment within 6 hours of admission in the first episode of care, and then at least weekly; it may need to be more frequent depending on the patient's condition (NICE 2005). Assessment of the patient should address the following:

Physical factors

In addition to assessment of patients' general health prior to admission to hospital, a thorough nutritional assessment should be undertaken using a recognised tool, such as the Malnutrition Universal Screening Tool (MUST) (see p. 152). Patients whose diet is lacking in protein, vitamins B and C, and zinc and iron are more susceptible to pressure ulcer development. Reduced nutritional status restricts the body's ability to build and repair tissue and impairs the elasticity of the skin, and skin that is dry (due to a poor or reduced fluid intake) is more susceptible to pressure damage.

When considering the patient's level of mobility, the nurse should consider the following: activity level (e.g ability to walk, reposition independently, and move from chair to bed), presence of paralysis and restrictions to mobility (e.g. wound drains, intravenous infusions, traction or plaster) and whether these restrictions are temporary or permanent. Patients' general awareness, level of anxiety and the existence of pain should also be assessed.

Assessment of skin should consider whether it is healthy, papery, dry, clammy, sweaty or oedematous. Skin hydration should be noted and any evidence of previous ulceration, broken skin or any pre-existing skin condition or discoloration. Excessive moisture should be considered as this may increase the body's susceptability to shear and friction forces (e.g sweating, (perspiration) and bathing). Assessing skin with a darker pigmentation needs to be undertaken very carefully, as discoloration tends to be less noticeable.

Patients' continence status should be also considered. Incontinence of urine and faeces, which are acidic, can lead to skin maceration and constant washing can remove the natural oils, thus drying the skin.

Medical/surgical history

Patients' previous medical or surgical history will indicate risk factors that impact on tissue perfusion and oxygenation of the tissues. Examples are diabetes, cardiovascular disease, respiratory disease and anaemia. Any surgery including the length of time on the operating table, type of anaesthetic (e.g. epidural, spinal, general) should be noted. Medications should be considered, particularly noting antibiotics, steroids, sedatives, anti-inflammatory and cytotoxic drugs or insulin.

Psychological factors

Assessment of patients' emotional status is important (e.g. whether grieving or depressed), as this may affect their motivation.

Lifestyle factors

Whether a patient smokes should be noted, as this may impact on respiratory function. When considering patients' weight and build, a note should be made of whether they are overweight or underweight (see p. 152, calculation of body mass index).

Age

The age of the patient should be considered in conjunction with general health. Factors that impact on older patients (nutrition, skin elasticity, fragility, the presence of chronic illnesses) may not be significant for those who are younger.

Calculating the risk

Each of the factors above is allocated a score on the chosen assessment tool. The total indicates the level of vulnerability, which in turn should indicate the nature of the prevention plan. However, the allocation of scores for increased vulnerability or elevated risk conditions or behaviours is not consistent across the assessment tools. In some tools a low total score indicates a high risk of pressure ulcer development, but in others, the opposite is true. There is considerable discussion in the literature as to the advantages and disadvantages of each tool. However, the NICE (2005) guidelines stress that the assessment tool should only be used as an *aide memoire* and should not replace clinical judgement. The risk assessment should be documented in the nursing records along with preventative strategies. The assessment must be repeated at weekly or as dictated by any changes in the patient's condition, e.g. following surgery.

12.3 Prevention of pressure ulcers

Principles

Prevention of pressure ulcers will not be achieved unless the predisposing factors are controlled or alleviated for each patient. Generic risk factors were previously identified, but it is the particular combination of these in each patient that determines how high the risk is. Nevertheless, there are general principles to follow when planning preventative strategies.

Careful positioning

Positioning when in bed and sitting in a chair is crucial. All patients who are vulnerable to pressure ulcers should as a minimum be placed on a high-specification (low tech) foam mattresses as they aim to redistribute pressure over a large contact area (NICE 2005). There is little research evidence to suggest that alternating pressure (Figure 12.1) or other high-tech pressure-relieving systems are more effective than low-tech devices. However, they should be considered for those patients who are identified as having: a high risk of developing pressure ulcers, a history of pressure damage or a clinical condition that indicates their use, although the effectiveness of the various types is the subject of much debate (NICE 2005). What is important is that friction and shear can be difficult to eliminate on alternating pressure-relieving mattresses and therefore, additional preventative strategies need to be used, e.g sliding sheets.

Regular repositioning

Frequent repositioning is essential whether the patient is in bed or in a chair. A useful yardstick is 2 hours, although this should be adjusted for the individual patient's need. Some patients, particularly those who are elderly, may need to be repositioned more regularly. The repositioning regimen must be rigorously implemented and in some cases can be supported by a repositioning chart, e.g. a 24-hour turning chart.

The use of a pressure-relieving mattress does not remove the need to adjust the patient's position. The 30° tilt position is recommended to help evenly distribute the body weight. Using the right side, back, left side regime also prevents any direct

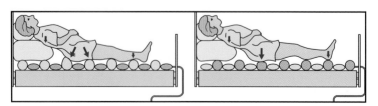

Figure 12.1 Alternating pressure mattress.

pressure on the sacrum or trochanter (EPUAP/NPUAP 2010). This is thought to allow pressure to be tolerated for up to three times longer than over bony prominences (Gebhardt 2002). However, it is important to discuss and agree any repositioning regime with the patient to ensure concordance and comfort. Bedclothes should be loose and sheets not wrinkled. Pillows can be used to support patients in the desired positions to prevent further deterioration brought about by incorrect positioning of limbs.

When seated in chairs patients should not be left for more than 2 hours regardless of the device being used. The chair must be of appropriate dimensions to promote good posture. There is little evidence that cushions are clinically effective for acutely ill patients, but may have some benefit for those who are wheel-chair bound or have a chronic risk of developing pressure ulcers. Self-repositioning is equally important for patients who sit for a prolonged time in a wheelchair. It is recommended that they move to relieve pressure every 15–30 minutes (Stockton and Flynn 2009a).

Exercise

Passive and active exercise is essential in maintaining and encouraging mobilisation and limiting the impact of some of the predisposing factors.

Safe moving and handling

When moving and handling patients, it is essential that appropriate manual handling equipment is used to prevent shear or friction e.g. sliding sheet, hoist. Positioning patients to prevent them sliding down the bed is important in preventing shear. Chairs are one of the main culprits in encouraging shearing forces if they fail to promote and maintain a good posture (Dealey 2005).

Nutrition and hydration

Consideration of patients' nutrition and hydration is important in order to maintain healthy skin and provide assistance with eating and drinking where necessary. Maintaining a food and fluid balance chart may be useful.

Skin care

Continuous assessment of the skin is vital. This can be undertaken when attending to the patient's hygiene needs. Skin should be inspected for persistent erythema, non-blanching hyperaemia, blisters, localised heat, oedema, induration, purplish/bluish localised areas and localised coolness if tissue death occurs. The skin should be kept clean and dry especially if the patient is incontinent, has a high temperature or is sweating excessively. However, caution should be exercised in the overuse of soap and detergents as they are the commonest cause of stripping of the epidermal protective barrier (Butcher 2005). Consideration should be given to the use of non-soap skin cleansers. Emollients in the bath or creams are useful for dry skin and a barrier cream for moist skin may be useful. They do, however, interfere with the use of adhesives on the skin and may also affect the absorptive properties of dressings and continence products (Butcher 2005).

Grading pressure ulcers

If the patient does develop a pressure ulcer it should be graded so that appropriate treatment can be given (NICE 2005). In 2009, the EPUAP and NPUAP published new guidelines and definitions for the prevention, classification and treatments for pressure ulcers. These are now referred to as the International EPUAP/NPUAP Pressure ulcer classification system (see Table 12.1). NICE (2005) recommend the following:

- All pressure ulcers graded 2 and above should be documented as a local clinical incident.

- Patients with grade 1–2 pressure ulcers should be closely observed for skin changes and, as a minimum, placed on a pressure reducing foam mattress/ cushion.

- Patients with grade 3–4 pressure ulcers require a high specification foam mattress with an alternating foam overlay or a 'sophisticated low pressure system' such as a low air loss system (NICE 2005).

For more information on the prevention and management of pressure ulcers see RCN (2005).

Table 12.1 International EPUA/NPUAP pressure ulcer classification system

Category/grade 1	Category/grade 2	Category/grade 3	Category/grade 4
• *Non-blanchable erythema of intact skin* of a localised area, usually over a bony prominence • Discolouration of the skin, warmth, oedema, hardness or pain may also be present • Darkly pigmented skin may not have visible blanching	• *Partial thickness skin loss or blister*. Partial thickness loss of dermis, presenting as a shallow open ulcer with a red/ pink wound bed without slough • May also present as an intact or open/ ruptued serum filled or sero-sanginous filled blister	• *Full thickness skin loss.* Subcutaneous fat may be visible but bone, muscle and tendon are not exposed • Some slough may be present. • May include undermining and tunnelling	• *Full thickness tissue loss.* Involves exposed bone, tendon or muscle • Slough or eschar may be present • Often include undermining and tunnelling

12.4 Complications of immobility

Complications of bed rest

Although fewer and fewer patients are now confined to bed for long periods, many of the patients you care for will be on partial or complete bed rest or sitting in chairs for long periods of time. This may be for a variety of reasons:

- To reduce cardiac effort e.g. flowing a heart attack
- To reduce respiratory effort e.g. asthma or pneumonia
- If the patient has a pyrexia (fever increases oxygen demand)
- To reduce pain e.g. after an operation or arthritis
- To prevent weight-bearing e.g. following knee replacement or a fracture
- Treatment of back pain or following surgery to relieve back pain
- During pregnancy to prevent miscarriage or in the event of pre-eclampsia
- To rest the patient e.g. after extensive abdominal surgery.

Although bed rest is clearly beneficial, there are a number of physical complications that can arise. Psychological complications such as depression and musculoskeletal complications such as contractures and muscular atrophy may also occur (Timmerman 2007). Nurses need to be alert to these and implement nursing interventions to minimise the risk. The four most common physical complications will be addressed here:

- Chest infection
- Pressure ulcers
- Deep vein thrombosis (DVT)
- Constipation.

Chest infection

Patients confined to bed are at risk of chest infection due to a reduction in chest expansion. If lying down, the pressure of abdominal contents against the diaphragm reduces lung volume and if coughing is painful or difficult, that can lead to accumulation of secretions in the lungs and a risk of a chest infection developing.

Prevention of chest infection

Positioning the patient upright (see p. 336) will help lung expansion and turning the patient from side-to-side will encourage expansion of the lung that is uppermost. Encouraging deep breathing and coughing and administering analgesics to control pain will help to clear the secretions. If the patient is receiving oxygen, humidification (see p. 342) will make it easier for the patient to expectorate secretions.

Pressure ulcers

There are many risk factors that make patients with reduced mobility more likely to develop pressure ulcers (e.g. incontinence, malnutrition see p. 377) but there are three causes: pressure, shearing and friction.

Pressure: a pressure ulcer will develop when there is localised pressure that is unrelieved, causing ischaemia (lack of blood supply) to an area of tissue. This occurs when the tissues become compressed between the bone and the surface of the bed or chair. The areas most at risk are the bony prominences such as the hips, shoulders, sacrum and heels.

Shearing: this is the damage to tissues caused when the skin 'sticks' to the surface of the bed or chair but the skeleton moves forward, for example when sliding down the bed. This causes stretching of the tissues and kinking or rupture of the capillaries leading to ischaemia.

Friction: rubbing the skin vigorously or constantly sliding down the bed or chair causes friction. Friction is increased when the skin is wet and this in turn causes shearing as the skin cannot slide easily over the bedclothes.

Pressure ulcer prevention (see also p. 380)

Regular changes of position are vital to prevent pressure ulcers. Patients confined to bed will require a pressure ulcer risk assessment (see p. 377) and those on long-term bed rest may require a pressure relieving mattress and/or other aids such as special cushions when sitting in a chair. In most organisations these are obtained by contacting the tissue viability nurse. It is also important to keep patients clean and dry as moisture increases the risk of damage due to friction and wet skin becomes less resilient and is more easily damaged.

Regular inspection (at least every 4 hours) of the patient's skin to assess the areas most at risk of pressure ulcers is crucial in order to detect any changes at an early stage. Almost all pressure ulcers are preventable; poor moving and handling techniques can increase the risk as can poor nutritional status. Nurses have a duty to protect their patients and ensure that risk assessment and regular position changes are carried out. Avoid leaving patients sitting in chairs for long periods of time; regular rests lying in bed will distribute the pressure over a larger area. Teach patients spending long periods in a chair/wheelchair to use their arms to raise themselves at regular intervals to relieve pressure and improve circulation.

Venous thromoembolism (VTE)

Venous thromboembolism (VTE) refers to deep vein thrombosis (DVT), which is a clot (thrombus) in the deep veins of the leg and pulmonary embolus. Immobility leads to venous stasis (slowing of blood flow) in the legs. This is because the muscles in the legs, which normally help to 'pump' blood back to the heart, are not active when lying in bed or immobile in a chair. Venous stasis is made worse if the patient is not able to breathe deeply and cough (see Chest Infection above), because the negative pressure that is created in the chest during inspiration also helps venous return to the heart.

Venous stasis means that clotting factors, which are normally quickly cleared from the circulation, remain active for longer and so make clot formation (thrombosis) more likely. If part of the clot breaks off it can travel in the bloodstream to the lungs and cause a pulmonary embolus, which can be fatal.

Prevention of VTE

VTE risk assessment is now part of most admission procedures and early mobilisation will reduce the risk of VTE. Prophylactic measures such as subcutaneous low molecular weight heparin and anti thrombolism stockings or a pneumatic compression device (see p. 389) will be prescribed and dehydration should be avoided if the patient's condition allows. It is important to remind the patient to exercise their legs by flexing the foot towards the knee and rotating the foot; this activates the calf muscles 'pump' to increase blood flow. If patients are unable to do this (e.g. unconscious patients) the nurse or physiotherapist will perform passive leg exercises to promote circulation and maintain muscle tone. Observe and teach patients to observe for signs of DVT: swelling, pain or tenderness, erythema and discolouration.

Constipation

Immobility leads to slowing of peristalsis in the large intestine, which means that faeces takes longer to pass through, allowing more water to be re-absorbed. This leads to drying and hardening of the faeces making them more difficult to pass. When accompanied by dehydration and a diet low in fibre, the risk of constipation in the immobile patient is even greater. Lack of fibre and fluid reduces the bulk of the faeces, which means that the bowel may not be sufficiently distended to stimulate the defaecation reflex.

If the patient is also embarrassed about using the commode or bedpan and 'busy' nurses do not respond quickly to requests to go to the toilet, patients may well ignore the urge to defaecate and become constipated.

Prevention and treatment of constipation

Monitor the bowel actions and if the patient's condition allows, increase oral fluids (2 litres a day if possible) and include fruit juices and vegetable soups to add fibre. If the patient is not on any fluid restriction or at risk of bowel obstruction encourage them to choose foods that are high in dietary fibre (fruit, vegetables, wholemeal bread and wholegrain cereals). Encourage increased mobility where possible, as this will increase peristalsis, and ensure privacy and dignity when using the commode or bed pan (see p. 231-234). Review all medication to see if there are any alternatives to medications known to cause constipation e.g. codeine based analgesics. Consider the use of laxatives if the above measures are unsuccessful.

12.5 Fitting anti-embolism stockings

Preparation

Patient

- All patients with reduced mobility or undergoing surgery are at risk of venous thromboembolism (VTE) but anti-embolism stockings are contraindicated for some patients ➡ **PFP1**
- Dehydration and hypotension increase the risk of venous thromboembolism

Equipment

- Tape measure and sizing chart
- Anti-embolism stockings of appropriate size and length (thigh or knee length) ➡ **PFP2**
- Pneumatic compression device may be prescribed instead ➡ **PFP3**

Nurse

- The hands should be clean
- An apron should be worn
- Additional protective clothing may be necessary if indicated by the patient's condition (see Ch. 1)

Procedure

1. Assess the patient's risk according to local policy using a VTE score such as the Wells Score (Table 12.2). Early mobilisation, if the patient's condition allows, reduces the risk of deep vein thrombosis (DVT).

2. Teach the patient foot and leg exercises before an operation or period of reduced mobility and encourage exercises at least hourly until fully mobile. Position the patient's legs during the operation and in bed so as to prevent calf compression. Discourage patients from crossing their legs in bed.

3. If the patient is unable to perform foot and leg exercises and does not have a pneumatic compression device, a nurse/physiotherapist should perform passive leg movements at least every 2 hours.

Table 12.2 The wells score for predicting probability of DVT	
Active cancer within last 6 months	1
Paralysis, paresis, recent plaster immobilisation	1
Recently bedridden >3 days, major surgery <12 weeks	1
Localised tenderness along distribution of deep veins	1
Entire leg swollen	1
Calf swelling >3 cm	1
Pitting oedema confined to symptomatic leg	1
Collateral superficial veins (non-varicose)	1
Previous documented DVT	1
Alternative diagnosis at least as likely as DVT	−2
Total score	
0 = low probability, 1–2 = moderate probability, >3 = high probability	

4. Deep breathing should be encouraged because the negative pressure that is created in the chest during inspiration helps venous return to the heart.

5. Observe the calves for swelling, heat, tenderness and erythema/discolouration (most commonly reddish purple) caused by venous engorgement and obstruction. Observe the patient for any of the contraindications to anti-embolism stockings ➡ **PFP1**

6. Measure the legs according to the manufacturer's instructions. It is crucial that the correct size stockings are used (Figure 12.2A & B).

7. Fit the anti-embolism stockings according to the manufacturer's instructions (Figure 12.2). Do not gather up the stocking as the bunching of the elastic makes it harder to put on. Place you hand inside and grasp the centre of the heel section (Figure 12.2C). Turn the stocking inside out as far as the heel section and carefully position the foot part over the foot (Figure 12.2E) and heel. Make sure that the heel part is correctly positioned over the heel (Figs 12.2D and G). Now pull the stocking over the foot and up the leg. Smooth out any wrinkles. The hole should be positioned under the toes and is designed to enable visual inspection of the toes and circulation (Figure 12.2F). Document the anti-embolism stockings according to local policy.

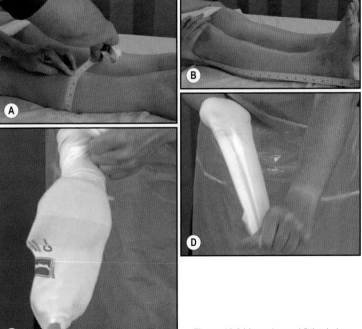

Figure 12.2 Measuring and fitting below knee anti-embolism stockings.

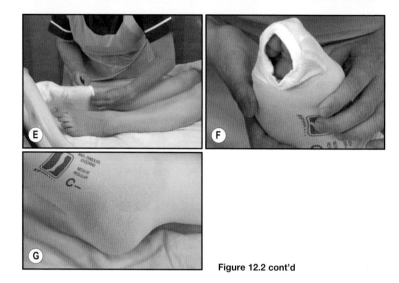

Figure 12.2 cont'd

8. If the patient's condition allows maintain adequate fluid intake (2 litres per day) and encourage mobilisation and/or leg exercises.

9. Remove anti-embolism stockings at least once daily, to inspect the skin, calves and feet for signs of VTE, pressure ulcers, colour changes etc. Check frequently that the stockings are not wrinkled or rolled down.

10. Ensure the patient understands the reason for the stockings and knows to report any signs of DVT and avoid activities that may increase the risk of VTE (e.g. dehydration, crossing legs).

11. Subcutaneous low molecular weight heparin may also be prescribed as a prophylactic measure and may be followed by oral anticoagulants.

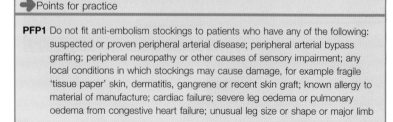

Points for practice

PFP1 Do not fit anti-embolism stockings to patients who have any of the following: suspected or proven peripheral arterial disease; peripheral arterial bypass grafting; peripheral neuropathy or other causes of sensory impairment; any local conditions in which stockings may cause damage, for example fragile 'tissue paper' skin, dermatitis, gangrene or recent skin graft; known allergy to material of manufacture; cardiac failure; severe leg oedema or pulmonary oedema from congestive heart failure; unusual leg size or shape or major limb deformity preventing correct fit. Use caution and clinical judgement when applying anti-embolism stockings over venous ulcers or wounds (NICE 2010).

PFP2 Thigh-length stockings can be more difficult to apply and may not be as effective if the thigh and calf are not in proportion; the stocking may be too tight or too loose in one area. Anti-embolism stockings work by promoting venous flow in the legs and preventing stasis. The stocking compression profile should be approximately: Ankle –18 mmHg; Mid calf – 14 mmHg; upper thigh – 8 mmHg (Hairon 2007).

PFP3 A pneumatic compression device is worn around the patient's legs or feet. They inflate automatically at regular intervals and apply pressure, which helps the blood in the legs to circulate. It should be used whilst the patient is in bed and when in a chair.

12.6 Falls prevention

Principles

Falls are a major cause of disability and the leading cause of death following injury in people over 75 years of age in the UK (NICE 2004). It is clear that falls have an impact on quality of life and although falls are not an inevitable result of ageing, they are a serious problem for many older people (NICE 2004). The Royal Society for the Prevention of Accidents (ROSPA) estimates that a third of those over 65 fall at least once a year and this figure rises to half of those over 80 years of age. The incidence of falls in nursing homes and hospitals is considerably greater than in a person's own home and complication rates are also higher (NICE 2004). Clearly falls prevention is an important part of the nursing care of older people.

In 2004 the Royal College of Nursing (RCN) published *Clinical practice guideline for the assessment and prevention of falls in older people*, which was commissioned by the National Institute for Clinical Excellence (NICE). The NICE guidelines (NICE 2004) promote a person-centred and multidisciplinary approach and recommend the following.

- Older people should routinely be asked about the frequency, context and characteristics of any falls within the previous year

- Patients and carers should be involved in shared decision making about falls prevention strategies

- It is important to respect the knowledge and experience of those who have been successfully self-managing this risk

- All members of the multidisciplinary team (MDT) should be aware of the guidelines and all care must be documented in the patient's records

- Nurses and other healthcare professionals need appropriate education to be able to assess risk and initiate and maintain preventative measures

- Staffing levels and skill mix should reflect the needs of patients at risk of falling.

Multifactorial falls risk assessment

Older people who are admitted following a fall or report recurrent falls and those who have an abnormal gait and/or problems with balance should be have a falls risk assessment. The risk factors for falling are diverse, and therefore assessment and prevention strategies need to be multifactorial i.e. have a number of components or interventions. According to NICE (2004) multifactorial assessment, which should be performed in the setting of a specialist falls service, may include assessment of the following:

- Falls history

- Assessment of gait, balance, mobility and muscle weakness

- Osteoporosis risk

- Functional ability and fear of falling
- Visual impairment
- Cognitive impairment and neurological examination
- Continence
- Hazards in the home
- Cardiovascular system and medication review.

Intervention programmes

Older people at risk of falls should be assessed to plan individualised interventions to promote independence and improve physical and psychological function. The following have been shown to lead to successful outcomes (NICE 2004):

- Strength and balance training
- Home hazard assessment and intervention
- Vision assessment and referral
- Medication review with modification/withdrawal
- Falls prevention programmes
- Education and information giving.

Strength and balance training

In hospitals the physiotherapists will design and monitor a muscle strengthening and balance programme. Age UK (formerly Age Concern and Help the Aged) also provide advice about exercises to improve strength and balance that are specifically designed for older people. They include gentle exercises to strengthen the arms, wrists, thighs and upper back and improve standing from a chair. There are also exercises to improve balance: side stepping, heel raises, toe raises, leg swinging and marching on the spot (Age UK 2011).

Home hazard assessment and intervention

Assessment of hazards in the home is only effective if the assessment is followed up and appropriate interventions are instigated (NICE 2004). Prior to discharge from hospital a home visit by an occupational therapist will identify any modifications required. This will take time to organise and so needs to be planned well in advance. Age UK (www.ageuk.org.uk) provide useful advice on possible modifications such as door ramps, intercom systems if answering the door is difficult and getting up and down stairs. They also provide information about sources of funding if modifications are required.

Vision assessment and referral

There is an inevitable decline in vision as we age and this is due to changes in the eye, rather than in the neural conduction system from the eye to the brain. With age it is common for the lens to become more opaque and some older people suffer from cataracts (Holman 2011). Gillespie et al. (2009) found that in participants with severe visual impairment a home safety programme significantly reduced the incidence of falls. However, if vision assessment leads to new spectacles, this was shown to actually increase the rate of falls. Older, frail people may need a considerable period of time to adjust to new spectacles and may be at greater risk of falling during this time (Gillespie 2010).

Medication review with modification/withdrawal

NICE (2004) recommend that older people on psychotropic medication should have it reviewed and, if possible, discontinued to reduce their risk of falls. However, Gillespie et al. (2009) argue that the evidence for withdrawal of psychotropic medicines and reduction in the risk of falls is limited. Vitamin D does not appear to prevent falls in older people although there is provisional evidence that it may reduce the risk of falls in older people with vitamin D deficiency (Gillespie et al. 2009).

Falls prevention programmes

In order to encourage participation in falls prevention programmes it is important to have a person-centred approach and discuss what changes the older person is willing to make. The programme should address issues such as low self-esteem and fear of falling as these may become barriers to participation. Programmes need to be sufficiently flexible to accommodate differing needs and should promote the benefits of social interaction with others (NICE 2004).

Education and information giving

Education and training are needed to ensure that all staff are knowledgeable and able to implement the guidelines. Older people at risk of falling should be given information both orally and in writing and this should include information about the preventable nature of some falls and how to prevent them, the benefits of exercises to improve strength and balance, and the physical and psychological benefits of reducing the risk of falls. Programmes should also include ways to cope if the older person does fall and how to summon help.

Bibliography/Suggested reading

Moving and handling

Royal College of Nursing, 2003. Manual handling assessment in hospital and the community: an RCN guide. RCN Revised, London [online]. Available from: www.rcn.org.uk (accessed 24.1.12.).

Provides practical advice on risk assessment in moving and handling

Edlich, R.F., Hudson, M.A., Britt, L.D., Long, W.B., 2004. Preventing of disabling back injuries in nurses by the use of mechanical patient lifting systems. Journal of Long Term Effects of Medical Implants 14 (6), 521–533.

Although this article is American, it has relevance to patient handling activities in the UK. The article confirms the risks associated with patient handling and its direct link to musculoskeletal disorders. It also discusses the benefits of using mechanical equipment to reduce these risks, and includes the anatomy and physiology, risk factors and associated legal issues

Smith, J., (Ed.), 2011. The guide to the handling of people, a systems approach, sixth ed. BackCare, Teddington.

This is the latest edition of The guide to the handling of patients published by BackCare in association with the RCN and National Back Exchange. It is widely recognised as the most comprehensive resource available for moving and handling.

Health and Safety at Work Act, 1974. [online]. Available from: http://www.hse.gov.uk/legislation/hswa.htm (accessed: 26.1.12.).

This website provides an overview of the moving and handling in health. It provides guidance for those involved in moving and handling and includes risk assessment, use of equipment and the law

Manual Handling Operations Regulations, 2004. [online]. Available for free download from: http://www.hse.gov.uk/pubns/books/l23.htm and www.nhsemployers.org (accessed: 26.1.12.)

This is a useful website that covers many of the healthcare issues in the NHS today, and includes information on musculoskletal disorders in relation to the workplace

Pressure ulcers

Butcher, M., 2005. Prevention and management of superficial pressure ulcers. British Journal of Community Nursing 10 (6) Suppl S16, S18–S20.

This article examines superficial pressure ulcers, those involving the upper layers of the skin. The article presents a practical approach for nurses in preventing pressure damage with a strong emphasis on skin care and reduction of friction

Dealey, C., 2005. The care of wounds, third edn. Blackwell, London.

This book addresses all aspects of wound assessment and management including pressure ulcers

Elliot, J., 2010. Strategies to improve the prevention of pressure ulcers. Nursing Older People 22 (9), 31–36.

This articles examines the implementation of best practice guidelines for the prevention of pressure ulcers in one Trust. The article presented the small study that was underatken and reports on the improved percentage of prevalence in the practice area

European Pressure Ulcer Advisory Panel and National Pressure Ulcer Advisory Panel, 2009. Pressure Ulcer Treatment Guidelines. [online]. Available from: www.epuap.org and www.npuap.org (accessed 24.01.12.).

European Pressure Ulcer Advisory Panel and National Pressure Ulcer Advisory Panel, 2010. Pressure Ulcer Prevention Guidelines. [online]. Available from: www.epuap.org and www.npuap.org (accessed 24.01.12.).

The European Pressure Ulcer Advisory Panel web site provides latest research and most recent guidelines for the prevention of pressure ulcers. These can be downloaded.

Gebhardt, K., 2002. Prevention of pressure ulcers - Part 3 Prevention strategies. Nursing Times 98 (13), 37–40.

Although aspects of the debate have now been superseded by the NICE clinical guideline 29, this article outlines the benefits and limitations of the tools used to assess pressure ulcers and the aids used to relieve pressure relief. Areas of further research identified

National Institute for Clinical Excellence (NICE), 2005. The prevention and treatment of pressure ulcers (Clinical Guideline 29). NICE, London. [online]. Available from: www.nice.org.uk (accessed 24.01.12.).

Norton, D., McLaren, R., Exton-Smith, A., 1975. An investigation of geriatric nursing problems in hospital. Churchill Livingstone, Edinburgh.

This is the original research that led to the development of the first pressure ulcer risk assessment tool, the Norton score designed to be used with elderly patients

Royal College of Nursing, 2005. The management of pressure ulcers in primary and secondary care. [online]. Available from: www.rcn.org.uk (accessed 24.01.12.).

This online document is the result of a collaboration between the RCN and NICE and is the result of a large UK consultation. This comprehensive document includes holistic assessment of pressure ulcer risk, grading of ulcers, the use of pressure-relieving aids, mobility and positioning, types of dressings, nutritional support and surgical and other treatments

Stockton, L., Flynn, M., 2009a. Sitting and pressure areas 1: risk factors, self-repositioning and other interventions. Nursing Times 105 (24), 12–14.

First in a series of two articles. This article provides an overview of the impact prolonged sitting has on the development of pressure ulcers, and includes some of the stategies that can prevent this

Stockton, L., Flynn, M., 2009b. Sitting and pressure ulcers 2: ensuring good posture and other preventative techniques. Nursing Times 105 (25), 16–18.

This is the second article that examines the posture technique when sitting in a chair and identifes the areas of concern in the development of pressure ulcers, and the techniques for preventing these

Thompson, D., 2005. An evaluation of the Waterlow pressure ulcer risk-assessment tool. British Journal of Nursing 14 (8), 455–458.

This article reviews studies related to the reliability and validity of the Waterlow pressure ulcer risk-assessment tool and concludes that whilst it has not been developed on scientific principles, it is a useful and practical way of systematically evaluating and re-evaluating individual patients' vulnerability to developing pressure ulcers

Waterlow, J., 2005. From costly treatment to cost-effective prevention: using Waterlow. British Journal of Community Nursing 10 (9) Suppl, S25–S30.

This is an updated article outlining the use of the Waterlow pressure ulcer risk-assessment tool. Waterlow describes the recent update to the system and explains how pressure ulcer risk assessments should be undertaken

Royal College of Nursing, 2001. Pressure ulcer risk assessment and prevention - clinical practice guidelines. RCN, London [online]. Available from: www.rcn.org (accessed 24.01.12.).

Complications of immobility

Goldhill, D.R., Imhoff, M., McLean, B., Waldmann, C., 2007. Rotational bed therapy to prevent and treat respiratory complications: a review and meta-analysis. American Journal of Critical Care 16 (1), 50–61.

This article reports a meta-analysis of the literature available regarding prevention and treatment of respiratory complications of immobility, in particular the use of rotational bed therapy

Holman, C., Roberts, S., Nicol, M., 2008. Preventing and treating constipation in later life. Nursing Older People 20 (5), 22–23.

This article discusses the increased risk of constipation in older patients and measures to prevent constipation. It also discusses bowel medications and ahow they work

Norton, C., 2006. Eliminating. In: Redfern, S.J., Ross, F.M., (Eds.), Nursing older people, fourth ed. Churchill Livingstone Elsevier, Edinburgh.

This comprehensive chapter addresses physical, psychological and social aspects relating to elimination as well as urinary and faecal continence and prevention and management of constipation

Timmerman, R.A., 2007. A mobility protocol for critically ill adults. Dimensions of Critical Care Nursing 26 (5), 175–179.

This article gives a good overview of the complications of immobility and discusses the use of a mobility protocol to prevent unnecessary periods of bed rest

Falls prevention

Age, U.K., 2011. [online]. Available from: www.ageuk.org.uk/Documents/EN-GB/strength_and_balance_training_PDF.pdf?dtrk=true (accessed 18.2.11.).

In 2009 Age Concern and Help the Aged merged to become Age UK. This website provides lots of helpful advice for older people and their carers including advice about preventing falls, exercises to improve strength, balance and nutrition

Gillespie, L.D., Robertson, M.C., Gillespie, W.J., Lamb, S.E., Gates, S., Cumming, R.G., et al., (2009) Interventions for preventing falls in older people living in the community (Review). The Cochrane Collaboration and published in *The Cochrane Library*, 2009, Issue 2. [online]. Available from: http://www.thecochranelibrary.com (accessed 24.01.12.).

A systematic review of interventions for preventing falls and the evidence to support them. Makes recommendations about which are effective

Holman, C., 2011. Nursing older people. In: Brooker, C., Nicol, M., (Eds.), Alexander's nursing practice, fourth ed. Mosby Elsevier, Edinburgh, Ch 34.

This chapter discusses physiological changes due to ageing, health promotion and nursing management of older people. It also reviews key UK policies and frameworks related to older people

National Institute for Health and Clinical Excellence, 2004. Clinical Guideline 21: The assessment and prevention of falls in older people. Published by NICE and available from: http://publications.nice.org.uk/falls-cg21/guidance (accessed 10.4.12).

UK national guidelines for best practice in the assessment and prevention of falls in older people. It addresses all of the key risk factors and provides good advice and examples of best practice.

Royal College of Nursing, 2004. Clinical practice guideline for the assessment and prevention of falls in older people (commissioned by NICE). RCN, London [online]. Available from: www.rcn.org.uk (accessed 24.01.12.).

An excellent practice guideline that is the basis of the NICE (2004) guidelines. It addresses risk factors, assessment and prevention of falls in older people

Venous thromboembolism

Department of Health, 2010. Risk assessment for venous thromboembolism. [online]. Available from: www.dh.gov.uk (accessed 24.01.12.).

Summarises the risk factors into a risk assessment tool that links with the guidance on VTE prophylaxis issued by NICE (see below)

Hairon, N., 2007. Prevention of venous thromboembolism in patients. Nursing Times 103 (18), 23–24.

This article summarises the NICE (2007) guidelines and includes the incidence of VTE, prevention and treatment and explains mechanical and pharmacological prophylaxis

NICE, 2010. Venous thromboembolism: reducing the risk. CG92. [online]. Available from: www.nice.org.uk (accessed 24.01.12.).

Comprehensive guidance on the prevention and treatment of VTE in all patient groups. Updated regularly on the web site

Normal values

The values below represent an 'average' reference range, in adults, for blood, cerebrospinal fluid, urine and faeces. These ranges should be used as a guide only. Reference ranges vary between individual laboratories and readers should consult their own laboratory for those used locally. This is especially important where reference values depend upon the analytical equipment and temperatures used.

©2012 Elsevier Ltd.

Blood (haematology)

Test	Reference range
Activated partial thromboplastin time (APTT)	26–36 s
Bleeding time (Ivy)	less than 8 min
Erythrocyte sedimentation rate (ESR)	
Adult women	3–15 mm/h
Adult men	0–10 mm/h
Fibrinogen	1.5–4.0 g/l
Folate (serum)	5.0–20 μg/l
Haemoglobin	
Women	115–165 g/L (115–165 g/dl)
Men	130–180 g/L (13–18 g/dl)
Haptoglobins	0.4–2.4 g/l
Mean cell haemoglobin (MCH)	27–32 pg
Mean cell volume (MCV)	78–98 fl
Packed cell volume (PCV) or haematocrit	
Women	0.37–0.47
Men	0.4–0.54
Platelets (thrombocytes)	$150–350 \times 10^9$/l
Prothrombin time	10.5–13.5 s
Red cells (erythrocytes)	
Women	$3.8–5.8 \times 10^{12}$/l
Men	$4.5–6.5 \times 10^{12}$/l
Reticulocytes (newly formed red cells in adults)	$25–85 \times 10^9$/l
White cells total (leucocytes)	$4.0–11.0 \times 10^9$/l
D-dimers	
To detect venous thromboembolism (VTE)	<500 μg/l
To detect disseminated intravascular coagulation (DIC)	<200 μg/l

Blood-venous plasma (biochemistry)

Test	Reference range
Alanine aminotransferase (ALT)	10–40 U/l
Albumin	36–47 g/l
Alkaline phosphatase	40–125 U/l
Amylase	<100 U/L

Test	Reference range
Aspartate aminotransferase (AST)	10–45 U/l
Bicarbonate (arterial)	21–7.5 mmol/l
Bilirubin (total)	2–17 μmol/l
Caeruloplasmin	0.2–0.6 g/l
Calcium	2.1–2.6 mmol/l
Chloride	95–107 mmol/l
Cholesterol (total) level varies and depends upon other cardiovascular risk factors	Ideally below 5.2 mmol/l
HDL – Cholesterol	>1.0 mmol/L
$PaCO_2$ (arterial)	4.4–6.1 kPa
Copper	13–24 μmol/l
Creatine kinase (total)	
Women	30–135 U/l
Men	55–170 U/l
Creatinine	55–120 μmol/l
Gamma-glutamyl-transferase (GGT)	
Women	5–35 U/l
Men	10–55 U/l
Glucose (venous blood, fasting)	3.6–5.8 mmol/l
Glycated haemoglobin (HbA1c)	4–6%
Hydrogen ion concentration (arterial)	35–44 nmol/l (ph 7.36–7.44)
Iron	10–30 μmol
Iron-binding capacity total (TIBC)	45–72 μmol/l
Lactate venous whole blood	0.6–2.2 mmol/l
Lactate dehydrogenase (total)	230–460 U/l
Lead (adults, whole blood)	<0.1 μmol/l
Magnesium	0.75–1.0 mmol/l
PaO_2 (arterial)	12–15 kPa
Oxygen saturation (arterial)	>97%
pH	7.36–7.42
Phosphate (fasting)	0.8–1.4 mmol/l
Potassium (serum)	3.6–5.0 mmol/l
Protein (total)	60–80 g/l
Sodium	136–145 mmol/l
Transferrin	2–4 g/L
Triglycerides (fasting)	0.6–1.7 mmol/l
Urate	
Women	0.12–0.36 mmol/l
Men	0.12–0.42 mmol/l
Urea	2.5–6.5 mmol/l
Vitamin B_{12}	251–900 mg/l
Zinc	11–22 μmol/l

Cerebrospinal fluid

Test	Reference range
Cells	<5 cells/mm^3
Glucose	2.5–4.0 mmol/l
Total protein	140–450 mg/l

Urine

Test	Reference range
Albumin/creatinine ration (ACR)	Less than 3.5 mg albumin/mmol creatinine
Calcium (diet dependent)	Up to 7.5 mmol/24 h (normal diet)
Copper	Up to 0.6 µmol/24 h
Cortisol	25–250 nmol/24 h
Creatinine	10–0 mmol/24 h
5-Hydroxyindale-3-acetic acid (5HIAA)	10–42 µmol/24 h
Oxalate	0.04–0.49 mmol/24 h
pH	4–8
Phosphate	15–50 mmol/24 h
Potassium (depends on intake)	25–100 mmol/24 h
Protein (total)	Up to 0.3 g/l
Sodium (depends on intake)	100–200 mmol/24 h
Urea	170–600 mmol/24 h

Index

NB: Page numbers followed by "f" indicate figures, "t" indicate tables, and "b" indicate boxes.

LIBRARY, UNIVERSITY OF CHESTER